calories
and
carbohydrates

calories
and
carbohydrates

by Barbara Kraus
Foreword by Edward B. Greenspan, M.D.

GROSSET & DUNLAP, INC.

A NATIONAL GENERAL COMPANY

Publishers • New York

For Rebecca K. Pecot

FOREWORD

Well-documented actuarial statistics indicate that one out of every five adult Americans is overweight. (If we include overweight children in the figure, the number of Americans suffering from obesity is staggering.)

Why is this statistic so important? Because obesity has come to be regarded by the medical profession as a forerunner of some diseases. Quite simply, your chances of being afflicted with a serious ailment, such as heart disease, are greater if you are overweight.

Scientific study of the metabolisms of obese patients reveal two important facts about the way fat accumulates: 1) the ingestion of more calories than energy expended will lead to an increase in weight. 2) an excess of carbohydrates or other calorie-yielding nutrients (such as protein or fat) causes the formation of fat in the body. Clearly, it is important for each one of us to keep a close watch on the foods we eat — especially in a society so fond of rich foods, desserts, alcoholic beverages and soft drinks.

This extraordinary compilation by Barbara Kraus reveals the caloric and carbohydrate content of foods, both natural and processed, and should prove an invaluable aid not only to dietitians and physicians, but also to all individuals who wish to maintain, gain or lose weight.

Edward B. Greenspan, M.D.
Mount Sinai Hospital

CONTENTS

INTRODUCTION

This dictionary of foods lists several thousand brand-name products and basic foods with their caloric and carbohydrate content. The calorie yield of your diet versus the amount of energy you expend is the key to whether you maintain your ideal weight, gain too many pounds or lose weight.

Because of the relationship of weight to health, many individuals are "counting calories" at every meal. Interest has also been directed to the carbohydrate content of the diet in relation to weight control. Comprehensive information on these values in basic foods and brand-name products is not readily available in any one source. Nor is the information regularly reported in portions that are usually eaten or bought at the grocery store. To compound the problem, hundreds of new food items appear in our stores every year.

Arrangement of this Book

Foods are listed alphabetically by brand name or by the name of the food. The singular form is used for the entries, that is, blackberry instead of blackberries. Most items are listed individually though a few are grouped (see p. xii), for example, all candies are listed together so that if you are looking for *Mars* bar, you look first under Candy, then under *M* in alphabetical order. But, if you are looking for a breakfast food such as Oatmeal, you will find it under *O* in the main alphabet. Many cross references are included to assist in finding items called by different names.

Under the main headings, it was often not possible nor even desirable to follow an alphabetical arrangement. For basic foods such as apricots, for example, the first entries are for the fresh product weighed with seeds as it is purchased in the store, then the fruit in small portions as they may be eaten or measured. These entries are followed by the processed products, canned (although it may actually be a bottle or jar), dehydrated, dried and frozen. This basic plan, with adaptations where necessary, was followed for fruits, vegetables and meats.

In almost all entries where data were available the U.S. Department of Agriculture figures are shown first. The Department values represent averages from several manufacturers and are shown for comparison with the values from individual companies or for use where particular brands are not available.

All brand-name products have been italicized and company names appear in parentheses.

Portions Used

The portion column is a most important one to read and note. Common household measures are used insofar as possible. For some items, the amounts given are those commonly purchased in the store, such as 1 pound of meat, or a 15-ounce package of cake mix. These quantities can be divided into the number of servings used in the home and the nutritive values available to each person served can then be readily determined. Of course, any ingredients added in preparing such products must also be taken into account.

The smaller portions given are for foods as served or measured in moderate amounts, such as ½ cup of juice reconstituted, or 4 ounces of meat. Be sure to adjust the calories and carbohydrates to the actual portions you use. For example, if you serve 1 cup of juice instead of ½ cup, multiply the calories and carbohydrates shown for the smaller amount by 2.

Don't fool yourself about the size of portions you use. If you are serious about controlling the calories and carbohydrates in your diet, weigh your foods until you can accurately gauge the weight visually. Remember, the calories and carbohydrates go up with any increase in the weight of foods. Remember, too, that 4 ounces by weight may be very different from ½ cup or 4 fluid ounces. Ounces in the table are always ounces by weight unless specified as fluid ounces, or fractions of a cup or other volumetric measure. Foods that are fluffy in texture, such as flaked coconut and bean sprouts vary greatly in weight per cup depending on how tightly they are packed into the cup. Such foods as canned green beans also vary when weighed with and without liquid, for example, canned green beans with liquid weigh 4.2 ounces for ½ cup, but drained beans weigh 2.5 ounces for the same ½ cup. Check the weights of your serving portions regularly. Bear in mind that you can cut calories and carbohydrates by cutting the serving size.

It was impossible to convert all the portions to a uniform basis. Some sources were only able to report data in terms of weights with no information on cup or other volumetric measures. We have shown small portions in quantities that might reasonably be expected to be served or measured in the home or institution. Package sizes are useful to show the composition of products as they are purchased and may be divided into the number of serving portions prepared from the entire product, taking into account any added ingredients.

You will find in the portion column the phrases "weighed with bone," or "weighed with skin and seeds" or other inedible parts. These descriptions apply to the products as you purchase them in the markets but the caloric values and the carbohydrate content as shown are for the amount of edible food after you discard the bone, skin, seed or other inedible part. The weight given in the "measure or quantity" column is to the nearest gram or fraction of an ounce.

Data on the composition of foods are constantly changing for many reasons. Better sampling and analytical methods, improvements in marketing procedures and changes in formulas of mixed products, all may alter values for carbohydrates and other nutrients as well as caloric values. Weights of packaged foods are frequently changed. It is essential to read label information to be informed about these matters and to make intelligent use of food tables.

Calories

What is a calorie? It is not a nutrient nor is it a good guide to the nutritive value of a food. It is more like a yardstick to measure the energy that a food will yield in the body. You need energy for your body functions as well as for exercise. If your diet contains more calories than your body uses for these purposes, the extra "energy" will be stored as fat. One pound of fat is equal to 3500 calories. Add this number of calories to those you need to balance your energy requirements and you will gain one pound; subtract it, and you will lose a pound.

Carbohydrates

The carbohydrate column shows the amount of this nutrient in grams for the quantities of foods indicated in the portion column. Some dietitians are giving special attention to this nutrient at present in connection with weight control. Carbohydrates include sugars, starches, acids and other nutrients. The values in this book are total carbohydrates, by difference, the basis on which calories from carbohydrates are calculated in the U.S. diet.

Other Nutrients

Do not forget that other nutrients are extremely important in diet planning — protein, fat, minerals and vitamins. Calories yielded by alcohol must also be considered in diet planning. From a nutrition viewpoint, perhaps the best advice that can be given to the dieter is to eat a varied diet with all classes of foods represented. Meat, fish, chicken, fats and oils, milk, vegetables, fruits and grain products are all important sources of essential nutrients and some foods from each of these classes of foods should be included in the diet every day. With the great abundance and variety of foods on the grocer's shelves, there is no reason why the dieter should not enjoy a tasty, nutritious and attractive diet. Just eat in moderation and there is no need to eliminate any one food altogether, except in special conditions under a doctor's directions. Choose wisely and eat well.

Sources of Data

Values in this dictionary are based on publications issued by the U.S. Department of Agriculture and on data submitted by manufacturers and processors. The U.S. Department of Agriculture issues basic tables on food composition for use in the United States. The commercial products from U.S.D.A. publications represent average values obtained on products of more than one company. The figures designated "home recipe" are based on recipes on file with the Department of Agriculture. Data on commercial products listed by brand name in this publication are based on values supplied by manufacturers and processors for their own individual products. Super-market brand names, such as A & P's *Ann Page*, or private labels could not be included in this book inasmuchas they are not usually analysed under these trade names. Every care has been taken to interpret the data and the descriptions supplied by the companies as fully and accurately as possible. Many values have been recalculated to different portions from those submitted in order to bring about greater uniformity among similar items.

Calories in these different sources are not always on a strictly uniform basis. In the Department of Agriculture, calories are calculated using specific factors, which make allowances for losses in digestion and metabolism. The technical explanation of these factors is given in Handbook 74 of the United States Department of Agriculture. Most manufacturers use average factors of 4, 9 and 4 for calories yielded by each gram of protein, fat and carbohydrates respectively; a factor of 7 is used as an average value to calculate the calories from one gram of alcohol. These differences in procedure will give somewhat different results for products of similar composition. Some manufacturers have adopted the values from U.S. Department of Agriculture publications as representative of their own products. In these cases, it will be apparent in the table that the data from the companies match exactly those from U.S.D.A. publications.

Analyses of foods to provide information on nutritive values are extremely expensive to conduct. Many small companies cannot afford to have their products analyzed and thus were unable to provide data for this book or were able to provide only the calories or only the carbohydrates. Other companies have simply never gotten around to having the analysis done.

Bear in mind that small differences in calorie values on similar products of the same weight are not important in diet planning. They may be due to different methods of calculating the calories or to small differences in the nutritive values of the samples analyzed because no two foods ever have exactly the same composition. Some differences may also be due to the way the food was measured as noted in the case of green beans earlier.

Carbohydrates in this book are usually total carbohydrates by difference. A few manufacturers reported only "available carbohydrates." These values were omitted.

Foods Listed by Groups

Foods in the following classes are reported together rather than as individual items in the main alphabet: Baby Food; Bread; Cake Icing; Cake Icing Mix; Candy; Cheese; Cookie; Cookie Mix; Cracker; Gravy; Salad Dressing; and Sauce.

BARBARA KRAUS

ABBREVIATIONS AND SYMBOLS

(USDA) = United States Department
of Agriculture
* = Prepared as package directs[1]
< = less than
& = and
″ = inch
D.N.A. = data not available
fl. = fluid
liq. = liquid
lb. = pound

med. = medium
oz. = ounce
pkg. = package
pt. = pint
qt. = quart
sq. = square
T. = tablespoon
Tr. = trace
tsp. = teaspoon
wt. = weight

EQUIVALENTS

By Weight

1 pound = 16 ounces
1 ounce = 28.35 grams
3.52 ounces = 100 grams

By Volume

1 quart = 4 cups
1 cup = 8 fluid ounces
1 cup = ½ pint
1 cup = 16 tablespoons
2 tablespoons = 1 fluid ounce
1 tablespoon = 3 teaspoons
1 pound butter = 4 sticks or 2 cups

[1]If the package directions call for whole or skim milk, the data given here is for whole milk, unless otherwise stated.

Food and Description	Measure or Quantity	Calories	Carbo-hydrates (grams)

A

ABALONE:
Raw, meat only (USDA)	4 oz.	111	3.9
Canned (USDA)	4 oz.	91	2.6

ABISANTE LIQUEUR (Leroux):
100 proof	1 fl. oz.	87	1.0
120 proof	1 fl. oz.	104	1.0

AC'CENT   1 gram   3   0.

ACEROLA, fresh (USDA):
Fruit	½ lb. (weighed with seeds)	52	12.6
Juice	½ cup (4.3 oz.)	28	5.8

ALBACORE, raw, meat only
(USDA)	4 oz.	201	0.

ALCOHOLIC BEVERAGES (See individual listings)

ALEWIFE (USDA):
Raw, meat only	4 oz.	144	0.
Canned, solids & liq.	4 oz.	160	0.

ALMOND:
In shell:
(USDA)	4 oz. (weighed in shell)	346	11.3
(USDA)	1 cup (2.8 oz.)	239	7.8

Shelled:
Plain:
Whole (USDA)	½ cup (2.5 oz.)	425	13.8
Whole (USDA)	1 oz.	170	5.5
Whole (USDA)	13-15 almonds	105	3.4
Chopped (USDA)	1 cup (4.5 oz.)	759	24.8
(Blue Diamond)	1 oz.	176	5.5
Blanched (Blue Diamond) salted or slivered	1 oz.	176	5.5

Chocolate-covered (See **CANDY**)

(USDA): United States Department of Agriculture
DNA: Data Not Available
*Prepared as Package Directs

Food and Description	Measure or Quantity	Calories	Carbo-hydrates (grams)
Flavored (Blue Diamond) barbecue, cheese, French-fried, onion-garlic or smokehouse-style	1 oz.	179	9.5
Roasted:			
Diced (Blue Diamond)	1 oz.	176	5.5
Dry (Planters)	1 oz.	187	4.8
Salted (USDA)	1 cup (5.5 oz.)	984	30.6
Salted (USDA)	1 oz.	178	5.5
ALMOND EXTRACT (Ehlers)	1 tsp.	5	D.N.A.
ALMOND MEAL, partially defatted (USDA)	1 oz.	116	8.2
ALPHABET SOUP MIX:			
*(Golden Grain)	1 cup	54	9.0
(Lipton) vegetable	1 pkg. (2 oz.)	205	36.6
ALPHA-BITS, oat cereal (Post)	1 cup (1 oz.)	110	23.0
AMARANTH, raw (USDA):			
Untrimmed	1 lb. (weighed untrimmed)	103	18.6
Trimmed	4 oz.	41	7.4
AMBROSIA, chilled bottled (Kraft)	4 oz.	86	17.8
ANCHOVY PASTE, canned (Crosse & Blackwell)	1 T.	20	1.0
ANCHOVY, PICKLED, canned with & without added oil (USDA)	1 oz.	50	.1
ANESONE LIQUEUR (Leroux) 90 proof	1 fl. oz.	86	2.8
ANGEL FOOD CAKE:			
Home recipe (USDA)	$\frac{1}{12}$ of 8″ cake (1.4 oz.)	108	24.1
Loaf (Van de Kamp's)	10-oz. loaf	1006	D.N.A.
Ring, chocolate iced (Van de Kamp's)	7½″ cake	2528	D.N.A.

(USDA): United States Department of Agriculture
DNA: Data Not Available
*Prepared as Package Directs

Food and Description	Measure or Quantity	Calories	Carbo-hydrates (grams)
ANGEL FOOD CAKE MIX:			
(USDA)	4 oz.	437	100.4
*(USDA)	2-oz. serving	147	33.7
(Betty Crocker):			
1 step	1-lb. pkg.	1664	392.0
2 step	15-oz. pkg.	1590	361.5
Confetti	1-lb. 1-oz. pkg.	1768	416.5
Lemon custard	1-lb. pkg.	1664	392.0
Strawberry	1-lb. 1-oz. pkg.	1768	416.5
*(Duncan Hines)	1 cake	1272	288.0
(Pillsbury) raspberry swirl	1 oz.	102	23.6
(Pillsbury) white	1 oz.	102	23.3
*(Swans Down)	1/15 of cake	106	24.5
ANISE EXTRACT (Ehlers)	1 tsp.	12	D.N.A.
ANISETTE LIQUEUR:			
(Bols) 50 proof	1 fl. oz.	111	13.9
(Garnier) 54 proof	1 fl. oz.	82	9.3
(Hiram Walker) 60 proof, red or white	1 fl. oz.	92	10.8
(Leroux) 60 proof, red or white	1 fl. oz.	89	9.9
(Old Mr. Boston) 42 proof	1 fl. oz.	64	8.0
(Old Mr. Boston) 60 proof	1 fl. oz.	90	7.5
APPLE, any variety:			
Fresh (USDA):			
Eaten with skin	1 lb. weighed with skin & core)	242	60.5
Eaten with skin	1 med., 2½″ dia. (about 3 per lb.)	80	20.0
Eaten without skin	1 lb. (weighed without skin & core)	211	55.0
Eaten without skin	1 med., 2½″ dia. (about 3 per lb.)	70	18.2
Pared, diced	1 cup (3.8 oz.)	59	15.4
Pared, quartered	1 cup (4.3 oz.)	66	17.2
Dehydrated:			
Uncooked (USDA)	1 oz.	100	26.1
Cooked, sweetened (USDA)	½ cup (4.2 oz.)	91	23.5
Slices (Vacu-Dry)	1 oz.	100	26.1
Dried (USDA):			
Uncooked	4 oz.	312	81.4
Cooked, unsweetened	½ cup (4.3 oz.)	94	24.6
Cooked, sweetened	½ cup (4.3 oz.)	136	35.3

(USDA): United States Department of Agriculture
DNA: Data Not Available
*Prepared as Package Directs

Food and Description	Measure or Quantity	Calories	Carbohydrates (grams)
Frozen, sweetened, slices, not thawed (USDA)	4 oz.	106	27.5
APPLE BROWN BETTY, home recipe (USDA)	1 cup (8.1 oz.)	347	68.3
APPLE BUTTER:			
(USDA)	½ cup (5 oz.)	262	66.0
(USDA)	1 oz.	53	13.0
(USDA)	1 T.	33	8.4
(Musselman's)	1 T.	33	D.N.A.
(White House)	1 T.	28	7.6
APPLE CIDER (Indian Summer)	6 fl. oz.	78	19.5
APPLE CRISPS, dehydrated snack (Epicure)	1 oz.	87	22.7
APPLE DRINK (Hi-C)	6 fl. oz.	87	22.2
APPLE FRUIT ROLL, frozen (Chun King)	1 oz.	64	10.1
APPLE JACKS, cereal (Kellogg's)	1 cup (1 oz.)	112	25.5
APPLE JELLY:			
Sweetened (White House)	1 T.	46	13.0
Dietetic or low calorie:			
(Dia-Mel) fresh pressed, old fashioned, or mint	1 T.	22	5.4
(Diet Delight)	1 T.	6	1.2
(Kraft)	1 oz.	13	3.1
(Slenderella)	1 T.	21	5.4
(Tillie Lewis)	1 T.	9	2.1
APPLE JUICE, canned:			
(USDA)	½ cup (4.4 oz.)	58	14.8
(Heinz)	5½-oz. can	69	16.8
(Musselman's)	½ cup	62	D.N.A.
(Seneca)	½ cup	56	13.6
(White House)	½ cup	58	15.0
APPLE-PAPAYA FRUIT SPREAD, low calorie (Vita)	1 T.	9	D.N.A.

Food and Description	Measure or Quantity	Calories	Carbo-hydrates (grams)
APPLE PIE:			
Home recipe (USDA)	⅙ of 9″ pie (5.6 oz.)	404	60.2
(Tastykake)	4-oz. pie	380	58.6
French apple (Tastykake)	4½-oz. pie	451	64.3
Frozen:			
Unbaked (USDA)	5 oz.	298	47.1
Baked (USDA)	5 oz.	361	56.8
(Banquet)	5 oz.	351	49.5
(Morton)	⅙ of 20-oz. pie	255	36.2
(Mrs. Smith's)	⅙ of 8″ pie	303	43.1
(Mrs. Smith's) Dutch apple	⅙ of 8″ pie	326	47.3
(Mrs. Smith's) tart	⅙ of 8″ pie	266	44.0
APPLE PIE FILLING:			
(Lucky Leaf)	8 oz.	248	60.8
(Musselman's)	1 cup	283	D.N.A.
APPLESAUCE, canned:			
Sweetened:			
(USDA)	½ cup (4.5 oz.)	116	30.5
(Musselman's)	½ cup	92	D.N.A.
(Seneca) cinnamon	½ cup	134	30.2
(Seneca) 100% McIntosh	½ cup	116	30.2
(Stokely-Van Camp)	½ cup	119	30.9
(White House)	½ cup (4.5 oz.)	110	28.2
Unsweetened, dietetic or low calorie:			
(USDA)	½ cup (4.3 oz.)	50	13.2
(Blue Boy)	4 oz.	49	11.7
(Diet Delight)	½ cup (4.3 oz.)	54	10.7
(Lucky Leaf)	4 oz.	49	11.6
(S and W) *Nutradiet*	4 oz.	54	13.1
(Tillie Lewis)	½ cup (4.2 oz.)	49	12.2
(White House)	½ cup (4.3 oz.)	48	12.2
APPLESAUCE CAKE MIX:			
*Raisin (Duncan Hines)	1 cake	1693	315.0
Spice (Pillsbury)	1 oz.	117	22.7
APPLE TURNOVER, frozen			
(Pepperidge Farm)	1 turnover (3.2 oz.)	290	30.0
APRICOT:			
Fresh (USDA):			
Whole	1 lb. (weighed with pits)	217	54.6

(USDA): United States Department of Agriculture
DNA: Data Not Available
*Prepared as Package Directs

APRICOT (Continued)

Food and Description	Measure or Quantity	Calories	Carbo-hydrates (grams)
Whole	3 apricots (about 12 per lb.)	54	13.6
Halves	1 cup (5.5 oz.)	80	20.0
Canned:			
Heavy syrup:			
Halves & syrup (USDA)	½ cup (4.4 oz.)	108	27.7
Halves & syrup (USDA)	4 med. halves with 2 T. syrup (4.3 oz.)	105	26.8
(Hunt's)	4 oz.	98	24.9
(Stokely-Van Camp)	4 med. halves with 2 T. syrup	105	26.8
Juice pack (USDA)	4 oz.	61	15.4
Unsweetened or low calorie:			
Water pack, halves & liq. (USDA)	4 oz.	43	10.9
Water pack, halves & liq. (USDA)	½ cup (4.3 oz.)	46	11.7
(Del Monte)	4 oz.	43	10.9
(Diet Delight) halves	½ cup (4.3 oz.)	43	8.0
(Diet Delight) whole, peeled	½ cup (4.3 oz.)	34	7.1
(Libby's)	4 oz.	40	10.9
(S and W) Nutradiet	4 halves (3.5 oz.)	38	8.7
Dehydrated:			
Uncooked (USDA)	4 oz.	376	95.9
Cooked, fruit & liq., sugar added (USDA)	½ cup (4.3 oz.)	145	37.2
Slices (Vacu-Dry)	1 oz.	94	24.0
Dried:			
Uncooked:			
(USDA)	1 lb.	1179	301.6
(USDA)	14 large halves (½ cup or 2.8 oz.)	210	53.8
(USDA)	10 small halves (¼ cup or 1.3 oz.)	99	25.3
Cooked (USDA):			
Sweetened	½ cup with liq. (4.3 oz.)	149	38.3
Unsweetened	½ cup with liq. (5 oz.)	121	30.7
Frozen, sweetened, not thawed (USDA)	4 oz.	111	28.5
APRICOT-APPLE JUICE DRINK, canned (BC)	6 fl. oz.	96	D.N.A.

(USDA): United States Department of Agriculture
DNA: Data Not Available
*Prepared as Package Directs

[6]

Food and Description	Measure or Quantity	Calories	Carbo-hydrates (grams)
APRICOT, CANDIED (USDA)	1 oz.	96	24.5
APRICOT JAM, low calorie (Slenderella)	1 T.	21	5.4
APRICOT LIQUEUR:			
(Bols) 60 proof	1 fl. oz.	96	8.9
(Hiram Walker) 60 proof	1 fl. oz.	82	8.2
(Leroux) 60 proof	1 fl. oz.	85	8.9
APRICOT NECTAR, canned:			
Sweetened:			
(USDA)	½ cup (4.2 oz.)	68	17.6
(Dewco)	½ cup	68	D.N.A.
(Heinz)	5½-oz. can	81	19.3
Low calorie (Diet Delight)	½ cup (4.3 oz.)	29	5.4
APRICOT-ORANGE PIE (Tastykake)	4-oz. pie	377	54.8
APRICOT PIE FILLING (Lucky Leaf)	8 oz.	316	77.6
APRICOT & PINEAPPLE NECTAR, unsweetened (S and W) *Nutradiet*	4 oz. (by wt.)	35	8.3
APRICOT & PINEAPPLE PRESERVE, dietetic or low calorie:			
(Dia-Mel)	1 T.	22	5.4
(Diet Delight)	1 T.	6	1.2
(Tillie Lewis)	1 T.	9	2.1
APRICOT PRESERVE, dietetic or low calorie:			
(Dia-Mel)	1 T.	22	5.4
(Polaner)	1 T.	6	.3
AQUAVIT (Leroux) 90 proof	1 fl. oz.	75	Tr.
ARTICHOKE, Globe or French (See also **JERUSALEM ARTICHOKE**):			

(USDA): United States Department of Agriculture
DNA: Data Not Available
*Prepared as Package Directs

Food and Description	Measure or Quantity	Calories	Carbo-hydrates (grams)
Raw, whole (USDA)	1 lb. (weighed untrimmed)	85	19.2
Boiled, drained (USDA)	4 oz.	50	11.2
Frozen, hearts (Birds Eye)	5-6 hearts (3 oz.)	22	4.0
ASPARAGUS:			
Raw, whole spears (USDA)	1 lb. (weighed untrimmed)	66	12.7
Boiled, cut spears, drained (USDA)	1 cup (5.1 oz.)	29	3.2
Canned, regular pack:			
Green:			
Spears & liq. (USDA)	4 oz.	20	3.3
Spears & liq. (USDA)	1 cup (8.6 oz.)	44	7.1
Spears only (USDA)	1 cup (7.6 oz.)	45	7.3
Spears only (USDA)	6 med. spears (3.4 oz.)	20	3.3
Liq. only (USDA)	2 T.	3	<.1
Spears & liq. (Green Giant)	4 oz.	20	3.3
Spears only (Stokely-Van Camp)	6 med. spears	20	3.2
Cut, drained solids (Cannon)	4 oz.	24	3.9
White:			
Spears & liq. (USDA)	4 oz.	20	3.8
Spears & liq. (USDA)	1 cup (8.4 oz.)	43	7.8
Spears only (USDA)	1 cup (7.6 oz.)	47	7.7
Spears only (USDA)	6 med. spears (3.4 oz.)	21	3.4
Liq. only (USDA)	2 T.	3	.8
Spears only (Stokely-Van Camp)	6 med. spears	21	3.4
Canned, dietetic pack:			
Green:			
Spears & liq. (USDA)	4 oz.	18	3.0
Spears & liq. (Blue Boy)	4 oz.	20	3.2
Spears & liq. (Diet Delight)	½ can (2.6 oz.)	9	1.6
(S and W) *Nutradiet*	5 whole spears (3.5 oz.)	16	2.0
(Tillie Lewis)	½ cup (4.2 oz.)	19	2.6
White, spears and liq. (USDA)	4 oz.	18	3.4
Frozen:			
Cuts & tips, not thawed (USDA)	4 oz.	26	4.1

Food and Description	Measure or Quantity	Calories	Carbo-hydrates (grams)
Cuts & tips, boiled, drained (USDA)	½ cup (3.2 oz.)	20	3.2
Cuts & tips, boiled, drained (USDA)	4 oz.	25	4.0
Cuts (Birds Eye)	½ cup (3.3 oz.)	21	3.4
Cuts (Stokely-Van Camp)	½ cup	20	3.2
Spears, not thawed (USDA)	4 oz.	27	4.4
Spears, boiled, drained (USDA)	4 oz.	26	4.3
Spears (Birds Eye)	5 spears (3.3 oz.)	23	3.7
Spears in butter sauce (Green Giant) boil-in-the-bag	4 oz.	83	4.3
ASPARAGUS CRISPS, dehydrated snack (Epicure)	1 oz.	78	12.2
ASPARAGUS SOUP, Cream of, canned:			
Condensed (USDA)	8 oz. (by wt.)	123	19.1
*Prepared with equal volume water (USDA)	1 cup (8.5 oz.)	65	10.1
*Prepared with equal volume milk (USDA)	1 cup (8.5 oz.)	144	16.3
Condensed (Campbell)	8 oz. (by wt.)	159	21.3
ASTI WINE (Gancia) 9% alcohol	3 fl. oz.	126	18.0
AUNT JEMIMA SYRUP	1 T.	53	13.0
AVOCADO, peeled, pitted (USDA):			
All commercial varieties:			
Whole	1 lb. (weighed with skin & pit)	568	21.4
Diced	½ cup (2.6 oz.)	124	4.7
Mashed	½ cup (4.1 oz.)	194	7.3
California varieties, mainly Fuerte:			
Whole	½ avocado (3⅛" dia.)	185	6.5
½" cubes	½ cup (2.7 oz.)	130	4.6
Florida varieties:			
Whole	½ avocado (3⅝" dia.)	195	13.4
½" cubes	½ cup (2.7 oz.)	97	6.7

(USDA): United States Department of Agriculture
DNA: Data Not Available
*Prepared as Package Directs

Food and Description	Measure or Quantity	Calories	Carbo-hydrates (grams)
AWAKE (Birds Eye)	½ cup (4 oz.)	51	12.6
AYDS:			
Chocolate or chocolate-mint	1 piece	26	5.5
Vanilla caramel	1 piece	26	5.6

B

BABY FOOD:
Apple:

& apricot, junior (Beech-Nut)	7¾ oz.	208	51.0
& apricot, strained (Beech-Nut)	4¾ oz.	129	31.7
& cranberry, junior (Heinz)	7¾ oz.	245	59.4
& cranberry, strained (Heinz)	4¾ oz.	143	35.2
& pear, junior (Heinz)	7¾ oz.	180	43.7
& pear, strained (Heinz)	4½ oz.	104	25.4
Dutch, dessert, junior (Gerber)	7¾ oz.	231	47.1
Dutch, dessert, strained (Gerber)	4¾ oz.	141	28.7
Apple-apricot juice, strained (Heinz)	4¼ fl. oz.	92	22.0
Apple Betty (Beech-Nut):			
Junior	7¾ oz.	254	59.8
Strained	4¾ oz.	156	36.8
Apple-cherry juice:			
Strained (Beech-Nut)	4⅕ fl. oz.	68	16.9
Strained (Gerber)	4⅕ fl. oz.	69	17.0
Strained (Heinz)	4¼ fl. oz.	79	18.6
Apple gel, strained (Beech-Nut)	4½ oz.	85	21.0
Apple-grape juice:			
Strained (Beech-Nut)	4⅕ fl. oz.	88	21.2
Strained (Heinz)	4¼ fl. oz.	93	21.0
Apple juice:			
Strained (Beech-Nut)	4⅕ fl. oz.	61	15.1
Strained (Gerber)	4⅕ fl. oz.	60	15.1
Strained (Heinz)	4¼ fl. oz.	93	21.4
Apple-pineapple juice, strained (Heinz)	4¼ fl. oz.	93	21.2
Apple-prune juice, strained (Heinz)	4¼ fl. oz.	93	21.0
Applesauce:			
Junior (Beech-Nut)	7¾ oz.	184	45.0
Junior (Gerber)	7¾ oz.	180	44.2
Junior (Heinz)	7¾ oz.	182	44.7

(USDA): United States Department of Agriculture
DNA: Data Not Available
*Prepared as Package Directs

Food and Description	Measure or Quantity	Calories	Carbo-hydrates (grams)
Strained (Beech-Nut)	4¾ oz.	108	27.0
Strained (Gerber)	4⁷⁄₁₀ oz.	117	28.4
Strained (Heinz)	4¼ oz.	76	17.7
& apricots, junior (Gerber)	7¾ oz.	187	45.8
& apricots, junior (Heinz)	7¾ oz.	216	52.3
& apricots, strained (Gerber)	4⁷⁄₁₀ oz.	121	29.1
& apricots, strained (Heinz)	4¾ oz.	128	30.7
& cherries, junior (Beech-Nut)	7¾ oz.	186	45.8
& cherries, strained (Beech-Nut)	4¾ oz.	114	28.2
& cranberries, junior (Beech-Nut)	7¾ oz.	208	51.2
& cranberries, strained (Beech-Nut)	4¾ oz.	127	31.4
& pineapple, junior (Beech-Nut)	7¾ oz.	195	48.0
& pineapple, junior (Gerber)	7¾ oz.	167	40.9
& pineapple, strained (Beech-Nut)	4¾ oz.	119	29.3
& pineapple, strained (Gerber)	4⁷⁄₁₀ oz.	103	24.8
& raspberries, junior (Beech-Nut)	7¾ oz.	219	53.8
& raspberries, strained (Beech-Nut)	4¾ oz.	134	32.8
Apricot with tapioca:			
Junior (Beech-Nut)	7¾ oz.	193	47.3
Junior (Gerber)	7¾ oz.	180	43.8
Junior (Heinz)	7¾ oz.	216	41.6
Strained (Beech-Nut)	4¾ oz.	112	27.7
Strained (Gerber)	4⁷⁄₁₀ oz.	110	26.7
Strained (Heinz)	4¾ oz.	147	36.1
Banana:			
Strained (Heinz)	4½ oz.	108	24.8
& pineapple junior (Heinz)	7¾ oz.	167	40.6
& pineapple with tapioca, junior (Beech-Nut)	7¾ oz.	197	48.5
& pineapple with tapioca, junior (Gerber)	7¾ oz.	185	44.4
& pineapple with tapioca, strained (Beech-Nut)	4¾ oz.	133	32.6
& pineapple with tapioca, strained (Gerber)	4⁷⁄₁₀ oz.	110	27.3
Dessert, junior (Beech-Nut)	7¾ oz.	199	49.0
Pudding, junior (Gerber)	7¾ oz.	202	46.9
With tapioca, strained (Beech-Nut)	4¾ oz.	118	29.1

Food and Description	Measure or Quantity	Calories	Carbo-hydrates (grams)
With tapioca, strained (Gerber)	4⁷⁄₁₀ oz.	114	27.3
Bean, green:			
Junior (Beech-Nut)	7¼ oz.	55	10.4
Strained (Beech-Nut)	4½ oz.	35	6.6
Strained (Gerber)	4½ oz.	32	6.0
Strained (Heinz)	4½ oz.	35	6.1
Creamed with bacon, junior (Gerber)	7½ oz.	146	19.7
With potatoes & ham, casserole, toddler (Gerber)	6 oz.	143	16.6
Beef:			
Junior (Beech-Nut)	3½ oz.	114	0.
Junior (Gerber)	3½ oz.	107	0.
Junior (Heinz)	3½ oz.	92	0.
Strained (Beech-Nut)	3½ oz.	116	0.
Strained (Gerber)	3½ oz.	97	0.
Strained (Heinz)	3½ oz.	89	.4
Beef & beef heart:			
Junior (Beech-Nut)	3½ oz.	116	0.
Strained (Beech-Nut)	3½ oz.	110	0.
Strained (Gerber)	3½ oz.	99	.1
Beef dinner:			
Junior (Beech-Nut)	4½ oz.	106	7.5
Strained (Beech-Nut)	4½ oz.	105	7.3
& noodles, junior (Beech-Nut)	7½ oz.	117	15.8
& noodles, junior (Gerber)	7½ oz.	102	13.1
& noodles, strained (Beech-Nut)	4½ oz.	56	11.7
& noodles, strained (Gerber)	4½ oz.	60	9.1
With vegetables, junior (Gerber)	4½ oz.	108	7.6
With vegetables, strained (Gerber)	3½ oz.	105	6.9
With vegetables & cereal, junior (Heinz)	4¾ oz.	96	6.2
With vegetables & cereal, strained (Heinz)	4¾ oz.	97	6.3
Beef lasagna with sauce, toddler (Gerber)	6 oz.	137	16.8
Beef liver:			
Junior (Beech-Nut)	3⁵⁄₁₆ oz.	100	2.2
Strained (Beech-Nut)	3⁵⁄₁₆ oz.	75	2.0
Strained (Gerber)	3½ oz.	94	2.4
Beef liver soup, strained (Heinz)	4½ oz.	50	4.9
Beef stew, toddler (Gerber)	6 oz.	120	14.0

(USDA): United States Department of Agriculture
DNA: Data Not Available
*Prepared as Package Directs

Food and Description	Measure or Quantity	Calories	Carbo-hydrates (grams)
Beet:			
Strained (Beech-Nut)	4½ oz.	59	13.1
Strained (Gerber)	4½ oz.	55	9.3
Strained (Heinz)	4½ oz.	54	11.0
Biscuits, teething (Gerber)	1 biscuit (.4 oz.)	43	8.5
Butterscotch pudding, strained (Gerber)	4½ oz.	131	22.3
Carrot:			
Junior (Beech-Nut)	7½ oz.	70	16.0
Junior (Gerber)	7½ oz.	61	13.1
Junior (Heinz)	7¾ oz.	87	15.8
Strained (Beech-Nut)	4½ oz.	41	9.3
Strained (Gerber)	4½ oz.	36	7.7
Strained (Heinz)	4½ oz.	20	3.0
In butter sauce, junior (Beech-Nut)	7½ oz.	85	15.7
In butter sauce, strained (Beech-Nut)	4½ oz.	51	10.6
Cereal, dry:			
Barley (Gerber)	3 T. (¼ oz.)	26	4.9
Barley, instant (Heinz)	1 oz.	89	17.6
High protein (Gerber)	3 T. (¼ oz.)	26	3.2
High protein, instant (Heinz)	1 oz.	99	13.9
Hi-protein (Beech-Nut)	1 oz.	102	12.2
Mixed (Beech-Nut)	1 oz.	105	18.8
Mixed (Gerber)	3 T. (¼ oz.)	27	4.9
Mixed (Heinz)	1 oz.	100	20.1
Oatmeal (Beech-Nut)	1 oz.	108	17.9
Oatmeal (Gerber)	3 T. (¼ oz.)	28	4.6
Oatmeal, instant (Heinz)	1 oz.	104	17.8
Rice (Beech-Nut)	1 oz.	102	22.2
Rice (Gerber)	3 T. (¼ oz.)	26	5.5
Rice, instant (Heinz)	1 oz.	100	22.3
Wheat (Beech-Nut)	1 oz.	101	19.8
Cereal, or mixed cereal:			
With applesauce & banana, strained (Beech-Nut)	4¾ oz.	116	27.3
With applesauce & banana, strained (Gerber)	4⁷⁄₁₀ oz.	109	23.7
With egg yolks & bacon, junior (Beech-Nut)	7½ oz.	184	17.0
With egg yolks & bacon, junior (Gerber)	7½ oz.	159	15.3

Food and Description	Measure or Quantity	Calories	Carbo-hydrates (grams)
With egg yolks & bacon, junior (Heinz)	7½ oz.	162	13.2
With egg yolks & bacon, strained (Beech-Nut)	4½ oz.	118	11.2
With egg yolks & bacon, strained (Gerber)	4½ oz.	93	9.2
With egg yolks & bacon, strained (Heinz)	4½ oz.	102	6.5
Oatmeal with applesauce & banana, strained (Beech-Nut)	4¾ oz.	102	22.9
Oatmeal with applesauce & banana, strained (Gerber)	4⁷⁄₁₀ oz.	103	20.9
Rice, with applesauce & banana, strained (Gerber)	4⁷⁄₁₀ oz.	92	22.2
Cheese:			
Cottage, with banana, junior (Heinz)	7¾ oz.	169	36.3
Cottage, with banana, strained (Heinz)	4½ oz.	96	20.2
Cottage, creamed, with pineapple, junior (Beech-Nut)	7¾ oz.	184	39.6
Cottage, creamed, with pineapple, strained (Gerber)	4½ oz.	181	23.0
Cottage, creamed, with pineapple juice, strained (Beech-Nut)	4¾ oz.	121	26.0
Cherry gel, strained (Beech-Nut)	4½ oz.	133	33.0
Cherry vanilla pudding (Gerber):			
Junior	7¾ oz.	235	57.0
Strained	4¾ oz.	143	34.7
Chicken:			
Junior (Beech-Nut)	3½ oz.	112	D.N.A.
Junior (Gerber)	3½ oz.	153	0.
Junior (Heinz)	3½ oz.	108	0.
Strained (Beech-Nut)	3½ oz.	116	0.
Strained (Gerber)	3½ oz.	151	.2
Strained (Heinz)	3½ oz.	137	0.
Chicken dinner:			
Junior (Beech-Nut)	4½ oz.	111	11.6
Strained (Beech-Nut)	4½ oz.	135	10.2
Noodle, junior (Beech-Nut)	7½ oz.	76	15.6
Noodle, junior (Gerber)	7½ oz.	95	15.3
Noodle, junior (Heinz)	7½ oz.	119	12.6
Noodle, strained (Beech-Nut)	4½ oz.	53	10.6

(USDA): United States Department of Agriculture
DNA: Data Not Available
*Prepared as Package Directs

Food and Description	Measure or Quantity	Calories	Carbo-hydrates (grams)
Noodle, strained (Gerber)	4½ oz.	58	9.3
Noodle, strained (Heinz)	4½ oz.	65	7.2
With vegetables, junior (Gerber)	4½ oz.	111	8.1
With vegetables, junior (Heinz)	4¾ oz.	151	6.1
With vegetables, strained (Gerber)	4½ oz.	101	7.0
With vegetables, strained (Heinz)	4¾ oz.	160	8.1
Chicken soup:			
Junior (Beech-Nut)	7½ oz.	85	17.2
Junior (Heinz)	7½ oz.	121	11.7
Strained (Beech-Nut)	4½ oz.	54	10.5
Strained (Heinz)	4½ oz.	61	6.7
Cream of, junior (Gerber)	7½ oz.	131	18.4
Cream of, strained (Gerber)	7½ oz.	79	11.1
Chicken stew, toddler (Gerber)	6 oz.	119	13.8
Chicken sticks:			
Junior (Beech-Nut)	2½ oz.	179	1.4
Junior (Gerber)	3½ oz.	148	1.9
Cookie, animal-shaped (Gerber)	1 cookie (.2 oz.)	28	4.2
Corn, creamed:			
Junior (Gerber)	7½ oz.	146	25.9
Junior (Heinz)	7½ oz.	136	29.9
Strained (Beech-Nut)	4½ oz.	109	25.0
Strained (Gerber)	4½ oz.	81	15.4
Strained (Heinz)	4½ oz.	82	17.8
Custard:			
Junior (Beech-Nut)	7¾ oz.	204	47.0
Junior (Heinz)	7¾ oz.	213	35.6
Strained (Beech-Nut)	4½ oz.	115	26.6
Strained (Heinz)	4½ oz.	120	25.8
Chocolate, junior (Gerber)	7¾ oz.	207	40.9
Chocolate, strained (Beech-Nut)	4½ oz.	126	28.9
Chocolate, strained (Gerber)	4½ oz.	123	22.7
Vanilla, junior (Gerber)	7½ oz.	197	38.6
Vanilla, strained (Gerber)	4½ oz.	123	22.7
Dutch apple dessert (See Apple, Dutch, dessert)			
Egg yolk:			
Strained (Beech-Nut)	3⅓ oz.	193	.1
Strained (Gerber)	3½ oz.	204	.1
Strained (Heinz)	3¼ oz.	182	.6
& bacon, strained (Beech-Nut)	3⅓ oz.	196	.1
& ham, strained (Gerber)	3½ oz.	196	0.

(USDA): United States Department of Agriculture
DNA: Data Not Available
*Prepared as Package Directs

BABY FOOD (Continued)

Food and Description	Measure or Quantity	Calories	Carbo-hydrates (grams)
Franks, junior (Beech-Nut)	2½ oz.	170	.9
Fruit dessert:			
Junior (Gerber)	7¾ oz.	185	44.9
Junior (Heinz)	7¾ oz.	180	42.2
Strained (Gerber)	4¾ oz.	121	29.3
Strained (Heinz)	4½ oz.	115	24.8
Tropical, junior (Beech-Nut)	7¾ oz.	219	54.1
With tapioca, junior (Beech-Nut)	7¾ oz.	204	50.4
With tapioca, strained (Beech-Nut)	4¾ oz.	126	31.0
Fruit gel, mixed fruit, strained (Beech-Nut)	4½ oz.	99	23.3
Fruit juice:			
Mixed, strained (Beech-Nut)	4⅕ fl. oz.	72	20.5
Mixed, strained (Gerber)	4⅕ fl. oz.	66	16.0
Ham:			
Strained (Beech-Nut)	3½ oz.	116	1.6
Strained (Gerber)	3½ oz.	123	.8
Ham dinner:			
Junior (Beech-Nut)	4½ oz.	129	9.8
Strained (Beech-Nut)	4½ oz.	149	11.0
With vegetables, junior (Gerber)	4½ oz.	99	7.7
With vegetables, strained (Gerber)	4½ oz.	109	7.7
With vegetables & cereal, junior (Heinz)	4¾ oz.	135	8.4
With vegetables & cereal, strained (Heinz)	4⅗ oz.	160	12.0
Lamb:			
Junior (Beech-Nut)	3½ oz.	114	0.
Junior (Gerber	3½ oz.	99	0.
Junior (Heinz)	3½ oz.	104	.3
Strained (Beech-Nut)	3½ oz.	116	0.
Strained (Gerber)	3½ oz.	104	0.
Strained (Heinz)	3½ oz.	109	.8
& noodles, junior (Beech-Nut)	7½ oz.	134	18.6
Liver, strained (Heinz)	3½ oz.	91	1.8
Macaroni:			
Alphabets & beef casserole, toddler (Gerber)	6 oz.	157	16.6
& bacon with vegetables, junior (Beech-Nut)	7½ oz.	170	22.7

(USDA): United States Department of Agriculture
DNA: Data Not Available
*Prepared as Package Directs

Food and Description	Measure or Quantity	Calories	Carbo-hydrates (grams)
& beef with vegetables, junior (Beech-Nut)	7½ oz.	112	17.8
With tomato, beef & bacon, junior (Gerber)	7½ oz.	140	20.4
With tomato, beef & bacon, junior (Heinz)	7½ oz.	141	19.0
With tomato, beef & bacon, strained (Gerber)	4½ oz.	78	11.0
With tomato, beef & bacon, strained (Heinz)	4½ oz.	84	11.2
With tomato sauce, beef & bacon dinner, strained (Beech-Nut)	4½ oz.	94	14.4
Meat sticks, junior (Gerber)	3½ oz.	109	1.2
Noodles & beef, junior (Heinz)	7½ oz.	102	12.8
Orange-apple juice, strained:			
(Beech-Nut)	4⅕ fl. oz.	83	20.3
(Gerber)	4⅕ fl. oz.	67	15.8
Orange-apple-banana juice, strained:			
(Gerber)	4⅕ fl. oz.	81	19.3
(Heinz)	4¼ fl. oz.	87	21.0
Orange-apricot juice, strained:			
(Beech-Nut)	4⅕ fl. oz.	107	26.1
(Gerber)	4⅕ fl. oz.	83	19.1
Orange-apricot juice drink, strained (Heinz)	4¼ fl. oz.	63	15.0
Orange-banana juice, strained (Beech-Nut)	4⅕ fl. oz.	104	25.4
Orange gel, strained (Beech-Nut)	4½ oz.	100	24.4
Orange juice, strained:			
(Beech-Nut)	4⅕ fl. oz.	71	17.1
(Gerber)	4⅕ fl. oz.	60	14.4
(Heinz)	4¼ fl. oz.	76	16.0
Orange-pineapple dessert, strained (Beech-Nut)	4¾ oz.	140	34.4
Orange-pineapple juice, strained:			
(Beech-Nut)	4⅕ fl. oz.	108	26.4
(Gerber)	4⅕ fl. oz.	62	14.9
(Heinz)	4¼ fl. oz.	68	15.8
Orange pudding, strained:			
(Gerber)	4¾ oz.	125	26.7
(Heinz)	4½ oz.	114	26.5

(USDA): United States Department of Agriculture
DNA: Data Not Available
*Prepared as Package Directs

Food and Description	Measure or Quantity	Calories	Carbohydrates (grams)
Pablum cereal (Drackett):			
Barley	1 oz.	100	21.7
High-protein	1 oz.	105	13.0
Mixed	1 oz.	105	19.7
Oatmeal	1 oz.	105	18.1
Rice	1 oz.	100	22.9
Pea, creamed:			
Junior (Heinz)	7¾ oz.	184	29.5
Strained (Heinz)	4½ oz.	101	15.5
Pea, split (See Split pea)			
Pea, strained:			
(Beech-Nut)	4½ oz.	83	14.5
(Gerber)	4½ oz.	60	9.2
Peach:			
Junior (Beech-Nut)	7¾ oz.	186	44.6
Junior (Gerber)	7¾ oz.	176	41.6
Junior (Heinz) freestone	7½ oz.	247	60.1
Strained (Beech-Nut)	4¾ oz.	112	27.1
Strained (Gerber)	4⁷⁄₁₀ oz.	117	27.6
Strained (Heinz)	4½ oz.	110	26.2
Peach cobbler, strained (Gerber)	4¾ oz.	134	27.5
Pear:			
Junior (Beech-Nut)	7½ oz.	138	33.6
Junior (Gerber)	7¾ oz.	139	33.2
Junior (Heinz)	7¾ oz.	167	40.0
Strained (Beech-Nut)	4¾ oz.	86	21.2
Strained (Gerber)	4⁷⁄₁₀ oz.	91	22.0
Strained (Heinz)	4½ oz.	83	19.6
Pear & pineapple:			
Junior (Beech-Nut)	7½ oz.	153	37.2
Junior (Gerber)	7¾ oz.	154	36.7
Junior (Heinz)	7¾ oz.	158	38.0
Strained (Beech-Nut)	4¾ oz.	95	23.3
Strained (Gerber)	4⁷⁄₁₀ oz.	98	23.7
Pineapple dessert, strained (Beech-Nut)	4¾ oz.	128	31.2
Pineapple-grapefruit juice drink, strained (Gerber)	4⅕ fl. oz.	72	17.3
Pineapple juice, strained (Heinz)	4¼ fl. oz.	68	14.9
Pineapple-orange:			
Junior (Heinz)	7¾ oz.	152	34.1
Strained (Heinz)	4½ oz.	109	26.4
Pineapple-orange dessert, strained (Heinz)	4½ oz.	120	28.8

(USDA): United States Department of Agriculture
DNA: Data Not Available
*Prepared as Package Directs

Food and Description	Measure or Quantity	Calories	Carbo-hydrates (grams)
Plum with tapioca:			
Junior (Beech-Nut)	7¾ oz.	208	51.1
Junior (Gerber)	7¾ oz.	225	54.9
Strained (Beech-Nut)	4¾ oz.	129	32.0
Strained (Gerber)	4⁷⁄₁₀ oz.	127	30.9
Strained (Heinz)	4½ oz.	150	36.0
Pork:			
Junior (Beech-Nut)	3½ oz.	117	0.
Junior (Gerber)	3½ oz.	124	0.
Strained (Beech-Nut)	3½ oz.	116	0.
Strained (Gerber)	3½ oz.	117	0.
Strained (Heinz)	3½ oz.	104	.5
Potatoes, creamed, with ham & bacon, toddler (Gerber)	6 oz.	197	17.2
Prune-orange juice, strained:			
(Beech-Nut)	4⅕ fl. oz.	99	24.3
(Gerber)	4⅕ fl. oz.	92	21.6
Prune-orange juice drink, strained (Heinz)	4¼ fl. oz.	71	16.8
Prune with tapioca:			
Junior (Beech-Nut)	7¾ oz.	206	50.0
Junior (Gerber)	7¾ oz.	202	48.1
Strained (Beech-Nut)	4¾ oz.	122	29.5
Strained (Gerber)	4⁷⁄₁₀ oz.	119	28.4
Strained (Heinz)	4¾ oz.	142	33.8
Spaghetti & meat balls with sauce, toddler (Gerber)	6 oz.	135	20.0
Spaghetti, tomato sauce & beef:			
Junior (Beech-Nut)	7½ oz.	136	21.2
Junior (Gerber)	7½ oz.	138	25.4
Junior (Heinz)	7½ oz.	175	23.2
Strained (Heinz)	4½ oz.	90	13.1
Spinach, creamed:			
Junior (Beech-Nut)	7½ oz.	93	17.3
Junior (Gerber)	7½ oz.	87	11.9
Strained (Beech-Nut)	4½ oz.	63	12.0
Strained (Gerber)	4½ oz.	51	6.9
Strained (Heinz)	4½ oz.	61	10.5
Split pea with bacon, junior (Gerber)	7½ oz.	170	24.4
Split pea, vegetables & bacon:			
Junior (Heinz)	7½ oz.	215	22.8
Strained (Heinz)	4½ oz.	107	11.8

Food and Description	Measure or Quantity	Calories	Carbo-hydrates (grams)
Split pea, vegetables & ham, junior (Beech-Nut)	7½ oz.	134	25.0
Squash:			
Junior (Beech-Nut)	7½ oz.	70	16.1
Junior (Gerber)	7½ oz.	53	10.6
Strained (Beech-Nut)	4½ oz.	40	8.6
Strained (Gerber)	4½ oz.	32	6.8
Strained (Heinz)	4½ oz.	33	6.9
In butter sauce, junior (Beech-Nut)	7½ oz.	89	16.2
In butter sauce, strained (Beech-Nut)	4½ oz.	54	8.8
Sweet potato:			
Junior (Beech-Nut)	7¾ oz.	144	34.6
Junior (Gerber)	7¾ oz.	156	35.6
Strained (Beech-Nut)	4¾ oz.	83	19.3
Strained (Gerber)	4½ oz.	98	22.4
Strained (Heinz)	4½ oz.	69	15.6
In butter sauce, junior (Beech-Nut)	7¾ oz.	149	33.5
In butter sauce, strained (Beech-Nut)	4¾ oz.	91	20.5
Tuna with noodles, strained (Heinz)	4½ oz.	53	8.4
Turkey:			
Junior (Beech-Nut)	3½ oz.	121	0.
Strained (Beech-Nut)	3½ oz.	116	0.
Strained (Gerber)	3½ oz.	132	.2
Turkey dinner:			
Junior (Beech-Nut)	4½ oz.	98	13.0
Strained (Beech-Nut)	4½ oz.	94	11.9
With rice, junior (Beech-Nut)	7½ oz.	76	15.8
With rice, strained (Beech-Nut)	4½ oz.	59	12.8
With vegetables, junior (Gerber)	4½ oz.	93	8.1
With vegetables, strained (Gerber)	4½ oz.	96	7.2
With vegetables, strained (Heinz)	4¾ oz.	128	8.6
Tutti frutti dessert (Heinz):			
Junior	7¾ oz.	191	44.2
Strained	4½ oz.	106	24.7
Veal:			
Junior (Beech-Nut)	3½ oz.	118	0.
Junior (Gerber)	3½ oz.	103	0.

(USDA): United States Department of Agriculture
DNA: Data Not Available
*Prepared as Package Directs

Food and Description	Measure or Quantity	Calories	Carbo-hydrates (grams)
Junior (Heinz)	3½ oz.	92	0.
Strained (Beech-Nut)	3½ oz.	116	0.
Strained (Gerber)	3½ oz.	98	0.
Strained (Heinz)	3½ oz.	67	.1
Veal dinner:			
Junior (Beech-Nut)	4½ oz.	87	8.1
Strained (Beech-Nut)	4¼ oz.	90	8.8
With vegetables, junior (Gerber)	4½ oz.	82	8.3
With vegetables, strained (Gerber)	4½ oz.	81	6.8
With vegetables & cereal, strained (Heinz)	4¾ oz.	97	5.9
Vegetables:			
Garden, strained (Beech-Nut)	4½ oz.	53	9.5
Garden, strained (Gerber)	4½ oz.	44	7.0
Mixed, junior (Gerber)	7½ oz.	83	17.2
Mixed, junior (Heinz)	7½ oz.	83	18.5
Mixed, strained (Gerber)	4½ oz.	52	11.0
Vegetables & bacon:			
Junior (Beech-Nut)	7½ oz.	123	17.7
Junior (Gerber)	7½ oz.	134	18.9
Junior (Heinz)	7½ oz.	153	14.7
Strained (Beech-Nut)	4½ oz.	72	11.3
Strained (Gerber)	4½ oz.	95	12.4
Strained (Heinz)	4½ oz.	82	9.2
Vegetables & beef:			
Junior (Beech-Nut)	7½ oz.	106	16.4
Junior (Gerber)	7½ oz.	119	15.9
Junior (Heinz)	7½ oz.	96	16.2
Strained (Beech-Nut)	4½ oz.	67	10.5
Strained (Gerber)	4½ oz.	77	9.0
Strained (Heinz)	4½ oz.	67	7.4
Vegetables & chicken (Gerber):			
Junior	7½ oz.	108	21.2
Strained	4½ oz.	56	9.0
Vegetables, dumplings, beef & bacon:			
Junior (Heinz)	7½ oz.	125	24.9
Strained (Heinz)	4½ oz.	74	10.9
Vegetables, egg noodles & chicken:			
Junior (Heinz)	7½ oz.	102	13.0
Strained (Heinz)	4½ oz.	70	9.0
Vegetables, egg noodles & turkey:			
Junior (Heinz)	7½ oz.	100	12.8

(USDA): United States Department of Agriculture
DNA: Data Not Available
*Prepared as Package Directs

Food and Description	Measure or Quantity	Calories	Carbo-hydrates (grams)
Strained (Heinz)	4½ oz.	54	7.4
Vegetables & ham:			
Strained (Beech-Nut)	4½ oz.	71	11.5
Junior (Heinz)	7½ oz.	136	14.9
With bacon, junior (Gerber)	7½ oz.	121	17.0
With bacon, strained (Gerber)	4½ oz.	93	9.7
With bacon, strained (Heinz)	4½ oz.	91	10.4
Vegetables & lamb:			
Junior (Beech-Nut)	7½ oz.	119	15.6
Junior (Gerber)	7½ oz.	117	15.5
Junior (Heinz)	7½ oz.	102	14.5
Strained (Beech-Nut)	4½ oz.	69	9.9
Strained (Gerber)	4½ oz.	68	8.6
Strained (Heinz)	4½ oz.	73	9.6
Vegetables & liver:			
Junior (Beech-Nut)	7½ oz.	87	15.9
Strained (Beech-Nut)	4½ oz.	51	9.3
With bacon, junior (Gerber)	7½ oz.	102	16.3
With bacon, strained (Gerber)	4½ oz.	76	7.9
Vegetable soup:			
Junior (Beech-Nut)	7½ oz.	80	17.6
Junior (Heinz)	7½ oz.	98	16.8
Strained (Beech-Nut)	4½ oz.	49	10.8
Strained (Heinz)	4½ oz.	54	10.6
Vegetables & turkey (Gerber):			
Junior	7½ oz.	83	15.7
Strained	4½ oz.	49	8.6
Toddler	6 oz.	164	14.6
BACO NOIR BURGUNDY WINE			
(Great Western) 12% alcohol	3 fl. oz.	78	2.1
BAC*O CHIPS (General Mills)	1 oz.	129	8.1
BAC*O'S (General Mills)	1 oz.	122	3.8
BACON, cured:			
Raw:			
(USDA) sliced	1 lb.	3016	4.5
(USDA) sliced	1 oz.	188	.2
(Oscar Mayer)	1 slice	53	D.N.A.
(Wilson)	3 oz.	506	.9
(Wilson) *Corn King*	3 oz.	531	.9

(USDA): United States Department of Agriculture
DNA: Data Not Available
*Prepared as Package Directs

Food and Description	Measure or Quantity	Calories	Carbo-hydrates (grams)
Broiled or fried, drained (USDA):			
Thin slice	1 slice (5 grams)	31	.2
Medium slice	1 slice (8 grams)	46	.2
Thick slice	1 slice (12 grams)	73	.4
Canned (USDA)	3 oz.	582	.9
BACON BITS (McCormick)	1 oz.	113	7.7
BACON, CANADIAN:			
Unheated:			
(USDA)	1 oz.	61	Tr.
(Wilson)	1 oz.	42	.3
Broiled or fried (USDA)	1 oz.	79	Tr.
BAGEL (USDA):			
Egg	3″ dia. (1.9 oz.)	165	28.0
Water	3″ dia. (1.9 oz.)	165	30.0
BAKING POWDER:			
Phosphate (USDA)	1 tsp.	6	1.4
SAS (USDA)	1 tsp.	5	1.1
Tartrate (USDA)	1 tsp.	3	.7
(Royal)	1 tsp.	4	1.0
BAKON DELITES (Wise):			
Regular	½ cup (8 grams)	44	0.
Barbecue flavored	½ cup (8 grams)	42	0.
BALI HAI WINE (Italian Swiss Colony–Gold Medal) 11% alcohol	3 fl. oz.	89	9.2
BAMBOO SHOOT, raw, whole (USDA)	½ lb. (weighed untrimmed)	18	3.4
BANANA (USDA):			
Common:			
Fresh:			
Whole	1 lb. (weighed with skin)	262	68.5
Small size	4.9-oz. banana (7¾″ x 1¹¹⁄₃₂″)	81	21.1
Medium size	6.2-oz. banana (8¾″ x 1¹³⁄₃₂″)	101	26.4
Large size	7-oz. banana (9¾″ x 1⁷⁄₁₆″)	116	30.2

(USDA): United States Department of Agriculture
DNA: Data Not Available
*Prepared as Package Directs

Food and Description	Measure or Quantity	Calories	Carbo-hydrates (grams)
Mashed	1 cup (about 2 med.)	189	49.3
Sliced	1 cup (1¼ med.)	124	32.4
Dehydrated or powder	1 oz.	96	25.1
Red, fresh, whole	1 lb. (weighed with skin)	278	72.2

BANANA, BAKING (see PLANTAIN)

BANANA CAKE MIX:
(Betty Crocker) *Chiquita Banana*	1-lb. 2.5-oz. pkg.	1814	365.5
(Betty Crocker) *Chiquita Banana*	1 oz.	117	23.0
(Pillsbury)	1 oz.	120	22.7
(Pillsbury) loaf cake	1 oz.	117	22.6

BANANA CREAM PIE:
(Tastykake)	4-oz. pie	485	82.4
Frozen (Banquet)	2½ oz.	185	25.0
Frozen (Mrs. Smith's)	⅙ of 8″ pie	193	23.1

*BANANA CREAM PIE FILLING MIX (Jell-O) — ½ cup (5.3 oz.) — 179 — 31.0

BANANA CREAM PUDDING MIX:
*Instant (Jell-O)	½ cup (5.3 oz.)	177	30.5
*Instant (Royal)	½ cup (5 oz.)	175	30.2
*Regular (Jell-O)	½ cup (5.3 oz.)	179	31.0
Regular (My-T-Fine)	1 oz.	122	26.9

BANANA CRISPS, dehydrated snack (Epicure) — 1 oz. — 74 — 19.2

BANANA CUSTARD PIE, home recipe (USDA) — ⅙ of 9″ pie — 336 — 46.7

BANANA LIQUEUR (Leroux):
56 proof	1 fl. oz.	92	11.4
100 proof	1 fl. oz.	116	9.2

*BANANA PUDDING MIX, regular (Royal) — ½ cup (5 oz.) — 165 — 27.2

(USDA): United States Department of Agriculture
DNA: Data Not Available
*Prepared as Package Directs

Food and Description	Measure or Quantity	Calories	Carbo-hydrates (grams)
BANANA SOFT DRINK (Yoo-Hoo):			
Regular	6 fl. oz.	90	18.0
High-protein	6 fl. oz.	114	24.6
BARBADOS CHERRY (See **ACEROLA**)			
BARBECUE SAUCE (See **SAUCE**, Barbecue)			
BARBECUE SEASONING (Lawry's):			
Bar-B-Q	1 pkg. (4½ oz.)	408	97.8
Sweet 'N Sour	1 pkg. (4½ oz.)	394	88.4
BARBERA WINE (Louis M. Martini) 12½% alcohol	3 fl. oz.	90	.2
BARDOLINO WINE, Italian red (Antinori) 12% alcohol	3 fl. oz.	84	6.3
BARLEY:			
Pearled, dry, light:			
(USDA)	¼ cup (1.8 oz.)	174	39.4
(Albers)	¼ cup	177	40.0
(Quaker-Scotch) regular or quick	¼ cup (1.7 oz.)	171	37.0
Pot or Scotch, dry (USDA)	2 oz.	197	43.8
BARRACUDA, raw, meat only (USDA)	4 oz.	128	0.
BASS (USDA):			
Black sea:			
Raw, meat only	4 oz.	106	0.
Baked, stuffed, home recipe	4 oz.	294	12.9
Smallmouth & largemouth, raw:			
Whole	1 lb. (weighed whole)	146	0.
Meat only	4 oz.	118	0.
Striped:			
Raw, whole	1 lb. (weighed whole)	205	0.

(USDA): United States Department of Agriculture
DNA: Data Not Available
*Prepared as Package Directs

Food and Description	Measure or Quantity	Calories	Carbo-hydrates (grams)
Raw, meat only	4 oz.	119	0.
Oven-fried	4 oz.	222	7.6
White, raw, meat only	4 oz.	111	0.
B & B LIQUEUR, (Julius Wile) 86 proof	1 fl. oz.	94	5.7
BAVARIAN PIE FILLING (Lucky Leaf)	8 oz.	306	51.8
BAVARIAN PIE or PUDDING MIX:			
Cream (My-T-Fine)	1 oz.	122	26.8
*Custard, *Rice-A-Roni*	½ cup (3.5 oz.)	126	21.7
BAVARIAN-STYLE VEGE-TABLES (Birds Eye) frozen	⅓ pkg. (3⅓ oz.)	138	11.9
BEAN, BAKED:			
Canned:			
(B & M) New England-style sauce	½ cup (4½ oz.)	180	30.2
(Heinz) in molasses sauce	½ cup	166	29.7
Canned with pork:			
(Campbell)	4 oz.	130	21.3
(Cannon)	4 oz.	138	21.5
(Hunt's)	4 oz.	138	21.5
Canned with pork & molasses sauce:			
(USDA)	1 cup (4.5 oz.)	192	27.0
(Green Giant)	½ cup (4.4 oz.)	154	24.1
(Heinz) Boston-style	½ cup	184	31.5
Canned with pork & tomato sauce:			
(USDA)	½ cup (4.5 oz.)	156	24.3
(Green Giant)	½ cup (4.4 oz.)	140	23.1
(Heinz)	½ cup	150	21.4
Canned with tomato sauce:			
(USDA)	½ cup (4.5 oz.)	154	29.4
(Heinz) *Campside*, smoky beans	½ cup	180	25.5
(Heinz) vegetarian	½ cup	135	25.6
(Morton House)	11-oz. can	460	D.N.A.
BEAN, BARBECUE (Campbell)	4 oz.	143	25.5
BEAN, BAYO, dry (USDA)	4 oz.	385	69.4

(USDA): United States Department of Agriculture
DNA: Data Not Available
*Prepared as Package Directs

Food and Description	Measure or Quantity	Calories	Carbo-hydrates (grams)
BEAN, BLACK, dry (USDA)	4 oz.	385	69.4
BEAN, BROWN, dry (USDA)	4 oz.	385	69.4
BEAN, CALICO, dry (USDA)	4 oz.	396	72.2
BEAN, CHILI (See **CHILI**)			
BEAN & FRANKFURTER, canned:			
(Campbell)	4 oz.	181	17.8
(Heinz)	4 oz.	184	18.0
BEAN & FRANKFURTER DINNER, frozen:			
(Banquet)	10¾-oz. dinner	687	70.5
(Morton)	11-oz. dinner	428	57.6
(Swanson)	11½-oz. dinner	610	70.1
BEAN, GREEN or SNAP: Fresh (USDA):			
Whole	1 lb. (weighed untrimmed)	128	28.3
1½″ to 2″ pieces	½ cup (1.8 oz.)	17	3.8
French-style	½ cup (1.4 oz.)	12	2.8
Boiled, drained, whole (USDA)	½ cup (2.2 oz.)	15	3.5
Boiled, drained, 1½″ to 2″ pieces (USDA)	½ cup (2.4 oz.)	17	3.7
Canned, regular pack:			
Solids & liq. (USDA)	½ cup (4.2 oz.)	22	5.0
Drained solids, whole (USDA)	4 oz.	27	5.9
Drained solids, cut (USDA)	½ cup (2.5 oz.)	17	3.6
Drained liq. (USDA)	4 oz.	11	2.7
Drained solids (Butter Kernel)	½ cup	20	4.6
Blue Lake, drained solids (Cannon)	4 oz.	27	5.9
(Fall River)	½ cup	20	4.6
(Green Giant)	½ cup (3.8 oz.)	20	4.6
Solids & liq. (Stokely-Van Camp)	½ cup	22	5.0
Canned, dietetic pack:			
Solids & liq. (USDA)	4 oz.	18	4.1
Drained solids (USDA)	4 oz.	25	5.4
Drained liq. (USDA)	4 oz.	9	2.0

(USDA): United States Department of Agriculture
DNA: Data Not Available
*Prepared as Package Directs

Food and Description	Measure or Quantity	Calories	Carbo-hydrates (grams)
Cut, solids & liq. (Blue Boy)	4 oz.	22	5.5
Cut (Diet Delight)	½ cup (4.2 oz.)	18	3.2
Cut (S and W) *Nutradiet*	4 oz.	18	3.2
(Tillie Lewis)	½ cup (4.2 oz.)	19	3.6
Frozen:			
Cut, not thawed (USDA)	4 oz.	29	6.8
Cut, boiled, drained solids (USDA)	4 oz.	28	6.5
Cut, boiled, drained solids (USDA)	½ cup (2.8 oz.)	20	4.6
Cut (Birds Eye)	½ cup (3 oz.)	23	5.2
Cut (Stokely-Van Camp)	4 oz.	29	6.8
Whole (Birds Eye)	½ cup (3 oz.)	23	5.2
(Blue Goose)	4 oz.	35	6.4
French-style (Birds Eye)	½ cup (3 oz.)	23	5.2
French-style, with toasted almonds (Birds Eye)	½ cup (3 oz.)	52	5.9
French-style, with sautéed mushrooms (Birds Eye)	½ cup (3 oz.)	33	5.7
In butter sauce (Birds Eye)	½ cup (3 oz.)	48	4.5
In butter sauce, kitchen-sliced (Green Giant)	4 oz.	67	5.6
In mushroom sauce (Green Giant)	4 oz.	69	7.4
BEAN & GROUND BEEF, canned (Campbell)	4 oz.	129	17.4
BEAN, ITALIAN, frozen:			
(Birds Eye)	½ cup (3 oz.)	23	5.2
In butter sauce (Green Giant) boil-in-the-bag	4 oz.	70	5.3
BEAN, KIDNEY or RED:			
Dry:			
(USDA)	1 lb.	1556	280.8
(USDA)	½ cup (3.2 oz.)	319	57.6
(Sinsheimer)	1 oz.	99	17.6
Cooked (USDA)	4 oz.	134	24.3
Canned:			
Solids & liq. (USDA)	½ cup (4.6 oz.)	115	21.0
Drained solids (Butter Kernel)	½ cup	108	19.7
Red kidney or small red (Hunt's)	4 oz.	102	18.6

(USDA): United States Department of Agriculture
DNA: Data Not Available
*Prepared as Package Directs

Food and Description	Measure or Quantity	Calories	Carbo-hydrates (grams)
Red kidney & chili gravy (Nalley's)	4 oz.	113*	18.5
BEAN, LIMA, young:			
Raw, whole (USDA)	1 lb. (weighed in pod)	223	40.1
Raw, without shell (USDA)	1 lb. (weighed shelled)	558	100.2
Boiled, drained solids (USDA)	½ cup (3 oz.)	94	16.8
Canned, regular pack:			
Solids & liq. (USDA)	4 oz.	81	15.2
Drained solids (USDA)	4 oz.	109	20.8
Drained solids (USDA)	½ cup (3 oz.)	84	15.9
Drained liq. (USDA)	4 oz.	23	4.4
With ham (Nalley's)	4 oz.	125	14.3
Canned, dietetic pack:			
Solids & liq., low sodium (USDA)	4 oz.	80	15.0
Drained solids, low sodium (USDA)	4 oz.	108	20.1
Solids & liq., unseasoned (Blue Boy)	4 oz.	79	12.5
Frozen:			
Baby butter beans (Birds Eye)	½ cup (3.3 oz.)	313	57.9
Baby limas:			
(USDA)	4 oz.	138	26.0
Boiled, drained solids (USDA)	4 oz.	134	25.3
Boiled, drained solids (USDA)	½ cup (3 oz.)	102	19.2
(Birds Eye)	½ cup (3.3 oz.)	114	21.5
(Stokely-Van Camp)	4 oz.	138	26.0
In butter sauce (Green Giant)	4 oz.	136	18.1
Fordhooks:			
(USDA)	4 oz.	116	22.0
Boiled, drained solids (USDA)	4 oz.	112	21.7
Boiled, drained solids (USDA)	½ cup (3 oz.)	83	16.0
(Birds Eye)	½ cup (3.3 oz.)	96	18.3
BEAN, LIMA, MATURE:			
Dry:			
Baby (USDA)	½ cup (3.4 oz.)	331	61.4
Large (USDA)	½ cup (3.1 oz.)	304	56.3
(Sinsheimer)	1 oz.	92	17.5
Boiled, drained solids (USDA)	½ cup (3.4 oz.)	131	24.3

(USDA): United States Department of Agriculture
DNA: Data Not Available
*Prepared as Package Directs

Food and Description	Measure or Quantity	Calories	Carbo-hydrates (grams)
BEAN, MUNG, dry (USDA)	½ cup (3.7 oz.)	357	63.3
BEAN, PINTO, dry:			
(USDA)	4 oz.	396	72.2
(USDA)	½ cup (3.4 oz.)	335	61.2
(Sinsheimer)	1 oz.	99	17.6
*(Uncle Ben's) quick-cooked, including broth	½ cup	91	17.3
BEAN, RED (See BEAN, KIDNEY or BEAN, RED MEXICAN).			
BEAN, RED MEXICAN, dry (USDA)	4 oz.	396	72.2
BEAN, REFRIED, canned (Rosarita)	4 oz.	120	17.2
BEAN SOUP, canned:			
*(Manischewitz)	8 oz. (by wt.)	112	17.6
*(Wyler's)	1 cup	96	D.N.A.
With bacon, condensed (Campbell)	8 oz. (by wt.)	302	38.8
With pork, condensed (USDA)	8 oz. (by wt.)	304	39.3
*With pork, prepared with equal volume water (USDA)	1 cup (8.8 oz.)	168	21.8
With smoked ham (Heinz) *Great American*	1 cup	184	22.5
*With smoked pork (Heinz)	1 cup	165	19.1
BEAN SOUP, BLACK, canned:			
Condensed (Campbell)	8 oz. (by wt.)	181	27.7
(Crosse & Blackwell)	8 oz. (by wt.)	118	19.1
***BEAN SOUP, LIMA,** canned (Manischewitz)	8 oz. (by wt.)	93	15.3
BEAN SOUP, NAVY, dehydrated (USDA)	1 oz.	92	17.8
BEAN SPROUT:			
Mung:			
Raw (USDA)	½ lb.	80	15.0
Raw (USDA)	½ cup (1.6 oz.)	15	3.0

Food and Description	Measure or Quantity	Calories	Carbo-hydrates (grams)
Boiled, drained solids (USDA)	½ cup (2.2 oz.)	17	3.2
Soy:			
Raw (USDA)	½ lb.	104	12.0
Raw (USDA)	½ cup (1.9 oz.)	25	2.9
Boiled, drained solids (USDA)	4 oz.	43	4.2
Canned (Chun King)	4 oz.	22	2.8

BEAN, WAX (See **BEAN, YELLOW**)

BEAN, WHITE, dry:

Raw:			
Great Northern (USDA)	½ cup (3.2 oz.)	302	54.6
White (USDA)	1 oz.	96	17.4
Navy or pea (Sinsheimer)	1 oz.	99	17.6
Cooked:			
Great Northern (USDA)	½ cup (3 oz.)	100	18.0
White (USDA)	4 oz.	134	24.0
*(Uncle Ben's) quick-cooked, including broth	½ cup	88	15.7

BEAN, YELLOW or WAX:

Raw, whole (USDA)	1 lb. (weighed untrimmed)	108	24.0
Boiled, drained solids (USDA)	4 oz.	25	5.2
Boiled, drained solids (USDA)	½ cup (2.8 oz.)	18	3.8
Canned, regular pack:			
Solids & liq. (USDA)	4 oz.	22	4.8
Drained solids (USDA)	4 oz.	27	5.9
Drained liq. (USDA)	4 oz.	12	2.8
Drained solids (Butter Kernel)	½ cup	20	4.6
(Green Giant)	½ cup (3.8 oz.)	20	4.6
Solids & liq. (Stokely-Van Camp)	4 oz.	25	5.2
Canned, dietetic pack:			
Solids & liq. (USDA)	4 oz.	17	3.9
Drained solids (USDA)	4 oz.	24	5.3
Drained liq. (USDA)	4 oz.	8	1.6
Solids & liq. (Blue Boy)	4 oz.	18	3.3
Frozen:			
Cut, not thawed (USDA)	4 oz.	32	7.4
Boiled, drained solids (USDA)	4 oz.	31	7.0
Cut (Birds Eye)	½ cup (3 oz.)	25	5.5

(USDA): United States Department of Agriculture
DNA: Data Not Available
*Prepared as Package Directs

Food and Description	Measure or Quantity	Calories	Carbo-hydrates (grams)
BEAUJOLAIS WINE, French Burgundy:			
(Barton & Guestier) St. Louis, 11% alcohol	3 fl. oz.	60	.1
(Chanson) St. Vincent, 11% alcohol	3 fl. oz.	78	6.3
(Cruse) 12% alcohol	3 fl. oz.	72	D.N.A.
BEAUNE WINE:			
Clos des Feves, French Burgundy (Chanson) 12% alcohol	3 fl. oz.	84	6.3
St. Vincent, French Burgundy (Chanson) 12% alcohol	3 fl. oz.	84	6.3
BEAVER, roasted (USDA)	4 oz.	281	0.
BEECHNUT:			
Whole (USDA)	4 oz. (weighed in shell)	393	14.1
Shelled (USDA)	4 oz. (weighed shelled)	644	23.0
BEEF. Values for beef cuts are given below for "lean and fat" and for "lean only." Beef purchased by the consumer at the retail store usually is trimmed to about one-half inch layer of fat. This is the meat described as "lean and fat." If all the fat that can be cut off with a knife is removed, the remainder is the "lean only." These cuts still contain flecks of fat known as "marbling" distributed through the meat. Choice grade cuts (USDA):			
Brisket:			
Raw	1 lb. (weighed with bone)	1284	0.
Braised:			
Lean & fat	4 oz.	467	0.
Lean only	4 oz.	252	0.
Chuck:			
Raw	1 lb. (weighed with bone)	984	0.

(USDA): United States Department of Agriculture
DNA: Data Not Available
*Prepared as Package Directs

Food and Description	Measure or Quantity	Calories	Carbo-hydrates (grams)
Braised or pot-roasted:			
Lean & fat	4 oz.	371	0.
Lean only	4 oz.	243	0.
Dried (See **BEEF, CHIPPED**)			
Fat, separable, cooked	1 oz.	207	0.
Filet mignon. There are no data available on its composition. For dietary estimates, the data for sirloin steak, lean only, affords the closest approximation.			
Flank:			
Raw	1 lb.	653	0.
Braised	4 oz.	222	0.
Foreshank:			
Raw	1 lb. (weighed with bone)	531	0.
Simmered:			
Lean & fat	4 oz.	310	0.
Lean only	4 oz.	209	0.
Ground:			
Lean:			
Raw	1 lb.	812	0.
Raw	1 cup (8 oz.)	405	0.
Broiled	4 oz.	248	0.
Regular:			
Raw	1 lb.	1216	0.
Raw	1 cup (8 oz.)	606	0.
Broiled	4 oz.	324	0.
Heel of round:			
Raw	1 lb.	967	0.
Roasted:			
Lean & fat	4 oz.	296	0.
Lean only	4 oz.	204	0.
Hindshank:			
Raw	1 lb. (weighed with bone)	604	0.
Braised:			
Lean & fat	4 oz.	409	0.
Lean only	4 oz.	209	0.
Neck:			
Raw	1 lb. (weighed with bone)	820	0.
Pot-roasted:			
Lean & fat	4 oz.	332	0.

(USDA): United States Department of Agriculture
DNA: Data Not Available
*Prepared as Package Directs

Food and Description	Measure or Quantity	Calories	Carbohydrates (grams)
Lean only	4 oz.	222	0.
Plate:			
Raw	1 lb. (weighed with bone)	1615	0.
Simmered:			
Lean & fat	4 oz.	538	0.
Lean only	4 oz.	252	0.
Rib:			
Raw	1 lb. (weighed with bone)	1673	0.
Roasted:			
Lean & fat	4 oz.	499	0.
Lean only	4 oz.	273	0.
Round:			
Raw	1 lb. (weighed with bone)	863	0.
Broiled:			
Lean & fat	4 oz.	296	0.
Lean only	4 oz.	214	0.
Rump:			
Raw	1 lb. (weighed with bone)	1167	0.
Roasted:			
Lean & fat	4 oz.	393	0.
Lean only	4 oz.	236	0.
Steak, club:			
Raw	1 lb. (weighed without bone)	1724	0.
Broiled:			
Lean & fat	4 oz.	515	0.
Lean only	4 oz.	277	0.
One 8-oz. steak (weighed without bone before cooking) will give you:			
Lean & fat	5.9 oz.	754	0.
Lean only	3.4 oz.	234	0.
Steak, porterhouse:			
Raw	1 lb. (weighed with bone)	1603	0.
Broiled:			
Lean & fat	4 oz.	527	0.
Lean only	4 oz.	254	0.
One 16-oz. steak (weighed with			

(USDA): United States Department of Agriculture
DNA: Data Not Available
*Prepared as Package Directs

Food and Description	Measure or Quantity	Calories	Carbo-hydrates (grams)
bone before cooking) will give you:			
Lean & fat	10.2 oz.	1339	0.
Lean only	5.9 oz.	372	0.
Steak, ribeye, broiled:			
One 10-oz. steak (weighed before cooking without bone) will give you:			
Lean & fat	7.3 oz.	911	0.
Lean only	3.8 oz.	258	0.
Steak, sirloin, double-bone:			
Raw	1 lb. (weighed with bone)	1240	0.
Broiled:			
Lean & fat	4 oz.	463	0.
Lean only	4 oz.	245	0.
One 16-oz. steak (weighed before cooking with bone) will give you:			
Lean & fat	8.9 oz.	1028	0.
Lean only	5.9 oz.	359	0.
One 12-oz. steak (weighed before cooking with bone) will give you:			
Lean & fat	6.6 oz.	767	0.
Lean only	4.4 oz.	268	0.
Steak, sirloin, hipbone:			
Raw	1 lb. (weighed with bone)	1585	0.
Broiled:			
Lean & fat	4 oz.	552	0.
Lean only	4 oz.	272	0.
Steak, sirloin, wedge & round bone:			
Raw	1 lb. (weighed with bone)	1316	0.
Broiled:			
Lean & fat	4 oz.	439	0.
Lean only	4 oz.	235	0.
Steak, T-bone:			
Raw	1 lb. (weighed with bone)	1596	0.
Broiled:			
Lean & fat	4 oz.	536	0.

Food and Description	Measure or Quantity	Calories	Carbohydrates (grams)
Lean only	4 oz.	253	0.
One 16-oz. steak (weighed before cooking with bone) will give you:			
Lean & fat	9.8 oz.	1315	0.
Lean only	5.5 oz.	348	0.
BEEFARONI, canned (Chef Boy-Ar-Dee)	8 oz. (⅕ of 40-oz. can)	208	27.9
BEEF & BEEF STOCK (Bunker Hill)	15-oz. can.	920	0.
BEEF BOUILLON/BROTH, cubes or powder (see also **BEEF SOUP**):			
(Croyden House)	1 tsp.	12	2.3
(Herb-Ox)	1 cube	6	.5
(Herb-Ox) instant	1 packet	10	.7
(Knorr Swiss)	1 cube	13	D.N.A.
(Knorr Swiss)	1 tsp.	11	D.N.A.
(Maggi)	1 cube	7	.5
(Maggi) instant	1 tsp.	7	.5
(Wyler's)	1 cube	7	.4
(Wyler's) instant	1 tsp.	7	.4
BEEF, CHIPPED:			
Uncooked:			
(USDA)	½ cup (2.9 oz.)	167	0.
(USDA)	2 oz. (about ⅓ cup)	115	0.
(Armour Star)	1 oz.	48	0.
(Eckrich) *Slender Sliced*	1 oz.	40	D.N.A.
Cooked, creamed, home recipe (USDA)	4 oz.	175	8.1
Frozen, creamed (Banquet) cookin' bag	5 oz.	127	11.8
BEEF, CHOPPED, canned (Hormel)	12-oz. can	865	2.0
BEEF, CORNED (See **CORNED BEEF**)			

(USDA): United States Department of Agriculture
DNA: Data Not Available
*Prepared as Package Directs

Food and Description	Measure or Quantity	Calories	Carbo-hydrates (grams)
BEEF DINNER, frozen:			
(Banquet)	11-oz. dinner	295	20.2
(Morton)	11-oz. dinner	350	20.3
(Swanson)	11-oz. dinner	414	32.5
(Swanson) 3-course	16¼-oz. dinner	602	65.4
Chopped (Banquet)	11-oz. dinner	386	27.0
Chopped (Swanson)	10-oz. dinner	447	40.0
Pot Roast, includes potatoes, peas and corn (USDA)	10 oz.	300	17.3
Stew (Tom Thumb)	3-lb. 8-oz. tray	1375	97.3
BEEF GOULASH:			
Canned (Heinz)	7¾ oz.	183	17.6
Seasoning mix (Lawry's)	1 pkg. (1.7 oz.)	126	24.1
BEEF HASH, ROAST:			
Canned (Hormel) *Mary Kitchen*	15-oz. can	705	37.8
Frozen (Stouffer's)	11½-oz. pkg.	460	21.7
BEEF JERKY (Giant Snacks)	1 oz.	85	0.
BEEF KABOBS, frozen (Colonial Beef)	6 oz.	540	D.N.A.
BEEF PIE:			
Baked, home recipe (USDA)	4¼″ pie (8 oz. before baking)	558	42.7
Frozen:			
Commercial, unheated (USDA)	8 oz.	436	40.8
(Banquet)	8-oz. pie	411	40.5
(Morton)	8¼-oz. pie	429	37.6
(Stouffer's)	10-oz. pie	572	42.9
(Swanson)	8-oz. pie	443	37.0
(Swanson) deep dish	1-lb. pie	631	51.3
BEEF PUFFS, hors d'oeuvre, frozen (Durkee)	1 piece (½ oz.)	62	3.1
BEEF RAGOUT, frozen (Swanson)	8.5-oz. pkg.	177	13.7
BEEF, ROAST, canned (USDA)	4 oz.	254	0.

(USDA): United States Department of Agriculture
DNA: Data Not Available
*Prepared as Package Directs

Food and Description	Measure or Quantity	Calories	Carbo-hydrates (grams)
BEEF, SLICED, with barbecue sauce:			
Buffet (Banquet)	2 lb.	1115	81.8
Cookin' bag (Banquet)	5 oz.	174	12.8
BEEF SOUP, canned:			
Condensed (Campbell)	8 oz. (by wt.)	197	20.9
*Barley (Manischewitz)	8 oz. (by wt.)	83	11.3
*Barley, mix (Wyler's)	6 fl. oz.	54	10.0
Bouillon, condensed (USDA)	8 oz. (by wt.)	59	5.0
*Bouillon, prepared with equal volume water (USDA)	1 cup (8.5 oz.)	31	2.6
Broth:			
Condensed (USDA)	8 oz. (by wt.)	59	5.0
*Prepared with equal volume water (USDA)	1 cup (8.5 oz.)	31	2.6
Condensed (Campbell)	8 oz. (by wt.)	50	4.8
*Cabbage (Manischewitz)	8 oz. (by wt.)	62	9.1
Consommé, condensed (USDA)	8 oz. (by wt.)	59	5.0
*Consommé, prepared with equal volume water (USDA)	1 cup (8.5 oz.)	31	2.6
Noodle:			
Condensed (USDA)	8 oz. (by wt.)	129	13.2
*Prepared with equal volume water (USDA)	1 cup (8.5 oz.)	67	7.0
Condensed (Campbell)	8 oz. (by wt.)	132	16.3
(Heinz)	1 cup	68	5.5
*(Manischewitz)	8 oz. (by wt.)	64	8.0
With dumplings (Heinz) *Great American*	1 cup	100	10.2
*Vegetable (Manischewitz)	8 oz. (by wt.)	59	8.9
BEEF SOUP MIX, noodle:			
(USDA)	1 oz.	110	18.5
*(USDA)	1 cup (8.1 oz.)	64	11.0
(Lipton)	1 pkg. (2 oz.)	197	32.6
*(Wyler's)	6 fl. oz.	37	7.0
BEEF STEW:			
Home recipe (USDA)	1 cup (8.3 oz.)	209	14.6
Canned:			
(USDA)	8 oz.	179	16.1
(Armour Star)	24-oz. can	600	38.8
(Austex)	15½-oz. can	347	31.2

(USDA): United States Department of Agriculture
DNA: Data Not Available
*Prepared as Package Directs

Food and Description	Measure or Quantity	Calories	Carbo-hydrates (grams)
(B&M)	1 cup (9 oz.)	163	14.7
(Bounty)	8 oz.	179	15.9
(Bunker Hill)	15-oz. can	422	18.0
(Dinty Moore)	15-oz. can	307	21.2
(Heinz)	8-oz. can	182	14.1
(Morton House)	15-oz. can	570	D.N.A.
(Nalley's)	8 oz.	204	18.8
(Wilson)	8 oz.	177	15.9
Dietetic (Claybourne)	8-oz. can	272	18.3
Meatball (Hormel)	1-lb. 8-oz. can	631	27.9
Frozen, buffet (Banquet)	2-lb. pkg.	720	82.2

BEEF STEW SEASONING MIX:

(French's)	1⅞-oz. pkg.	91	13.9
(Lawry's)	1⅗-oz. pkg.	131	24.2

BEEF STROGANOFF (See **STROGANOFF**)

BEER, canned:
Regular:

(USDA) 4.5% alcohol	12 fl. oz.	151	13.7
Andeker	12 fl. oz.	165	D.N.A.
Buckeye, 4.6% alcohol	12 fl. oz.	144	11.0
Budweiser, 4.9% alcohol	12 fl. oz.	156	12.3
Budweiser, 3.9% alcohol	12 fl. oz.	137	11.9
Busch Bavarian, 4.9% alcohol	12 fl. oz.	156	12.3
Busch Bavarian, 3.9% alcohol	12 fl. oz.	137	11.9
Eastside Lager	12 fl. oz.	145	D.N.A.
Gold Medal	12 fl. oz.	160	9.6
Hamm's	12 fl. oz.	151	13.3
Knickerbocker, 4.6% alcohol	12 fl. oz.	160	13.7
Meister Brau Premium, 4.6% alcohol	12 fl. oz.	144	11.0
Meister Brau Premium Draft, 4.6% alcohol	12 fl. oz.	144	11.0
Michelob, 4.9% alcohol	12 fl. oz.	160	12.8
Narragansett, 4.7% alcohol	12 fl. oz.	155	14.4
North Star, regular	12 fl. oz.	165	14.9
North Star, 3.2 low gravity	12 fl. oz.	142	13.6
Pabst Blue Ribbon	12 fl. oz.	150	D.N.A.
Pfeifer, regular	12 fl. oz.	165	14.9
Pfeifer, 3.2 low gravity	12 fl. oz.	142	13.6
Rheingold, 4.6% alcohol	12 fl. oz.	160	13.7

(USDA): United States Department of Agriculture
DNA: Data Not Available
*Prepared as Package Directs

Food and Description	Measure or Quantity	Calories	Carbo- hydrates (grams)
Schlitz	12 fl. oz.	155	D.N.A.
Schmidt, regular	12 fl. oz.	165	14.9
Schmidt, extra special, regular	12 fl. oz.	165	14.9
Schmidt, 3.2 low gravity	12 fl. oz.	142	13.6
Utica Club	12 fl. oz.	150	D.N.A.
Yuengling Premium	12 fl. oz.	144	15.1
Low carbohydrate:			
Dia-beer	12 fl. oz.	145	4.3
Dia-beer	7 fl. oz.	85	2.5
Gablinger's, 4.5% alcohol	12 fl. oz.	99	.2
Meister Brau Lite, 4.6% alcohol	12 fl. oz.	96	1.4
BEER, NEAR:			
Select (Schmidt)	12 fl. oz.	78	D.N.A.
Zing (Heileman)	12 fl. oz.	55	D.N.A.
BEET:			
Raw (USDA)	1 lb. (weighed with skins, without tops)	137	31.4
Raw, diced (USDA)	½ cup (3 oz.)	28	6.6
Boiled, diced, drained solids (USDA)	½ cup (3.2 oz.)	27	6.1
Boiled, sliced, drained solids (USDA)	½ cup (3.6 oz.)	32	7.4
Canned, regular pack:			
Solids & liq. (USDA)	4 oz.	39	9.0
Solids & liq. (USDA)	½ cup (4.3 oz.)	42	9.7
Drained solids (USDA)	4 oz.	42	10.0
Drained solids, whole (USDA)	½ cup (2.8 oz.)	29	7.0
Drained solids, diced (USDA)	½ cup (2.8 oz.)	30	7.2
Drained solids, sliced (USDA)	½ cup (3.1 oz.)	32	7.7
Drained liq. (USDA)	4 oz.	29	7.0
Drained solids (Butter Kernel)	½ cup	38	9.1
Drained solids (Comstock-Greenwood)	4 oz.	39	10.0
(Fall River)	½ cup	38	9.1
Pickled, drained (Comstock-Greenwood)	1 oz.	14	3.5
Canned, dietetic pack:			
Solids & liq. (USDA)	4 oz.	36	8.8
Drained solids (USDA)	4 oz.	42	9.9
Drained liq. (USDA)	4 oz.	28	6.7
Whole (Blue Boy)	10 small (3.5 oz.)	35	7.5

(USDA): United States Department of Agriculture
DNA: Data Not Available
*Prepared as Package Directs

Food and Description	Measure or Quantity	Calories	Carbo-hydrates (grams)
Diced, solids & liq. (Blue Boy)	4 oz.	25	5.1
Sliced (Blue Boy)	10 slices (3½ oz.)	26	5.5
Sliced (S and W) *Nutradiet*	4 oz.	32	6.7
(Tillie Lewis)	½ cup (4.3 oz.)	46	9.0
Frozen, sliced, in orange flavor glaze (Birds Eye)	½ cup (3.3 oz.)	53	12.9
BEET GREENS (USDA):			
Raw, whole	1 lb. (weighed untrimmed)	61	11.7
Boiled, leaves & stems drained	4 oz.	20	3.7
Boiled, leaves & stems drained	½ cup (2.6 oz.)	13	2.4
BENEDICTINE LIQUEUR (Julius Wile) 86 proof	1 fl. oz.	112	10.3
BERNKASTELER, German Moselle wine, (Deinhard) 11% alcohol	3 fl. oz.	60	1.0
BERNKASTELER DOKTOR, 1966 German Moselle wine, (Deinhard) 11% alcohol	3 fl. oz.	60	1.0
BEVERAGE (See individual listings.)			
BIANCA DELLA COSTA TOSCANA, Italian white wine (Antinori) 12½% alcohol	3 fl. oz.	87	6.3
BIF (Wilson) canned luncheon meat	3 oz.	272	1.5
BIRCH BEER, soft drink:			
(Canada Dry)	6 fl. oz.	78	20.4
(Yukon Club)	6 fl. oz.	88	21.9
BISCUIT:			
Baking powder, home recipe (USDA)	1.3-oz. biscuit (2½″ dia.)	140	17.4
Egg (Stella D'oro):			
Dietetic	1 piece	42	6.6
Regular	1 piece	37	D.N.A.
Roman	1 piece	135	19.2
Sugared	1 piece	57	D.N.A.

(USDA): United States Department of Agriculture
DNA: Data Not Available
*Prepared as Package Directs

Food and Description	Measure or Quantity	Calories	Carbo-hydrates (grams)
BISCUIT DOUGH:			
Frozen, commerical (USDA)	1 oz.	92	13.8
Refrigerated:			
Commercial (USDA)	1 oz.	78	13.2
(Pillsbury) *Ballard*, ovenready	1 oz.	72	12.8
(Pillsbury) baking powder, Tenderflake:			
Regular	1 oz.	92	11.1
Buttermilk	1 oz.	94	11.1
(Pillsbury) buttermilk:			
Regular	1 oz.	72	12.8
Extra light	1 oz.	75	12.0
Hungry Jack, regular	1 oz.	77	12.2
Hungry Jack, flaky	1 oz.	97	10.9
Tenderflake	1 oz.	94	11.1
(Pillsbury) country style	1 oz.	72	12.8
(Pillsbury) Hungry Jack:			
Butter tastin'	1 oz.	101	10.4
Flaky	1 oz.	97	10.6
(Pillsbury) Tenderburst	1 oz.	95	11.0
BISCUIT MIX:			
Dry, with enriched flour (USDA)	1 oz.	120	19.5
*Baked from mix, with added milk (USDA)	1-oz. biscuit	92	14.8
Bisquick (Betty Crocker)	1-lb. 4-oz. pkg.	2380	390.0
New Bisquick (Betty Crocker)	1-lb. 4-oz. pkg.	2420	382.0
BI-SICLE (Popsicle Industries)	3 fl. oz.	116	D.N.A.
BITTER LEMON, soft drink:			
(Canada Dry)	6 fl. oz.	78	20.4
(Hoffmann)	6 fl. oz.	84	21.0
(Schweppes)	6 fl. oz.	96	23.4
BITTER ORANGE, soft drink			
(Schweppes)	6 fl. oz.	92	22.6
BITTERS (Angostura)	½ tsp.	7	1.0
BLACKBERRY (USDA):			
Fresh (includes boysenberry, dewberry, youngberry):			
With hulls	1 lb. (weighed untrimmed)	250	55.6

(USDA): United States Department of Agriculture
DNA: Data Not Available
*Prepared as Package Directs

Food and Description	Measure or Quantity	Calories	Carbo-hydrates (grams)
Hulled	4 oz. (weighed hulled)	66	14.6
Hulled	½ cup (2.6 oz.)	42	9.4
Canned, regular, solids & liq.:			
Juice pack	4 oz.	61	13.7
Light syrup	4 oz.	82	19.6
Heavy syrup	½ cup (4.6 oz.)	118	28.9
Extra heavy syrup	4 oz.	125	30.7
Canned, water pack:			
Solids & liq.	4 oz.	45	10.2
Solids & liq.	½ cup (4.3 oz.)	48	11.0
Frozen:			
Sweetened, not thawed	4 oz.	109	27.7
Unsweetened, not thawed	4 oz.	55	12.9
BLACKBERRY CRISPS, dehydrated snack (Epicure)	1 oz.	90	21.2
BLACKBERRY JAM dietetic:			
(Dia-Mel)	1 T.	22	5.4
(Diet Delight)	1 T.	6	.9
BLACKBERRY JELLY, low calorie (Slenderella)	1 T.	21	5.4
BLACKBERRY JUICE, canned, unsweetened (USDA)	½ cup (4.3 oz.)	46	9.6
BLACKBERRY LIQUEUR:			
(Bols) 60 proof	1 fl. oz.	96	8.9
(Hiram Walker) 60 proof	1 fl. oz.	100	12.8
BLACKBERRY PIE:			
Home recipe (USDA)	⅙ of 9″ pie (5.6 oz.)	384	54.4
(Tastykake)	4-oz. pie	386	60.1
Frozen (Banquet)	5-oz. serving	376	55.5
BLACKBERRY PIE FILLING (Lucky Leaf)	8 oz.	258	62.4
BLACKBERRY WINE (Mogen David) 12% alcohol	3 fl. oz.	135	18.7

(USDA): United States Department of Agriculture
DNA: Data Not Available
*Prepared as Package Directs

Food and Description	Measure or Quantity	Calories	Carbo-hydrates (grams)
BLACK-EYED PEA, frozen (See also **COWPEA**):			
Uncooked (USDA)	10-oz. pkg.	372	67.0
Cooked, drained solids (USDA)	½ cup	111	20.1
(Birds Eye)	⅓ pkg. (3.3 oz.)	122	20.8
BLANCMANGE (See VANILLA PUDDING)			
BLINTZE, frozen (Aunt Leah's):			
Apple, blueberry or cherry	1 blintze (2.5 oz.)	80	D.N.A.
Cheese	1 blintze (2.5 oz.)	70	D.N.A.
BLOOD PUDDING or SAUSAGE (USDA)	1 oz.	112	.1
BLOODY MARY MIX (Bar-Tender's)	1 serving (.3 oz.)	26	5.7
BLUEBERRY:			
Fresh, whole (USDA)	1 lb. (weighed untrimmed)	259	63.8
Fresh, trimmed (USDA)	½ cup (2.6 oz.)	45	11.2
Canned, solids & liq. (USDA):			
Syrup pack, extra heavy	½ cup (4.4 oz.)	126	32.5
Water pack	½ cup (4.2 oz.)	47	11.8
Frozen:			
Sweetened, solids & liq. (USDA)	½ cup (4 oz.)	120	30.2
Quick thaw (Birds Eye)	½ cup (5 oz.)	121	30.2
Unsweetened, solids & liq. (USDA)	4 oz.	62	15.0
Unsweetened, solids & liq. (USDA)	½ cup (2.9 oz.)	46	11.2
BLUEBERRY PIE:			
Home recipe (USDA)	⅙ of 9″ pie (5.6 oz.)	382	55.1
(Tastykake)	4-oz. pie	376	57.8
Frozen:			
(Banquet)	5-oz. serving	366	58.2
(Mrs. Smith's)	⅙ of 8″ pie	288	39.2
BLUEBERRY PIE FILLING:			
(Lucky Leaf)	8 oz.	256	61.4
(Musselman's)	1 cup	321	D.N.A.
BLUEBERRY PRESERVE, dietetic (Dia-Mel)	1 T.	22	5.4

(USDA): United States Department of Agriculture
DNA: Data Not Available
*Prepared as Package Directs

Food and Description	Measure or Quantity	Calories	Carbo-hydrates (grams)
BLUEBERRY SYRUP, dietetic (Dia-Mel)	1 T.	22	5.5
BLUEBERRY TURNOVER, frozen (Pepperidge Farm)	1 piece	294	D.N.A.
BLUEFISH (USDA):			
Raw, whole	1 lb. (weighed whole)	271	0.
Raw, meat only	4 oz.	133	0.
Baked or broiled	4 oz.	180	0.
Fried	4 oz.	232	5.3
BOCKWURST (USDA)	1 oz.	75	.2
BOLOGNA:			
All meat, very thin slice (USDA)	1 oz.	79	1.0
With cereal, very thin slice (USDA)	1 oz.	74	1.1
(Armour Star)	1 oz.	97	D.N.A.
(Eckrich):			
All meat	1 oz.	92	D.N.A.
All meat sandwich	1 oz.	84	D.N.A.
German brand	1 oz.	79	D.N.A.
Pure beef	1 oz.	64	D.N.A.
(Vienna)	1 oz.	67	.7
(Wilson)	1 oz.	89	.8
BONITO, raw (USDA):			
Whole	1 lb. (weighed whole)	442	0.
Meat only	4 oz.	191	0.
BORDEAUX, rouge (Cruse) 10½% alcohol	3 fl. oz.	63	D.N.A.
BORDEAUX WINE (See also individual regional, vineyard or brand names or **CLARET WINE**)			
BORSCHT:			
(Manischewitz)	8 oz. (by wt.)	72	17.5
*Concentrate, frozen (Aunt Leah's)	8 fl. oz.	46	D.N.A.

(USDA): United States Department of Agriculture
DNA: Data Not Available
*Prepared as Package Directs

Food and Description	Measure or Quantity	Calories	Carbo-hydrates (grams)
*Concentrate, frozen, diet (Aunt Leah's)	8 fl. oz.	25	D.N.A.
Lo-Cal (Manischewitz)	8 oz. (by wt.)	24	D.N.A.
Low calorie (Gold's)	8 oz.	24	D.N.A.
BOSCO (Best Foods)	1 T.	45	10.4
BOSTON BROWN BREAD (See **BREAD**)			
BOSTON CREAM PIE:			
Home recipe (USDA)	2-oz.	171	28.3
Mix (Betty Crocker)	15.5-oz. pkg.	1782	370.4
BOUILLON CUBE (See also individual flavors):			
(USDA) flavor not indicated	1 cube (½″)	5	Tr.
(Steero) flavor not indicated	1 cube	7	D.N.A.
(Steero) instant, flavor not indicated	1 tsp.	7	D.N.A.
BOURBON WHISKEY, Unflavored (See **DISTILLED LIQUOR**)			
BOURBON WHISKEY, PEACH FLAVORED (Old Mr. Boston) 70 proof	1 fl. oz.	100	8.0
BOYSENBERRY, fresh (See **BLACKBERRY,** fresh)			
BOYSENBERRY CRISPS, dehydrated snack (Epicure)	1 oz.	90	21.3
BOYSENBERRY JAM, low calorie (Slenderella)	1 T.	21	5.4
BOYSENBERRY PIE, frozen (Banquet)	5-oz.	344	54.2
BOYSENBERRY PRESERVE, low calorie (Tillie Lewis)	1 T.	9	2.1
BRAINS, all animals, raw (USDA)	4 oz.	142	.9

(USDA): United States Department of Agriculture
DNA: Data Not Available
*Prepared as Package Directs

Food and Description	Measure or Quantity	Calories	Carbo-hydrates (grams)
BRAN BREAKFAST CEREAL:			
Plain:			
All-Bran (Kellogg's)	1 cup (2 oz.)	192	42.8
Bran-Buds (Kellogg's)	1 cup (2 oz.)	196	45.0
40% bran flakes (USDA)	1 cup (1.2 oz.)	103	27.4
40% bran flakes (Kellogg's)	1 cup (1⅓ oz.)	139	30.1
40% bran flakes (Post)	1 cup (1½ oz.)	133	31.3
100% bran (Nabisco)	1 cup (2 oz.)	150	41.6
& prune flakes (Post)	1 cup (1⅓ oz.)	120	29.3
Raisin:			
(USDA)	1 cup (2 oz.)	164	45.2
(Kellogg's)	1 cup (1½ oz.)	150	33.6
(Post)	1 cup (2 oz.)	178	42.0
Chex (Ralston)	1 cup (1½ oz.)	123	29.2
BRANDY, Unflavored (See **DISTILLED LIQUOR**)			
BRANDY EXTRACT (Ehlers)	1 tsp.	7	D.N.A.
BRANDY, FLAVORED:			
Apricot:			
(Bols) 70 proof	1 fl. oz.	100	7.4
(Garnier) 70 proof	1 fl. oz.	86	7.1
(Hiram Walker) 70 proof	1 fl. oz.	88	7.5
(Leroux) 70 proof	1 fl. oz.	92	8.6
(Old Mr. Boston) 70 proof	1 fl. oz.	100	8.0
(Mr. Boston's) apricot & brandy, 42 proof	1 fl. oz.	75	8.0
Blackberry:			
(Garnier) 70 proof	1 fl. oz.	86	7.1
(Hiram Walker) 70 proof	1 fl. oz.	86	7.0
(Leroux) 70 proof	1 fl. oz.	91	8.3
(Leroux) Polish, 70 proof	1 fl. oz.	92	8.6
(Old Mr. Boston) 70 proof	1 fl. oz.	100	8.0
(Mr. Boston's) blackberry & brandy, 42 proof	1 fl. oz.	75	8.0
Cherry:			
(Garnier) 70 proof	1 fl. oz.	86	7.1
(Hiram Walker) 70 proof	1 fl. oz.	86	7.0
(Leroux) 70 proof	1 fl. oz.	91	8.3
(Old Mr. Boston) wild cherry, 70 proof	1 fl. oz.	100	8.0
(Mr. Boston's) wild cherry & brandy, 42 proof	1 fl. oz.	75	8.0

(USDA): United States Department of Agriculture
DNA: Data Not Available
*Prepared as Package Directs

Food and Description	Measure or Quantity	Calories	Carbo-hydrates (grams)
Coffee:			
(Garnier) 70 proof	1 fl. oz.	86	7.1
(Old Mr. Boston) 70 proof	1 fl. oz.	74	1.0
(Leroux) coffee & brandy, 70 proof	1 fl. oz.	91	8.3
Ginger:			
(Garnier) 70 proof	1 fl. oz.	74	4.0
(Hiram Walker) 70 proof	1 fl. oz.	72	3.5
(Leroux) 70 proof	1 fl. oz.	76	4.4
(Leroux) sharp, 70 proof	1 fl. oz.	77	4.7
(Old Mr. Boston) 70 proof	1 fl. oz.	74	1.0
(Mr. Boston's) ginger & brandy, 42 proof	1 fl. oz.	75	8.0
Peach:			
(Garnier) 70 proof	1 fl. oz.	86	7.1
(Hiram Walker) 70 proof	1 fl. oz.	87	7.2
(Leroux) 70 proof	1 fl. oz.	93	8.9
(Old Mr. Boston) 70 proof	1 fl. oz.	100	8.0
(Mr. Boston's) peach & brandy, 42 proof	1 fl. oz.	75	8.0
BRAUNSCHWEIGER:			
(USDA)	1 oz.	90	.6
(Eckrich) beef	1 oz.	71	D.N.A.
(Wilson)	1 oz.	90	.6
BRAZIL NUT (USDA):			
Whole	1 lb. (weighed in shell)	1424	23.7
Shelled	½ cup (2.4 oz.)	458	7.5
Shelled	4 nuts	115	2.0
BREAD (listed by type or brand name):			
Banana nut loaf (Van de Kamp's)	14-oz. loaf	1288	D.N.A.
Boston brown (USDA)	1 oz.	60	12.9
Cheese, 1-lb. loaf (Van de Kamp's)	.8-oz. slice	61	D.N.A.
Cinnamon raisin (Thomas')	1 slice	63	12.2
Corn and molasses (Pepperidge Farm)	.9-oz. slice	63	12.8
Cracked-wheat:			
(USDA)	1 lb.	1193	236.3
(USDA) 20 slices to 1 lb.	.8-oz. slice	60	12.0
(Pepperidge Farm)	.9-oz. slice	66	12.3

(USDA): United States Department of Agriculture
DNA: Data Not Available
*Prepared as Package Directs

Food and Description	Measure or Quantity	Calories	Carbo-hydrates (grams)
Daffodil Farm (Wonder)	1 slice	50	9.2
Date-nut loaf:			
(Thomas')	1 slice	100	18.8
(Van de Kamp's)	1-lb. 2-oz. loaf	1720	D.N.A.
Dutch Crunch, 1-lb. loaf (Van de Kamp's)	.8-oz. slice	63	D.N.A.
Dutch Egg (Arnold)	.9-oz slice	82	12.8
Egg sesame, 1-lb. loaf (Van de Kamp's)	.9-oz. slice	77	D.N.A.
English muffin loaf, 1-lb. loaf (Van de Kamp's)	1-oz. slice	65	D.N.A.
Finn Crisp	1 piece	23	5.0
Flat, Norwegian (Ideal)	1 double wafer	25	5.5
French:			
Enriched or unenriched (USDA)	1 lb.	1315	251.3
Brown & serve (Pepperidge Farm)	¾″ slice (1 oz.)	79	14.7
Giraffe	.8-oz. slice	70	11.2
Glutogen Gluten (Thomas')	1 slice	35	5.6
Hollywood, dark or light	1 slice	46	10.0
Honey bran, 1-lb. loaf (Van de Kamp's)	.7-oz. slice	77	D.N.A.
Italian:			
Enriched or unenriched (USDA)	1 lb.	1252	255.8
Brown & serve (Pepperidge Farm)	¾″ slice (1 oz.)	81	14.5
Low sodium, 1-lb. loaf (Van de Kamp's)	.8-oz. slice	66	D.N.A.
Oatmeal:			
(Arnold)	.8-oz. slice	64	10.7
(Pepperidge Farm)	.9-oz. slice	66	12.3
Irish, 1-lb. loaf (Van de Kamp's)	.9-oz. slice	69	D.N.A.
100% Milk 'n Butter, 1-lb. loaf (Van de Kamp's)	.9-oz. slice	71	D.N.A.
Orange raisin (Arnold)	.8-oz. slice	69	11.8
Panettone, wine fruit loaf (Van de Kamp's)	1½ lb.	2167	D.N.A.
Profile (Wonder)	1 slice	58	10.5
Protogen Protein (Thomas')	1 slice	45	8.6
Pumpernickel:			
(USDA)	1 lb.	1116	240.9
(Levy's)	1.1-oz. slice	70	12.4
Family (Pepperidge Farm)	1.1-oz. slice	79	15.1

(USDA): United States Department of Agriculture
DNA: Data Not Available
*Prepared as Package Directs

Food and Description	Measure or Quantity	Calories	Carbo-hydrates (grams)
(Van de Kamp's) 1-lb. loaf	.6-oz. slice	48	D.N.A.
Raisin:			
(USDA)	1 lb.	1188	243.1
Tea (Arnold)	.8-oz. slice	67	11.5
With cinnamon (Pepperidge Farm)	.9-oz. slice	76	14.1
Rite Diet (Thomas')	1 slice	56	9.3
Roman Light	.8-oz. slice	57	10.4
Roman Meal	.8-oz. slice	58	11.0
Rye:			
Light (USDA)	1 lb.	1102	236.3
Delicatessen (Arnold)	.8-oz. slice	61	10.2
Family (Pepperidge Farm)	1.1-oz. slice	88	17.0
Westchester, with or without caraway seeds (Levy's)	1.1-oz. slice	55	12.1
With or without caraway seeds (Levy's)	1.1-oz. slice	70	12.1
Salt rising (USDA)	1 lb.	1211	236.8
Salt rising (Van de Kamp's)	.9-oz. slice	67	D.N.A.
Slender Key (Arnold)	.8-oz slice	56	10.1
Soft sandwich, 1½-lb. loaf (Arnold)	.8-oz. slice	67	10.6
Toaster cake (See **TOASTER CAKE**)			
Vienna, enriched or unenriched (USDA)	1 lb.	1315	251.3
Wheat germ (Pepperidge Farm)	.9-oz. slice	63	11.6
White, enriched or unenriched:			
Prepared with 1-2% nonfat dry milk (USDA)	1 lb.	1220	228.6
Prepared with 3-4% nonfat dry milk (USDA)	1 lb.	1225	229.1
Prepared with 5-6% nonfat dry milk (USDA)	1 lb.	1247	227.7
Brick Oven (Arnold) 1-lb. loaf	.8-oz. slice	64	10.7
Brick Oven (Arnold) 2-lb. loaf	1.1-oz. slice	79	12.9
English Tea Loaf (Pepperidge Farm)	.9-oz. slice	71	12.4
Hearthstone (Arnold) 1-lb. loaf	.9-oz. slice	72	12.0
Hearthstone (Arnold) 30-oz. loaf	1.1-oz. slice	84	13.9
Hearthstone (Arnold) 2-lb. loaf	1.1-oz. slice	80	12.9
Large loaf (Pepperidge Farm)	.8-oz. slice	70	12.2
Oven-Crust (Levy's)	.8-oz. slice	73	12.0
Sandwich (Pepperidge Farm)	.8-oz. slice	64	11.6

(USDA): United States Department of Agriculture
DNA: Data Not Available
*Prepared as Package Directs

Food and Description	Measure or Quantity	Calories	Carbo- hydrates (grams)
(Thomas')	1 slice	64	12.2
(Van de Kamp's) 1-lb loaf	.9-oz. slice	69	D.N.A.
(Wonder)	1 slice	69	12.7
Wheat, 1-lb. loaf (Van de Kamp's)	1.1-oz. slice	69	D.N.A.
Whole-wheat:			
Prepared with 2% nonfat dry milk (USDA)	1 lb.	1102	216.4
Prepared with 2% nonfat dry milk (USDA)	.8-oz. slice	56	11.0
Prepared with water (USDA)	1 lb.	1093	223.6
Brick Oven, 1-lb. loaf (Arnold)	.8-oz. slice	64	9.8
Cap Sheaf (Freund)	1 slice	45	D.N.A.
Krinko, 1-lb. loaf (Van de Kamp's)	.9-oz. slice	63	D.N.A.
(Pepperidge Farm)	.9-oz. slice	61	10.8
(Thomas')	1 slice	65	11.2
BREAD, CANNED:			
Banana nut (Dromedary)	½″ slice (1 oz.)	71	11.0
Brown with raisins (B&M)	½″ slice (1.6 oz.)	90	16.3
Chocolate nut (Crosse & Blackwell)	½″ slice (1 oz.)	65	14.8
Chocolate nut (Dromedary)	½″ slice (1 oz.)	87	13.5
Date & nut (Crosse & Blackwell)	½″ slice (1 oz.)	65	12.6
Date & nut (Dromedary)	½″ slice (1 oz.)	75	11.7
Fruit & nut (Crosse & Blackwell)	½″ slice (1 oz.)	76	13.6
Orange nut (Crosse & Blackwell)	½″ slice (1 oz.)	76	15.4
Orange nut (Dromedary)	½″ slice (1 oz.)	77	12.8
Spice nut (Crosse & Blackwell)	½″ slice (1 oz.)	62	13.2
BREAD CRUMBS:			
Dry, grated (USDA)	1 cup (3.6 oz.)	400	74.9
Dry, grated (USDA)	1 T.	25	4.7
(Wonder)	1 oz.	108	20.5
BREAD PUDDING with raisins, home recipe (USDA)	4 oz.	212	32.2
BREAD STICK:			
Cheese (Keebler)	1 piece (2 grams)	10	1.8
Garlic (Keebler)	1 piece (2 grams)	11	1.9
Onion (Keebler)	1 piece (2 grams)	10	1.9
Onion (Stella D'oro)	1 piece	36	D.N.A.

(USDA): United States Department of Agriculture
DNA: Data Not Available
*Prepared as Package Directs

Food and Description	Measure or Quantity	Calories	Carbohydrates (grams)
Regular (Stella D'oro)	1 piece	40	D.N.A.
Salt:			
(USDA)	1 oz.	109	21.3
Vienna type (USDA)	1 oz.	86	16.4
(Keebler)	1 piece (2 grams)	10	1.9
Salt free (Stella D'oro)	1 piece	39	6.3
Sesame (Stella D'oro)	1 piece	38	D.N.A.
BREAD STUFFING MIX:			
Dry (USDA)	4 oz.	421	82.1
Dry (USDA)	1 cup (2½ oz.)	263	51.4
*Crumb type, prepared with water & fat (USDA)	4 oz.	406	40.4
*Crumb type, prepared with water & fat (USDA)	1 cup (5 oz.)	505	50.2
*Moist type, prepared with water, egg & fat (USDA)	4 oz.	236	22.3
*Moist type, prepared with water, egg & fat (USDA)	1 cup (7.2 oz.)	422	40.0
Corn bread, dry (Pepperidge Farm)	4 oz.	446	D.N.A.
Cube, dry (Pepperidge Farm)	4 oz.	438	D.N.A.
Herb seasoned, dry (Pepperidge Farm)	4 oz.	425	D.N.A.
BREADFRUIT, fresh (USDA):			
Whole	1 lb. (weighed untrimmed)	360	91.5
Peeled & trimmed	4 oz. (weighed trimmed)	117	29.7
BROCCOLI:			
Raw, whole (USDA)	1 lb. (weighed untrimmed)	89	16.3
Raw, large leaves removed (USDA)	1 lb. (weighed partially trimmed)	113	20.9
Boiled, drained solids (USDA)	½ cup (2.6 oz.)	20	3.5
Frozen:			
Chopped:			
Uncooked (USDA)	10-oz. pkg.	82	14.7
Boiled, drained solids (USDA)	½ cup (3.3 oz.)	25	4.3
(Birds Eye)	½ cup (3.3 oz.)	27	3.8
In cream sauce (Birds Eye)	½ cup (3.3 oz.)	114	9.6

(USDA): United States Department of Agriculture
DNA: Data Not Available
*Prepared as Package Directs

Food and Description	Measure or Quantity	Calories	Carbo-hydrates (grams)
Spears:			
Uncooked (USDA)	10-oz. pkg.	79	14.4
Boiled, drained solids (USDA)	4 oz.	29	5.3
Boiled, drained solids (USDA)	½ cup (3.2 oz.)	24	4.4
(Stokely-Van Camp)	4 oz.	32	5.8
Baby spears (Birds Eye)	⅓ pkg. (3.3 oz.)	26	3.7
In butter sauce (Birds Eye)	½ cup (3.3 oz.)	58	4.0
In butter sauce (Green Giant) boil-in-the-bag	4 oz.	71	5.6
In cheese sauce (Green Giant)	4 oz.	93	9.9
In Hollandaise sauce (Birds Eye)	½ cup (3.3 oz.)	100	3.2
BROTH & SEASONING (See also individual kinds):			
Beef (Maggi)	1 T.	32	4.6
Chicken (Maggi)	1 T.	34	5.4
Clam (Maggi)	1 T.	35	5.3
Golden (George Washington)	1 packet (4 grams)	5	1.0
Onion (Maggi)	1 T.	33	4.8
Rich brown (George Washington)	1 packet (4 grams)	5	1.2
Vegetable (Maggi)	1 T.	32	4.4
BROWNIE (See **COOKIE**)			
BRUSSELS SPROUT:			
Raw (USDA)	1 lb.	188	34.6
Boiled, drained solids (USDA)	½ cup (3.2 oz.)	32	5.8
Frozen:			
(USDA)	10-oz. pkg.	102	20.7
Boiled, drained solids (USDA)	4 oz.	37	7.4
Baby sprouts or full size (Birds Eye)	½ cup (3.3 oz.)	34	5.7
In butter sauce (Green Giant)	4 oz.	82	6.9
BUCKWHEAT FLOUR (See **FLOUR**)			
BUCKWHEAT GROATS:			
(Birkett)	1 oz.	98	20.4
(Pocono)	1 oz.	108	21.8

(USDA): United States Department of Agriculture
DNA: Data Not Available
*Prepared as Package Directs

Food and Description	Measure or Quantity	Calories	Carbohydrates (grams)
BUFFALOFISH, raw (USDA):			
Whole	1 lb. (weighed whole)	164	0.
Meat only	4 oz.	128	0.
BULGUR (from hard red winter wheat) (USDA):			
Dry	1 lb.	1605	343.4
Canned:			
Unseasoned (USDA)	4 oz.	191	39.7
Seasoned (USDA)	4 oz.	207	37.2
BULLHEAD, raw (USDA):			
Whole	1 lb. (weighed whole)	72	0.
Meat only	4 oz.	95	0.
BULLOCK'S-HEART (See **CUSTARD APPLE**)			
BUN (See **ROLL**)			
BURBOT, raw (USDA):			
Whole	1 lb. (weighed whole)	56	0.
Meat only	4 oz.	93	0.
BURGUNDY WINE (See also individual regional, vineyard, grape, or brand names):			
(Gallo) 13% alcohol	3 fl. oz.	52	.9
(Gallo) hearty, 14% alcohol	3 fl. oz.	48	1.2
(Gold seal) 12% alcohol	3 fl. oz.	82	.4
(Italian Swiss Colony-Gold Medal) Napa-Sonoma-Medocino 12.3% alcohol	3 fl. oz.	65	1.1
(Italian Swiss Colony-Gold Medal) 12.3% alcohol	3 fl. oz.	63	.7
(Italian Swiss Colony-Private Stock) 12% alcohol	3 fl. oz.	60	.2
(Louis M. Martini) 12½% alcohol	3 fl. oz.	90	.2
(Mogen David) American 12% alcohol	3 fl. oz.	24	1.8
(Taylor) 12.5% alcohol	3 fl. oz.	72	Tr.

(USDA): United States Department of Agriculture
DNA: Data Not Available
*Prepared as Package Directs

Food and Description	Measure or Quantity	Calories	Carbo-hydrates (grams)
BURGUNDY WINE, SPARKLING:			
(Barton & Guestier) French red, 12% alcohol	3 fl. oz.	69	2.2
(Chanson) French red	3 fl. oz.	72	3.6
(Gold Seal) 12% alcohol	3 fl. oz.	87	2.6
(Great Western) 12% alcohol	3 fl. oz.	88	5.0
(Italian Swiss Colony-Private Stock) 12% alcohol	3 fl. oz.	67	2.3
(Lejon) 12% alcohol	3 fl. oz.	67	2.3
(Taylor) 12.5% alcohol	3 fl. oz.	78	1.8
BURRITOS, frozen (Rosarita):			
Bean	8-oz. pkg.	486	D.N.A.
Green or red chili	7½-oz. pkg.	444	D.N.A.
BUTTER, salted or unsalted:			
(USDA)	4 oz.	812	.5
(USDA)	1 cup (8 oz.)	1625	1.0
(USDA)	1 T.	102	.1
(Breakstone)	1 T.	102	.1
(Hotel Bar)	1 T.	100	Tr.
(Land O'Lakes)	1 T.	102	.1
(Sealtest)	1 T.	100	.2
Whipped (Breakstone)	4 oz.	820	.9
Whipped (Breakstone)	1 T.	68	.1
BUTTER BEAN (See **BEAN, LIMA**)			
BUTTER BRICKLE CAKE MIX (Betty Crocker)	1-lb. 2.5-oz. pkg.	2202	420.0
BUTTER CAKE (Van de Kamp's)	1-lb. loaf	1284	D.N.A.
BUTTERFISH, raw (USDA):			
Gulf:			
Whole	1 lb. (weighed whole)	220	0.
Meat only	4 oz.	108	0.
Northern:			
Whole	1 lb. (weighed whole)	391	0.
Meat only	4 oz.	192	0.

(USDA): United States Department of Agriculture
DNA: Data Not Available
*Prepared as Package Directs

Food and Description	Measure or Quantity	Calories	Carbo-hydrates (grams)
BUTTER FLAVORING, imitation (Ehlers)	1 tsp.	7	D.N.A.
BUTTERMILK (See **MILK**)			
BUTTERNUT (USDA):			
Whole	1 lb. (weighed in shell)	399	5.3
Shelled	4 oz.	713	9.5
BUTTER OIL or dehydrated butter (USDA)	1 cup (7.2 oz.)	1787	0.
BUTTERSCOTCH MORSELS (Nestlé's)	6 oz.	900	102.1
BUTTERSCOTCH PIE:			
Home recipe (USDA)	⅙ of 9″ pie (5.4 oz.)	406	58.2
Frozen, cream (Banquet)	2½-oz. serving	187	27.0
BUTTERSCOTCH PIE FILLING MIX:			
*With whole milk, low calorie (D-Zerta)	½ cup (4.5 oz.)	99	9.8
*With nonfat milk, low calorie (D-Zerta)	½ cup (4.5 oz.)	60	10.0
(My-T-Fine)	1 oz.	122	26.8
BUTTERSCOTCH PUDDING:			
(Betty Crocker)	1-lb. 2-oz. can	666	115.2
(Betty Crocker)	4 oz.	148	25.6
(Bounty)	4 oz.	178	30.3
BUTTERSCOTCH PUDDING MIX:			
Sweetened:			
*Instant (Jell-O)	½ cup (5.3 oz.)	177	30.5
Instant (My-T-Fine)	1 oz.	82	20.6
*Instant (Royal)	½ cup (5.2 oz.)	185	29.6
Regular (My-T-Fine)	1 oz.	122	26.8
*Regular (Royal)	½ cup (5 oz.)	190	31.5
*(Thank You)	½ cup	169	29.2

(USDA): United States Department of Agriculture
DNA: Data Not Available
*Prepared as Package Directs

Food and Description	Measure or Quantity	Calories	Carbo-hydrates (grams)
Low calorie:			
*With whole milk (D-Zerta)	½ cup (4.5 oz.)	107	12.0
*With nonfat milk (D-Zerta)	½ cup (4.5 oz.)	71	12.0
B-V (Wilson)	1 tsp. (¼ oz.)	11	.6

C

CABBAGE:
White (USDA):
Raw:

Whole	1 lb. (weighed untrimmed)	86	19.3
Finely shredded	1 cup (3.7 oz.)	24	5.4

Boiled:

Shredded, in small amount of water, short time, drained solids	½ cup (2.6 oz.)	15	3.1
Wedges, in large amount of water, long time, drained solids	½ cup (3.2 oz.)	16	3.7
Dehydrated	1 oz.	87	20.9
Red, raw, whole (USDA)	1 lb. (weighed untrimmed)	111	24.7
Red, canned (Comstock-Greenwood)	1 oz.	18	4.5
Savoy, raw, whole (USDA)	1 lb. (weighed untrimmed)	86	16.5

CABBAGE, CHINESE or CELERY, raw (USDA):

Whole	1 lb. (weighed untrimmed)	62	13.2
1″ pieces, leaves with stalk	½ cup (1.8 oz.)	7	1.5

CABBAGE ROLLS, stuffed with beef, in tomato sauce, frozen (Holloway House)

	1 roll (7 oz.)	272	62.0

CABBAGE, SPOON or WHITE MUSTARD (USDA):

Raw	1 lb.	69	12.5
Boiled, drained solids	½ cup (2.6 oz.)	10	1.8

(USDA): United States Department of Agriculture
DNA: Data Not Available
*Prepared as Package Directs

Food and Description	Measure or Quantity	Calories	Carbo-hydrates (grams)
CABERNET SAUVIGNON WINE (Louis M. Martini) 12½% alcohol	3 fl. oz.	90	.2
CACTUS COOLER, soft drink (Canada Dry)	6 fl. oz.	85	22.2
CAKE. Most cakes are listed elsewhere by kind of cake such as **ANGEL FOOD** or **CHOCOLATE** or brand name, such as *YANKEE DOODLES.* (USDA):			
Plain, home recipe:			
Without icing	1.9-oz. piece (3" x 2" x 1½")	200	30.7
With chocolate icing	3.5-oz. piece (⅟₁₆ of 10" layer cake)	368	59.4
With boiled white icing	3.5-oz. piece (⅟₁₆ of 10" layer cake)	352	61.8
With uncooked white icing	3.5-oz. piece (⅟₁₆ of 10" layer cake)	367	63.3
White, home recipe:			
Without icing	1.9-oz. piece (3" x 2" x 1½")	206	29.7
With coconut icing	2 oz.	210	34.4
With uncooked white icing	2 oz.	212	35.6
Yellow, home recipe:			
Without icing	2 oz.	206	33.0
With caramel icing	2 oz.	206	34.8
With chocolate icing	2 oz.	206	34.2
CAKE DECORATOR, canned, any color (Pillsbury)	1 oz.	110	21.0
CAKE FROSTING (See **CAKE ICING & CAKE ICING MIX**)			
CAKE ICING:			
Butterscotch (Betty Crocker)	16.5-oz. can	1914	323.4
Caramel, home recipe (USDA)	4 oz.	408	86.8
Chocolate, home recipe (USDA)	4 oz.	426	76.4
Chocolate (Betty Crocker)	16.5-oz. can	1881	290.4
Chocolate (Q-T)	4 oz.	452	D.N.A.
Coconut, home recipe (USDA)	4 oz.	413	84.9

(USDA): United States Department of Agriculture
DNA: Data Not Available
*Prepared as Package Directs

Food and Description	Measure or Quantity	Calories	Carbo- hydrates (grams)
Dark Dutch fudge (Betty Crocker)	16.5-oz. can	1782	287.1
Milk chocolate (Betty Crocker)	16.5-oz. can	1898	316.8
Sunkist Lemon (Betty Crocker)	16.5-oz. can	1931	326.7
Vanilla (Betty Crocker)	16.5-oz. can	1931	325.1
White, boiled (USDA)	4 oz.	358	91.1
White, uncooked (USDA)	4 oz.	426	92.5

CAKE ICING MIX:

Food and Description	Measure or Quantity	Calories	Carbo- hydrates (grams)
Butter Brickle, creamy (Betty Crocker)	13.5-oz. pkg.	1620	344.2
Caramel, creamy (Betty Crocker)	13-oz. pkg.	1547	330.2
Cherry, creamy (Betty Crocker)	13-oz. pkg.	1547	332.8
Cherry fluff (Betty Crocker)	7-oz. pkg.	750	191.1
Cherry fudge, creamy (Betty Crocker)	13-oz. pkg.	1469	317.2
Chiquita Banana, creamy (Betty Crocker)	13-oz. pkg.	1547	328.9
Chocolate, fluffy, (Betty Crocker)	6.5-oz. pkg.	806	148.2
Chocolate fudge (USDA)	1 oz.	116	24.5
*Chocolate fudge (USDA)	4 oz.	429	76.0
Chocolate fudge, creamy (Betty Crocker)	14-oz. pkg.	1596	341.6
Chocolate malt, creamy (Betty Crocker)	13-oz. pkg.	1521	319.8
Chocolate, walnut, creamy (Betty Crocker)	13-oz. pkg.	1508	308.1
Coconut-pecan, creamy (Betty Crocker)	9-oz. pkg.	1188	190.8
Coconut, toasted, creamy (Betty Crocker)	13-oz. pkg.	1573	319.8
Dark chocolate fudge, creamy (Betty Crocker)	13-oz. pkg.	1508	278.2
Dole Pineapple, creamy (Betty Crocker)	13-oz. pkg.	1547	327.6
Fudge, creamy (USDA)	1 oz.	109	24.1
*Fudge, creamy, prepared with water (USDA)	4 oz.	384	84.6
*Fudge, creamy, prepared with water & fat (USDA)	4 oz.	434	74.7
*Fudge (Dromedary)	1″ x 1″ x ½″ piece (5 oz.)	55	9.9
Fudge nugget, creamy (Betty Crocker)	13-oz. pkg.	1482	318.5

(USDA): United States Department of Agriculture
DNA: Data Not Available
*Prepared as Package Directs

Food and Description	Measure or Quantity	Calories	Carbo-hydrates (grams)
Sour cream, chocolate fudge, creamy (Betty Crocker)	13-oz. pkg.	1495	317.2
Spice, creamy (Betty Crocker)	13-oz. pkg.	1547	325.0
Sunkist Lemon, creamy (Betty Crocker)	13-oz. pkg.	1547	330.2
Sunkist Lemon fluff (Betty Crocker)	6.5-oz. pkg.	689	176.8
Sunkist Orange, creamy (Betty Crocker)	13-oz. pkg.	1547	326.3
White, creamy (Betty Crocker)	14-oz. pkg.	1666	355.6
White, fluffy (Betty Crocker)	6.5-oz. pkg.	689	176.8

CAKE MIX. Most cake mixes are listed by kind of cake, such as **ANGEL FOOD CAKE MIX, CHOCOLATE CAKE MIX,** etc.

Food and Description	Measure or Quantity	Calories	Carbo-hydrates (grams)
White:			
(USDA)	1 oz.	123	22.2
(Betty Crocker)	1-lb. 2.5-oz. pkg.	2183	418.1
(Betty Crocker)	1 oz.	118	22.4
*Party White (Crutchfield's)	4 oz.	397	71.2
*(Duncan Hines)	1 cake	2222	384.0
*(Duncan Hines)	1/12 of cake (2.5 oz.)	185	32.0
(Pillsbury)	1 oz.	121	21.4
Loaf (Pillsbury)	1 oz.	122	21.8
Whipping cream (Pillsbury)	1 oz.	127	20.8
*(Swans Down)	1/12 of cake	177	36.2
*With chocolate icing (USDA)	2-oz.	199	35.6
Yellow:			
(USDA)	1 oz.	124	22.0
(Betty Crocker)	1-lb. 2.5-oz. pkg.	2202	420.0
(Betty Crocker)	1 oz.	119	23.2
Butter recipe (Betty Crocker)	1-lb. 2.5-oz. pkg.	2220	429.2
Butter recipe (Betty Crocker)	1 oz.	120	23.2
*Party Yellow (Crutchfield's)	4-oz.	381	65.3
*(Duncan Hines)	1 cake	2386	384.0
*(Duncan Hines)	1/12 of cake (2.5 oz.)	199	32.0
*Golden butter (Duncan Hines)	1 cake	3287	432.0
*Golden butter (Duncan Hines)	1/12 of cake (2.5 oz.)	274	36.0
(Pillsbury)	1 oz.	122	21.9
Butter flavor (Pillsbury)	1 oz.	122	21.9
Loaf (Pillsbury)	1 oz.	120	21.6
*(Swans Down)	1/12 of cake	187	36.2
*With chocolate icing (USDA)	2-oz.	191	32.6

(USDA): United States Department of Agriculture
DNA: Data Not Available
*Prepared as Package Directs

Food and Description	Measure or Quantity	Calories	Carbo-hydrates (grams)
CALYPSO COOLER, syrup, low calorie	1 oz.	<1	Tr.
CANADIAN WHISKY (See **DISTILLED LIQUOR**)			
CANDIED FRUIT (See individual kinds)			
CANDY. The following values of candies from the U.S. Department of Agriculture are representative of the types sold commercially. These values may be useful when individual brands or sizes are not known:			
Almond:			
Chocolate-coated	1 cup (6.3 oz.)	1024	71.2
Chocolate-coated	1 oz.	161	11.2
Sugar-coated or Jordan	1 oz.	129	19.9
Butterscotch	1 oz.	113	26.9
Caramel:			
Plain	1 oz.	113	21.7
Plain with nuts	1 oz.	121	20.0
Chocolate	1 oz.	113	21.7
Chocolate with nuts	1 oz.	121	20.0
Chocolate-flavored roll	1 oz.	112	23.4
Chocolate:			
Bittersweet	1 oz.	135	13.3
Milk:			
Plain	1 oz.	147	16.1
With almonds	1 oz.	151	14.5
With peanuts	1 oz.	154	12.6
Semisweet	1 oz.	144	16.2
Sweet	1 oz.	150	16.4
Chocolate discs, sugar-coated	1 oz.	132	20.6
Coconut center, chocolate-coated	1 oz.	124	20.4
Fondant, plain	1 oz.	103	25.4
Fondant, chocolate-covered	1 oz.	116	23.0
Fudge:			
Chocolate fudge	1 oz.	113	21.3
Chocolate fudge, chocolate-coated	1 oz.	122	20.7
Chocolate fudge with nuts	1 oz.	121	19.6
Chocolate fudge with nuts, chocolate-coated	1 oz.	128	19.1

(USDA): United States Department of Agriculture
DNA: Data Not Available
*Prepared as Package Directs

Food and Description	Measure or Quantity	Calories	Carbo-hydrates (grams)
Vanilla fudge	1 oz.	113	21.2
Vanilla fudge with nuts	1 oz.	120	19.5
With peanuts & caramel, chocolate-coated	1 oz.	130	16.6
Gum drops	1 oz.	98	24.8
Hard	1 oz.	109	27.6
Honeycombed hard candy, with peanut butter, chocolate-covered	1 oz.	131	20.0
Jelly beans	1 oz.	104	26.4
Marshmallows	1 oz.	90	22.8
Nougat & caramel, chocolate-covered	1 oz.	118	20.6
Peanut bar	1 oz.	146	13.4
Peanut brittle	1 oz.	119	23.0
Peanuts, chocolate-covered	1 oz.	159	11.1
Raisins, chocolate-covered	1 oz.	120	20.0
Vanilla creams, chocolate-covered	1 oz.	123	19.9

CANDY, COMMERCIAL (See also **CANDY, DIETETIC**):

Food and Description	Measure or Quantity	Calories	Carbo-hydrates (grams)
Air Bon (Whitman's)	1 piece	10	D.N.A.
Almond Cluster (Peter Paul)	10¢ bar (1¾₆ oz.)	171	19.8
Almond Joy (Peter Paul)	10¢ bar (1½ oz.)	198	24.1
Almonds, chocolate-covered:			
(Hershey's)	1 oz.	142	16.9
(Kraft)	1 piece (2 grams)	14	1.0
Babies, chocolate flavor (Heide)	1 oz.	101	D.N.A.
Baby Ruth (Curtiss)	1 oz.	135	21.0
Baffle Bar (Cardinet's)	1 bar (1¾ oz.)	189	10.9
Berries, French gum drop (Mason)	1 oz.	100	D.N.A.
Bit-O-Honey (Schutter)	1 oz.	116	D.N.A.
Black Crows (Mason)	1 oz.	100	D.N.A.
Brazil nuts, chocolate-covered (Kraft)	1 piece (6 grams)	32	1.7
Bridge Mix:			
Almond (Kraft)	1 piece (4 grams)	22	1.6
Caramelette (Kraft)	1 piece (2 grams)	12	1.9
Jelly (Kraft)	1 piece (2 grams)	12	2.0
Malted milk ball (Kraft)	1 piece (2 grams)	11	1.4
Mintette (Kraft)	1 piece (2 grams)	12	1.8
Peanut (Kraft)	1 piece (2 grams)	12	1.8
Peanut crunch (Kraft)	1 piece (5 grams)	25	3.4
Raisin (Kraft)	1 piece (1 gram)	5	.7

(USDA): United States Department of Agriculture
DNA: Data Not Available
*Prepared as Package Directs

Food and Description	Measure or Quantity	Calories	Carbo-hydrates (grams)
(Nabisco)	1 piece (2 grams)	8	1.4
Butter Chip Bar (Hershey's)	1 oz.	144	18.7
Butterfinger (Curtiss)	1 oz.	134	21.0
Butternut (Hollywood)	1¼ oz.	165	20.6
Candy Corn:			
(Brach's)	1 piece (1 gram)	4	.9
(Goelitz)	1 oz.	94	D.N.A.
(Heide)	1 oz.	101	D.N.A.
Caramel:			
(Curtiss)	1 oz.	119	24.1
Caramelette (Kraft)	1 piece (2 grams)	12	1.9
Chocolate (Kraft)	1 piece (8 grams)	32	5.9
Chocolate-covered (Brach's)	1 piece (8 grams)	33	5.9
Coconut chocolate (Kraft)	1 piece (8 grams)	38	5.7
Coconut vanilla (Kraft)	1 piece (8 grams)	32	5.5
Milk Maid (Brach's)	1 piece (.4 oz.)	45	8.4
Rum (Reed's)	1 piece	17	D.N.A.
Treats (Kraft)	1 piece (8 grams)	34	6.4
Vanilla, plain (Kraft)	1 piece (8 grams)	33	6.2
Vanilla, chocolate-covered (Kraft)	1 piece (9 grams)	39	6.3
Caravelle (Peter Paul)	10¢ bar (1½ oz.)	190	28.5
Carmallow (Queen Anne)	1 piece	83	D.N.A.
Cashew crunch, canned (Planters)	1 oz.	135	14.4
Charleston Chew:			
Bar	5¢ bar	125	D.N.A.
Bite-size	1 piece	28	D.N.A.
Cherry, chocolate-covered:			
(Brach's)	1 piece (.6 oz.)	66	13.2
Dark (Nabisco)	1 piece (⅔ oz.)	76	14.6
Milk (Nabisco)	1 piece (⅔ oz.)	72	15.5
Cherry-A-Let (Hoffman)	1 piece	215	D.N.A.
Chewees (Curtiss)	1 oz.	116	24.1
Chocolate bar:			
Milk chocolate:			
(Ghirardelli)	10¢ bar (1¼ oz.)	188	20.5
(Hershey's)	10¢ bar (1¾ oz.)	266	27.8
(Hershey's)	1 oz.	152	15.9
(Nestlé's)	1 oz.	148	13.1
Plain (Nestlé's) *Gala*	1 oz.	148	13.8
Sweet (Nestlé's) *Gala*	1 oz.	152	14.6
Mint chocolate (Ghirardelli)	10¢ bar (1¼ oz.)	189	20.6
Semisweet, (Hershey's)	1 oz.	147	17.5

(USDA): United States Department of Agriculture
DNA: Data Not Available
*Prepared as Package Directs

Food and Description	Measure or Quantity	Calories	Carbo-hydrates (grams)
Semisweet, (Nestlé's)	1 oz.	141	17.3
Chocolate bar with almonds:			
(Ghirardelli)	10¢ bar (1¼ oz.)	191	19.4
(Hershey's)	10¢ bar (1⅝ oz.)	250	22.4
(Hershey's)	1 oz.	154	13.8
(Nestlé's)	1 oz.	149	15.3
Chocolate blocks, milk:			
(Ghirardelli)	1 sq.	180	19.7
(Hershey's)	1 oz.	145	17.8
Chocolate Crisp Bar (Ghirardelli)	10¢ bar (1¼ oz.)	188	20.5
Chocolate Crunch Bar (Nestlé's)	1 oz.	140	17.8
Chocolate Drops (Nabisco)	1 piece (.4 oz.)	54	10.6
Chocolate Parfait (Pearson's)	1 piece	34	D.N.A.
Chocolate Sponge (Schutter)	1 oz.	122	D.N.A.
Choc-Shop (Hoffman)	1 piece	241	D.N.A.
Chuckles	1 oz.	92	23.0
Chunky	1 oz.	131	D.N.A.
Circlets (Curtiss)	1 oz.	108	26.1
Circus Peanuts (Brach's)	1 piece (7 grams)	27	6.4
Cluster:			
Almond (Kraft)	1 piece (.4 oz.)	63	4.6
Cashew, chocolate-covered			
(Kraft)	1 piece (.4 oz.)	58	4.9
Crispy (Nabisco)	1 piece (.6 oz.)	64	13.6
Peanut, chocolate-covered:			
(Brach's)	1 piece (.5 oz.)	79	7.0
(Hoffman)	1 cluster	204	D.N.A.
(Kraft)	1 piece (.4 oz.)	70	5.0
Royal Clusters (Nabisco)	1 piece (.6 oz.)	96	10.4
Coconut:			
(Welch's)	1 piece (1 oz.)	132	21.1
Bar (Curtiss)	1 oz.	126	21.0
Bon Bons (Brach's)	1 piece (.6 oz.)	70	12.6
Cream egg (Hershey's)	1 oz.	142	20.4
Neapolitan (Brach's)	1 piece (.4 oz.)	48	8.0
Squares (Nabisco)	1 piece (.5 oz.)	64	12.2
Coffee-ets (Saylor's)	1 piece	13	D.N.A.
Coffee Nips (Pearson's)	1 piece	26	D.N.A.
Coffee Time (F&F)	1 piece	10	D.N.A.
Cup-O-Gold (Hoffman)	1 piece	210	D.N.A.
Dainties, semisweet chocolate			
(Hershey's)	1 oz.	147	17.5
Dots (Mason)	1 oz.	100	D.N.A.
Eagle Bar (Ghirardelli)	1 sq.	151	16.7

(USDA): United States Department of Agriculture
DNA: Data Not Available
*Prepared as Package Directs

Food and Description	Measure or Quantity	Calories	Carbo-hydrates (grams)
Frappe (Welch's)	1 piece	115	21.4
5th Avenue Bar (Luden's):			
5¢ size	1 bar	71	D.N.A.
10¢ size	1 bar	129	D.N.A.
15¢ size	1 bar	179	D.N.A.
Fruit 'n Nut chocolate bar (Nestlé's)	1 oz.	140	16.5
Fudge:			
Bar (Nabisco)	1 piece (1.1 oz.)	130	22.8
Fudgies (Kraft)	1 piece (8 grams)	33	6.1
Nut, bar (Nabisco)	1 piece (.6 oz.)	84	3.6
Nut, square (Nabisco)	1 piece (.6 oz.)	84	3.6
Hard candy:			
(Bonomo)	1 oz.	112	D.N.A.
(H-B)	1 piece	12	2.9
(Peerless Maid)	1 piece	22	5.6
Butterscotch:			
(Reed's)	1 piece	17	D.N.A.
Disks (Brach's)	1 piece (6 grams)	23	5.7
Skimmers (Nabisco)	1 piece (6 grams)	22	5.4
Cherry, wild, drops, old fashioned (Nabisco)	1 piece (2 grams)	11	2.7
Cinnamon (Reed's)	1 piece	17	D.N.A.
Honey & horehound drops, old fashioned (Nabisco)	1 piece (2 grams)	11	2.7
Lemon drops (Brach's)	1 piece (4 grams)	15	3.8
Peppermint (Reed's)	1 piece	17	D.N.A.
Pops, assorted (Brach's)	1 piece (5 grams)	19	4.8
Root beer (Reed's)	1 piece	17	D.N.A.
Sherbit (F&F)	1 piece	9	2.2
Sour balls (Brach's)	1 piece (6 grams)	22	5.7
Spearmint (Reed's)	1 piece	17	D.N.A.
Wintergreen (Reed's)	1 piece	17	D.N.A.
Hershey-Ets, candy-coated	1 oz.	134	21.0
Hollywood	1½ oz.	185	24.1
Jelly (See also individual flavors and brand names in this section):			
Beans:			
(Brach's)	1 piece (3 grams)	11	2.8
(Heide)	1 oz.	90	D.N.A.
Big Ben Jellies (Brach's)	1 piece (8 grams)	26	6.8
Iced Jelly Cones (Brach's)	1 piece (4 grams)	15	3.4
Nougats (Brach's)	1 piece (.4 oz.)	43	10.0

(USDA): United States Department of Agriculture
DNA: Data Not Available
*Prepared as Package Directs

Food and Description	Measure or Quantity	Calories	Carbohydrates (grams)
Jube Jels (Brach's)	1 piece (3 grams)	11	2.7
Jujubes, assorted (Heide)	1 oz.	93	D.N.A.
Jujyfruits (Heide)	1 oz.	94	D.N.A.
Kisses, milk chocolate (Hershey's)	1 piece (5⁄16 oz.)	48	5.0
Krackel Bar (Hershey's)	1 oz.	148	15.0
Licorice:			
(Y&S)	1 oz.	100	D.N.A.
Diamond Drops (Heide)	1 oz.	94	D.N.A.
Pastilles (Heide)	1 oz.	96	D.N.A.
Twist (American Licorice Co.):			
Black	1 piece	27	6.4
Red	1 piece	33	7.3
Life Savers (Beech-Nut):			
Cl-O-Ve	1 piece	6	1.6
Pep-O-Mint	1 piece	6	1.6
Spear-O-Mint	1 piece	6	1.6
Wint-O-Green	1 piece	6	1.6
All other flavors	1 piece	9	2.2
Lozenges, mint or wintergreen (Brach's)	1 piece (3 grams)	11	2.9
Mallo Cup (Boyer):			
5¢ size	3⁄4- oz. cup	104	14.8
10¢ size	1¼-oz. cup	173	24.6
15¢ size	1⅝-oz. cup	225	32.3
Malted Milk Balls, milk chocolate-covered (Brach's)	1 piece (2 grams)	9	1.6
Malted Milk Crunch (Welch's)	1 piece (1 gram)	8	.9
Maple Nut Goodies (Brach's)	1 piece (6 grams)	29	4.0
Mars Almond Bar (M&M/Mars)	1 oz.	130	16.9
Marshmallow:			
(Campfire)	1 piece (¼ oz.)	25	5.8
Royal Marshmallow (Curtiss)	1 oz.	90	22.0
Chocolate (Kraft)	1 piece (5 grams)	18	4.2
Chocolate-covered (Kraft)	1 piece (7 grams)	31	4.7
Jet Puff (Kraft):			
Plain	1 piece (6 grams)	18	4.6
Chocolate-covered	1 piece (7 grams)	32	4.7
Flavored	1 piece (5 grams)	18	4.4
Macaroon	1 piece (8 grams)	30	4.9
Miniature	1 piece (<1 gram)	2	.5
Mary Jane (Miller):			
1¢ size	1 piece (.3 oz.)	31	5.6
5¢ size	1 piece (1.2 oz.)	125	21.8
Merrimints (Delson)	1 piece	30	D.N.A.

Food and Description	Measure or Quantity	Calories	Carbo-hydrates (grams)
Milk Shake (Hollywood)	1¼ oz.	150	26.8
Milky Way, milk or dark chocolate (M&M/Mars)	1 oz.	120	17.7
Mint:			
Anise, midget (Kraft)	1 piece (<1 gram)	3	.8
Anise, regular (Kraft)	1 piece (<1 gram)	7	1.8
Buttermint (Kraft)	1 piece (2 grams)	8	1.9
Candy-coated mint chocolate (Hershey's)	1 oz.	133	21.1
Chocolate-covered bar (Brach's)	1 piece (1 oz.)	124	23.0
Colored, mints, midget (Kraft)	1 piece (<1 gram)	3	.8
Colored, mints, regular (Kraft)	1 piece (2 grams)	7	1.8
Dessert (Brach's)	1 piece (<1 gram)	4	.9
Jamaica Mints (Nabisco)	1 piece (5 grams)	21	5.2
Liberty Mints (Nabisco)	1 piece (5 grams)	21	5.2
Mint Parfait (Pearson's)	1 piece	34	D.N.A.
Pattie, chocolate-covered:			
(Brach's)	1 piece (.4 oz.)	50	9.2
(Hoffman)	1 piece	120	D.N.A.
Junior Mint Pattie (Nabisco)	1 piece (2 grams)	8	2.1
Mason Mints	1 oz.	200	D.N.A.
Peppermint pattie (Nabisco)	1 piece (.6 oz.)	67	13.3
Sherbit pressed mints (F&F)	1 piece	7	1.8
Starlight Mints (Brach's)	1 piece (5 grams)	19	4.8
Swedish (Brach's)	1 piece (2 grams)	8	1.9
Thin (Delson)	1 piece	45	D.N.A.
Thin (Nabisco)	1 piece (.4 oz.)	44	8.7
White, midget (Kraft)	1 piece (<1 gram)	3	.8
White, regular (Kraft)	1 piece (<1 gram)	7	1.8
Mounds (Peter Paul)	10¢ pkg. (1⅝ oz.)	202	26.6
M&M's (M&M/Mars):			
Chocolate	1 oz.	140	18.1
Peanut	1 oz.	140	16.8
Mr. Goodbar (Hershey's)	1 oz.	153	12.5
Necco:			
Canada Mints	1 piece	13	D.N.A.
Necco Wafers	1 piece	7	D.N.A.
Wintergreen	1 piece	13	D.N.A.
North Pole (F&F)	1 bar (1⅜ oz.)	150	31.0
Nutty Crunch, bar (Nabisco)	1 piece (4 grams)	20	2.8
Nutty Crunch, squares (Nabisco)	1 piece (½ oz.)	71	10.1
Old Nick (Schutter)	1 oz.	134	D.N.A.
$100,000 Bar (Nestlé's)	1 oz.	121	18.9
Orange Slices (Brach's)	1 piece (.6 oz.)	55	14.4

(USDA): United States Department of Agriculture
DNA: Data Not Available
*Prepared as Package Directs

Food and Description	Measure or Quantity	Calories	Carbo-hydrates (grams)
Payday (Hollywood)	1¼ oz.	150	22.3
Peaks (Mason)	1 oz.	175	D.N.A.
Peanut:			
Chocolate-covered:			
(BB)	1 oz.	158	6.5
(Brach's)	1 piece (2 grams)	11	1.1
(Hershey's) candy-coated	1 oz.	139	17.9
(Kraft) bite-size	1 piece (9 grams)	43	7.6
(Kraft) boxed	1 piece (2 grams)	12	1.0
(Nabisco)	1 piece (4 grams)	23	1.6
French Burnt (Brach's)	1 piece (1 gram)	5	.6
Peanut Brittle:			
(Bonomo)	1 oz.	132	D.N.A.
(Kraft)	1 bar (1¼ oz.)	164	23.2
Coconut (Kraft)	1 oz.	122	22.3
Jumbo Peanut Block Bar			
(Planters)	1 oz.	140	14.0
Peanut Butter Cup:			
(Boyer):			
5¢ size	¾-oz. cup	130	10.8
10¢ size	1¼-oz. cup	216	17.9
15¢ size	1⅝-oz. cup	281	23.6
(Reese's)	1 oz.	143	15.4
Smoothie (Boyer):			
5¢ size	¾-oz. cup	135	10.8
10¢ size	1¼-oz. cup	224	17.9
15¢ size	1⅝-oz. cup	292	23.6
Peanut Butter Egg (Reese's)	1 oz.	135	12.4
P-Nut Butter Crunch			
(Pearson's)	1 piece	35	D.N.A.
Pom Poms (Nabisco)	1 piece	12	2.2
Poppycock	1 oz.	147	22.0
Raisin, chocolate-covered:			
(Brach's)	1 piece (1 gram)	4	.7
(Nabisco)	1 piece (<1 gram)	4	.6
Bar (Ghirardelli)	10¢ bar (1¼ oz.)	176	20.9
Raisinets (B&B)	5¢ box	140	15.4
Red Hot Dollars (Heide)	1 oz.	94	D.N.A.
Saf-T-Pops (Curtiss)	1 oz.	108	26.1
Snickers (M&M/Mars)	1 oz.	130	15.0
Spearmint Leaves (Brach's)	1 piece (7 grams)	23	5.9
Spicettes (Brach's)	1 piece (3 grams)	10	2.5
Sprigs, sweet chocolate			
(Hershey's)	1 oz.	136	18.3

Food and Description	Measure or Quantity	Calories	Carbo-hydrates (grams)
Sprint, chocolate wafer bar (M&M/Mars)	1 oz.	150	16.2
Stark Wafer Roll	5¢ roll (1¼ oz.)	132	32.9
Stars, chocolate:			
(Brach's)	1 piece (3 grams)	16	1.7
(Nabisco)	1 piece (2 grams)	9	1.0
Sugar Babies (Nabisco)	1 piece	4	.9
Sugar Daddy (Nabisco):			
Giant sucker	1 piece (1 lb.)	1806	398.2
Junior sucker	1 piece (.4 oz.)	42	9.3
Junior sucker, chocolate-flavored	1 piece (.4 oz.)	43	9.1
Nugget	1 piece (6 grams)	26	5.7
Sucker	1 piece (1.1 oz.)	129	28.4
Sugar Mama, pop (Nabisco)	1 piece (1 oz.)	121	22.6
Sugar Wafer (F&F)	1¼-oz. pkg.	180	26.0
Taffy:			
Salt water (Brach's)	1 piece (8 grams)	31	6.8
Turkish (Bonomo):			
Bar	1⅛ oz.	115	29.3
Bite-size	1 piece	19	4.6
Miniatures	1 piece	21	5.6
Nibbles, chocolate-covered	1 piece	9	1.7
Pop	1 piece	45	11.3
Roll	1¢ size	21	5.6
3 Musketeers Bar (M&M/Mars)	1 oz.	120	19.6
Toffee:			
Almond (Kraft)	1-oz. bar	142	7.9
Almond, chocolate-covered (Kraft)	1 piece (6 grams)	50	6.3
Assorted (Brach's)	1 piece (7 grams)	28	5.2
Chocolate (Kraft)	1 piece (6 grams)	36	5.0
Coffee (Kraft)	1 piece (6 grams)	36	5.2
Rum butter (Kraft)	1 piece (6 grams)	36	5.2
Vanilla (Kraft)	1 piece (6 grams)	36	5.2
Tootsie Roll:			
Regular:			
1¢ size or midgee	1 piece (.23 oz.)	27	5.0
2¢ size	1 piece (.37 oz.)	43	8.1
5¢ size	1 piece (1 oz.)	116	21.5
10¢ size	1 piece (1.75 oz.)	202	37.7
Vending-machine size	1 piece (.18 oz.)	21	3.9
Pop	1 piece (.5 oz.)	55	13.2
Pop-drop	1 piece (.16 oz.)	18	4.4

Food and Description	Measure or Quantity	Calories	Carbohydrates (grams)
Triple Decker bar (Nestlé's)	1 oz.	148	16.8
U-No (Cardinet's)	1 bar (⅞ oz.)	161	9.3
Virginia Nut Roll (Queen Anne)	10¢ size	250	D.N.A.
Walnut Hill (F&F)	1 bar (1⅜ oz.)	177	29.0
Wetem & Wearem (Heide)	1 oz.	94	D.N.A.
Whirligigs (Nabisco)	1 piece (4 grams)	14	3.0

CANDY, DIETETIC:

Food and Description	Measure or Quantity	Calories	Carbohydrates (grams)
Almondettes (Estee)	1 piece	22	1.0
Banana wafer chocolate bar (Estee)	1 bar (¾ oz.)	126	10.4
Chocolate, assorted:			
Bittersweet (Estee)	1 piece	51	3.0
Milk (Estee)	1 piece	53	2.9
Miniatures (Dia-Mel)	1 piece (8 grams)	37	4.4
Chocolate bar with almonds:			
(Estee)	1 section of 2-oz. bar	14	.9
(Estee)	1 section of 4-oz. bar	85	5.7
(Estee)	1 bar (¾ oz.)	128	8.5
Chocolate bar, bittersweet:			
(Estee)	1 bar (¾ oz.)	121	10.0
(Estee)	1 section of 4-oz. bar	80	6.7
(Estee)	1 section of 2-oz. bar	13	1.1
Chocolate bar, milk:			
(Estee)	1 section of 4-oz. bar	83	5.8
(Estee)	1 section of 2-oz. bar	14	1.0
White (Estee)	1 section of 4-oz. bar	79	6.1
With peppermint (Estee)	1 bar (¾ oz.)	125	8.7
Chocolate pops bar (Estee)	1 section of 2½-oz. bar	21	1.4
Chocolettes, almond (Estee)	1 piece	19	1.2
Chocolettes, milk (Estee)	1 piece	19	1.3
Coconut chocolate bar (Estee)	1 bar (¾ oz.)	127	8.1
Coffee & almond chocolate bar (Estee)	1 section of 2-oz. bar	14	D.N.A.

(USDA): United States Department of Agriculture
DNA: Data Not Available
*Prepared as Package Directs

Food and Description	Measure or Quantity	Calories	Carbo-hydrates (grams)
Coffee beans, milk chocolate-covered (Estee)	1 piece	4	.2
Creams, assorted (Estee)	1 piece	52	3.4
Gum drops:			
(Dia-Mel)	1 piece (2 grams)	3	0.
All flavors (Estee)	1 piece	2	.6
Hard candy:			
All flavors (Estee)	1 piece	12	3.0
Assorted flavors (Barton's)	1 piece	11	2.8
Coffee (Barton's)	1 piece	8	1.7
Coffee (Estee)	1 piece	13	2.8
Lollipops (Estee)	1 pop	14	3.6
Licorice (Dia-Mel)	1 piece (2 grams)	3	0.
Marshmallow (Dia-Mel)	1 piece (8 grams)	27	2.9
Mint:			
Butterscotch (Estee)	1 piece	4	1.0
Chocolate (Estee)	1 piece	4	1.0
Fruit flavors (Estee)	1 piece	4	1.0
Peppermint (Estee)	1 piece	4	1.0
Peppermint chocolette (Estee)	1 piece	19	1.3
Peppermint cream (Estee)	1 piece	52	3.4
Thin (Dia-Mel)	1 piece (6 grams)	22	1.5
Nut, milk chocolate-covered (Estee)	1 piece	49	2.8
Nut cluster (Estee)	1 piece	41	3.9
Peanut butter cup (Estee)	1 cup	42	2.7
Peanutette (Estee)	1 piece	4	.4
Petit fours (Estee)	1 piece	47	4.2
Raisin, chocolate-covered (Estee)	1 piece	4	.5
Soff Jells (Dia-Mel)	1 piece (2 grams)	3	0.
Stick, filled (Estee)	1 piece	38	4.1
Tri-Pak, chocolate-covered assorted bars (Dia-Mel)	3-oz. pkg.	305	34.0
Truffle, chocolate (Estee)	1 piece	51	2.7
TV mix (Estee)	1 piece	15	.8
Wafer bar (Estee):			
Bittersweet chocolate-covered	1 bar (¾ oz.)	123	10.4
Milk chocolate-covered	1 bar (¾ oz.)	124	10.6
CANE SYRUP (USDA)	1 T.	53	13.6
CANTALOUPE, fresh:			
Whole (USDA)	1 lb. (weighed whole)	68	17.0

(USDA): United States Department of Agriculture
DNA: Data Not Available
*Prepared as Package Directs

Food and Description	Measure or Quantity	Calories	Carbo-hydrates (grams)
Whole (USDA)	½ med. melon, 5″ dia. (13.6 oz.)	60	14.0
Cubed (USDA)	½ cup (2.8 oz.)	24	6.1
CAPE GOOSEBERRY (See **GROUND-CHERRY**)			
CAPERS (Crosse & Blackwell)	1 T.	6	1.0
CAPICOLA or CAPACOLA SAUSAGE (USDA)	1 oz.	141	0.
CAP'N CRUNCH, cereal (Quaker)	1 cup (1.3 oz.)	163	30.7
CAPPELLA WINE (Italian Swiss Colony-Gold Medal) 12.3% alcohol	3 fl. oz.	66	1.2
CARAMBOLA, raw (USDA):			
Whole	1 lb. (weighed whole)	149	34.1
Flesh only	4 oz.	40	9.1
CARAMEL CAKE, home recipe (USDA):			
Without icing	2-oz. serving	218	30.4
With caramel icing	2-oz. serving	215	33.5
CARAMEL CAKE MIX:			
*(Duncan Hines)	1 cake	2351	384.0
Pudding (Betty Crocker)	11-oz. pkg.	1276	267.3
*CARAMEL NUT PUDDING,** instant (Royal)	½ cup (5.2 oz.)	195	30.9
CARAWAY SEED (Information supplied by General Mills Laboratory)	1 oz.	72	12.3
CARISSA or NATAL PLUM, raw:			
Whole (USDA)	1 lb. (weighed whole)	273	62.4
Flesh only (USDA)	4 oz.	79	18.1

Food and Description	Measure or Quantity	Calories	Carbo-hydrates (grams)
CARNATION INSTANT BREAKFAST	1 envelope with 8 fl. oz. whole milk	290	35.1
CAROB FLOUR (See **FLOUR**)			
CAROUSEL WINE (Gold Seal):			
Pink or white, 13-14% alcohol	3 fl. oz.	125	9.8
Red, 13-14% alcohol	3 fl. oz.	104	5.2
CARP, raw (USDA):			
Whole	1 lb. (weighed whole)	156	0.
Meat only	4 oz.	131	0.
CARROT:			
Raw (USDA):			
Whole	1 lb. (weighed with full tops)	112	26.0
Partially trimmed	1 lb. (weighed without tops, with skins)	156	36.1
Trimmed	5½″ x 1″ carrot (1.8 oz.)	20	5.0
Trimmed	25 thin strips (1.8 oz.)	20	5.0
Chunks	½ cup (2.4 oz.)	28	6.6
Diced	½ cup (2.5 oz.)	30	7.0
Grated or shredded	½ cup (1.9 oz.)	22	5.2
Slices	½ cup (2.2 oz.)	26	6.2
Strips	½ cup (2 oz.)	24	5.6
Boiled (USDA):			
Chunks, drained	½ cup (2.8 oz.)	25	5.8
Diced, drained	½ cup (2.4 oz.)	22	5.0
Slices, drained	½ cup (2.6 oz.)	24	5.4
Canned, regular pack:			
Solids & liq. (USDA)	4 oz.	32	7.4
Diced, drained (USDA)	½ cup (2.8 oz.)	24	5.3
(Butter Kernel)	½ cup	29	7.0
(Fall River)	½ cup	29	7.0
Solids & liq. (Stokely-Van Camp)	4 oz.	32	7.4
Canned, dietetic pack:			
Low sodium, solids & liq. (USDA)	4 oz.	25	5.7

(USDA): United States Department of Agriculture
DNA: Data Not Available
*Prepared as Package Directs

Food and Description	Measure or Quantity	Calories	Carbohydrates (grams)
Low sodium, drained solids			
(USDA)	4 oz.	28	6.4
Diced, solids & liq. (Blue Boy)	4 oz.	25	5.2
Slices (S and W) *Nutradiet*	4 oz.	25	5.2
(Tillie Lewis)	½ cup (4.3 oz.)	27	5.4
Dehydrated (USDA)	1 oz.	97	23.0
Frozen (Birds Eye):			
Slices in butter sauce	½ cup (3.3 oz.)	70	7.7
With brown sugar glaze	½ cup (3.3 oz.)	78	15.5
CASABA MELON, fresh (USDA):			
Whole	1 lb. (weighed whole)	61	14.7
Flesh only	4 oz.	31	7.4
CASANOVE, Italian liqueur			
(Leroux) 80 proof	1 fl. oz.	104	9.5
CASHEW NUT:			
(USDA)	1 oz.	159	8.3
(USDA)	½ cup (2.5 oz.)	393	20.5
(USDA)	5 large or 8 med.	60	3.1
Dry roasted (Planters)	1 oz.	175	7.9
Dry roasted (Skippy)	1 oz.	166	8.4
Oil roasted (Planters)	1 oz.	180	7.8
Oil roasted (Skippy)	1 oz.	178	6.9
CATAWBA WINE:			
(Gold Seal) 13-14% alcohol	3 fl. oz.	125	9.8
(Great Western) pink, 13% alcohol	3 fl. oz.	116	11.0
(Mogen David) pink, New York			
State, 12% alcohol	3 fl. oz.	75	11.6
(Mogen David) red, New York			
State, 12% alcohol	3 fl. oz.	75	11.6
CATFISH, freshwater, raw, fillet			
(USDA)	4 oz.	117	0.
CATSUP:			
Regular pack:			
(USDA)	1 T.	18	4.3
(Heinz)	1 T.	21	4.9
(Hunt's)	1 oz.	30	7.2
(Nalley's)	1 oz.	28	6.9

(USDA): United States Department of Agriculture
DNA: Data Not Available
*Prepared as Package Directs

Food and Description	Measure or Quantity	Calories	Carbo-hydrates (grams)
(Smucker's)	1 oz.	52	D.N.A.
Dietetic pack:			
(Diet Delight)	1 T.	6	1.2
(Tillie Lewis)	1 T.	6	1.2
CAULIFLOWER:			
Fresh (USDA):			
Whole	1 lb. (weighed untrimmed)	48	9.2
Flowerbuds	1 lb. (weighed trimmed)	122	23.6
Slices	½ cup (1.4 oz.)	11	2.2
Boiled, flowerbuds, drained (USDA)	½ cup (2.2 oz.)	14	2.5
Frozen:			
(USDA)	4 oz.	24	4.8
Boiled, drained (USDA)	½ cup (3.2 oz.)	16	3.0
(Birds Eye)	½ cup (3.3 oz.)	21	3.3
(Stokely-Van Camp)	4 oz.	24	4.8
Au gratin (Stouffer's)	10-oz. pkg.	339	17.9
Buds, in butter sauce (Green Giant) boil-in-the-bag	4 oz.	74	5.8
In cheese sauce (Green Giant)	4 oz.	69	8.1
CAULIFLOWER CRISPS, dehydrated snack (Epicure)	1 oz.	82	15.9
CAULIFLOWER, SWEET PICKLED (Smucker's)	½ oz.	23	5.8
CAVIAR, STURGEON (USDA):			
Pressed	1 oz.	89	1.4
Whole eggs	1 oz.	74	.9
CELERIAC ROOT, raw (USDA):			
Whole	1 lb. (weighed unpared)	156	33.2
Pared	4 oz.	45	9.6
CELERY, all varieties (USDA):			
Raw:			
Whole	1 lb. (weighed untrimmed)	58	13.3
1 large outer stalk	8″ x 1½″ at root end (1.4 oz.)	7	1.6

(USDA): United States Department of Agriculture
DNA: Data Not Available
*Prepared as Package Directs

Food and Description	Measure or Quantity	Calories	Carbo- hydrates (grams)
Diced, chopped or cut in chunks	½ cup (2.1 oz.)	10	2.3
Slices	½ cup (1.8 oz.)	9	2.1
Boiled, drained solids:			
Diced or cut in chunks	½ cup (2.6 oz.)	11	2.4
Slices	½ cup (3 oz.)	12	2.6

CELERY CABBAGE (See
CABBAGE, CHINESE)

CELERY SOUP, Cream of:

Condensed (USDA)	8 oz. (by wt.)	163	16.8
*Prepared with equal volume water (USDA)	1 cup (8.4 oz.)	86	8.9
*Prepared with equal volume milk (USDA)	1 cup (8.4 oz.)	166	14.9
Condensed (Campbell)	8 oz. (by wt.)	150	14.5
*(Heinz)	1 cup	104	8.6

CEREAL BREAKFAST FOODS
(See kind of cereal such as **CORN
FLAKES** or brand name such as
KIX)

CERVELAT (USDA):

Dry	1 oz.	128	.5
Soft	1 oz.	87	.5

CERTS (Warner-Lambert)   1 piece   6   1.5

CHABLIS WINE:

(Barton & Guestier) 12% alcohol	3 fl. oz.	60	.1
(Chanson) St. Vincent, 11½% alcohol	3 fl. oz.	81	6.3
(Cruse) 11% alcohol	3 fl. oz.	66	D.N.A.
(Gallo) 12% alcohol	3 fl. oz.	50	.9
(Gallo) pink, 13% alcohol	3 fl. oz.	61	3.0
(Gold Seal) 12% alcohol	3 fl. oz.	82	.4
(Great Western) 12% alcohol	3 fl. oz.	76	1.7
(Italian Swiss Colony - Gold Medal) 11.6% alcohol	3 fl. oz.	59	.6
(Italian Swiss Colony - Gold Medal) Napa-Sonoma-Mendocino, 12% alcohol	3 fl. oz.	64	1.2

Food and Description	Measure or Quantity	Calories	Carbo- hydrates (grams)
(Italian Swiss Colony - Private Stock) 12% alcohol	3 fl. oz.	59	< .1
(Italian Swiss Colony - Gold Medal) gold or pink, 12.3% alcohol	3 fl. oz.	69	3.0
(Louis M. Martini) 12½% alcohol	3 fl. oz.	90	.2

CHAMPAGNE:

(Bollinger)	3 fl. oz.	72	3.6
(Gold Seal) brut, 12% alcohol	3 fl. oz.	85	1.4
(Gold Seal) brut *C.F.*, 12% alcohol	3 fl. oz.	82	.6
(Gold Seal) pink extra dry, 12% alcohol	3 fl. oz.	87	2.6
(Great Western) brut, 12% alcohol	3 fl. oz.	82	3.2
(Great Western) extra dry, 12% alcohol	3 fl. oz.	75	4.5
(Great Western) pink, 12% alcohol	3 fl. oz.	88	4.7
(Great Western) special reserve, 12% alcohol	3 fl. oz.	79	3.8
(Italian Swiss Colony - Private Stock) 12% alcohol	3 fl. oz.	69	2.8
(Italian Swiss Colony - Private Stock) pink, 12% alcohol	3 fl. oz.	69	2.6
(Lejon) extra dry, 12% alcohol	3 fl. oz.	68	2.4
(Lejon) pink, 12% alcohol	3 fl. oz.	69	2.6
(Mandia)	3 fl. oz.	75	D.N.A.
(Mogen David) American Concord red, 12% alcohol	3 fl. oz.	90	8.9
(Mogen David) American dry, 12% alcohol	3 fl. oz.	36	4.4
(Mumm's) Cordon Rouge brut, 12% alcohol	3 fl. oz.	65	1.4
(Mumm's) extra dry, 12% alcohol	3 fl. oz.	82	5.6
(Taylor) brut, 12.5% alcohol	3 fl. oz.	75	1.4
(Taylor) dry, 12.5%	3 fl. oz.	78	2.0
(Taylor) pink, 12.5%	3 fl. oz.	81	2.9
(Veuve Clicquot) 12.5% alcohol	3 fl. oz.	78	.6

CHARD, Swiss (USDA):

Raw, whole	1 lb. (weighed untrimmed)	104	19.2
Boiled, drained solids	½ cup (3.4 oz.)	17	3.2

(USDA): United States Department of Agriculture
DNA: Data Not Available
*Prepared as Package Directs

Food and Description	Measure or Quantity	Calories	Carbohydrates (grams)
CHARLOTTE RUSSE, with ladyfingers, whipped cream filling, home recipe (USDA)	4 oz.	324	38.0
CHATEAU LA GARDE CLARET, French red Bordeaux (Chanson) 11½% alcohol	3 fl. oz.	60	6.3
CHATEAUNEUF-DU-PAPE, French red Rhone:			
(Barton & Guestier) 13.5% alcohol	3 fl. oz.	70	.5
(Chanson) 13% alcohol	3 fl. oz.	90	6.3
(Cruse) 12% alcohol	3 fl. oz.	72	D.N.A.
CHATEAU OLIVIER BLANC, French white Graves (Chanson) 11½% alcohol	3 fl. oz.	60	6.3
CHATEAU OLIVIER ROUGE, French red Graves (Chanson) 11½% alcohol	3 fl. oz.	60	6.3
CHATEAU PONTET CANET (Cruse) 12% alcohol	3 fl. oz.	72	D.N.A.
CHATEAU RAUSAN SEGLA, French red Bordeaux (Chanson) 11½% alcohol	3 fl. oz.	60	6.3
CHATEAU ST. GERMAIN, French red Bordeaux (Chanson) 11½% alcohol	3 fl. oz.	60	6.3
CHATEAU VOIGNY, French Sauternes (Chanson) 13% alcohol	3 fl. oz.	96	7.5
CHAYOTE, raw, (USDA):			
Whole	1 lb. (weighed unpared)	108	27.4
Pared	4 oz.	32	8.1
CHEDDAR CHEESE SOUP, condensed (Campbell)	8 oz. (by wt.)	284	19.3
CHEERIOS, cereal (General Mills)	1¼ cup (1 oz.)	112	20.2

(USDA): United States Department of Agriculture
DNA: Data Not Available
*Prepared as Package Directs

Food and Description	Measure or Quantity	Calories	Carbo-hydrates (grams)
CHEESE:			
American or cheddar:			
Natural:			
(USDA)	1″ cube (.6 oz.)	68	.4
Diced (USDA)	1 cup (4.6 oz.)	521	2.8
Grated or shredded (USDA)	1 cup (3.9 oz.)	442	2.3
Grated or shredded (USDA)	1 T.	28	.1
(Borden)	1″ cube	70	.6
(Kraft)	1 oz.	113	.6
(Sealtest)	1 oz.	115	.6
Sharp cheddar (Gerber)	1 T.	50	1.5
Process:			
(USDA)	1 oz.	105	.5
(Borden)	1 oz.	105	.5
(Breakstone)	1 oz.	105	.5
Loaf or slice (Kraft)	1 oz.	105	.5
(Sealtest)	1 oz.	105	.5
With Brick cheese (Kraft)	1 oz.	101	.5
With Monterey (Kraft)	1 oz.	101	.5
With Muenster (Kraft)	1 oz.	100	.5
Dried, sharp cheddar (Information supplied by General Mills Laboratory)	1 oz.	171	1.7
Asiago (Frigo)	1 oz.	113	.6
Bakers Special (Kraft)	1 oz.	110	7.2
Bleu or blue:			
Natural (USDA)	1 oz.	104	.6
(Borden)	1 oz.	104	.6
(Foremost Blue Moon)	1 T.	52	Tr.
(Frigo)	1 oz.	99	.5
(Gerber)	1 T.	49	1.6
Natural (Kraft)	1 oz.	99	.5
(Stella)	1 oz.	113	.6
Bond-Ost, natural (Kraft)	1 oz.	104	.4
Brick:			
Natural (USDA)	1 oz.	105	.5
Natural (Kraft)	1 oz.	104	.3
Process, slices (Kraft)	1 oz.	102	.4
Camembert, domestic:			
Natural (USDA)	1 oz.	85	.5
(Borden)	1 oz.	85	.5
(Kraft)	1 oz.	85	.5
Caraway, natural (Kraft)	1 oz.	111	.6
Chantelle, natural (Kraft)	1 oz.	91	.3

(USDA): United States Department of Agriculture
DNA: Data Not Available
*Prepared as Package Directs

Food and Description	Measure or Quantity	Calories	Carbo- hydrates (grams)
Cheddar (See American)			
Ched-ett, process, cold pack (Kraft)	1 oz.	85	2.1
Colby, natural (Kraft)	1 oz.	111	.6
Cottage:			
Creamed, unflavored:			
(USDA)	1 cup (8.2 oz.)	247	6.8
(USDA)	1 T.	15	.4
(Borden)	1 cup	241	6.6
Lite Line, low fat (Borden)	1 cup	189	7.0
California (Breakstone)	4 oz.	115	2.9
Tangy small curd (Breakstone)	4 oz.	1·15	2.8
Tangy small curd (Breakstone)	1 T.	14	.4
Tiny soft curd (Breakstone)	4 oz.	115	2.8
Tiny soft curd (Breakstone)	1 T.	14	.4
(Foremost Blue Moon)	1 oz.	30	.4
(Kraft)	1 oz.	27	.9
(Sealtest)	1 cup	213	5.1
Light n' Lively, low fat (Sealtest)	1 cup	153	6.6
Creamed, flavored:			
Chive (Breakstone)	4 oz.	115	2.9
Chive (Breakstone)	1 T.	14	.4
Pineapple (Breakstone)	4 oz.	132	2.9
Pineapple (Breakstone)	1 T.	17	.4
Pineapple (Sealtest)	1 cup	204	13.0
Spring Garden Salad (Sealtest)	1 cup	210	8.1
Uncreamed:			
(USDA)	1 cup (7.9 oz.)	194	6.1
(USDA)	1 oz.	24	.8
(Borden)	1 cup	200	6.2
(Kraft)	1 oz.	26	.6
(Sealtest)	⅓ cup	60	1.0
Pot style (Breakstone)	4 oz.	85	1.9
Pot style (Breakstone)	1 T.	11	.2
Skim milk, no salt added (Breakstone)	4 oz.	88	2.2
Skim milk, no salt added (Breakstone)	1 T.	11	.3
Cream cheese:			
Plain, unwhipped:			
(USDA)	1 oz.	101	.6

(USDA): United States Department of Agriculture
DNA: Data Not Available
*Prepared as Package Directs

Food and Description	Measure or Quantity	Calories	Carbo-hydrates (grams)
(USDA)	1 T.	55	.3
(Borden)	1 oz.	105	1.0
(Breakstone)	1 oz.	99	.4
(Breakstone)	1 T.	50	.2
Glass or loaf (Kraft)	1 oz.	98	.6
(Sealtest)	1 oz.	98	.6
Plain, whipped (Breakstone):			
Temp-Tee	1 oz.	99	.4
Temp-Tee	1 T.	33	.2
Flavored, unwhipped (Kraft):			
With bacon & horseradish, glass	1 oz.	91	.5
With chive, glass or loaf	1 oz.	84	.8
With olive-pimento, glass	1 oz.	85	.8
With pimento, glass or loaf	1 oz.	85	.7
With pineapple	1 oz.	87	2.5
With relish, loaf	1 oz.	88	2.4
With Roquefort, glass	1 oz.	80	.7
Flavored, whipped (Kraft):			
Catalina	1 oz.	94	1.1
With bacon & horseradish	1 oz.	95	.7
With blue cheese	1 oz.	98	.7
With chive	1 oz.	92	1.0
With onion	1 oz.	93	1.5
With pimento	1 oz.	91	1.2
With Roquefort cheese	1 oz.	99	1.3
With salami	1 oz.	88	1.2
With smoked salmon	1 oz.	90	1.7
Edam (House of Gold)	1 oz.	105	.3
Edam, natural (Kraft)	1 oz.	105	.3
Farmer cheese, packaged (Breakstone)	1 T.	19	.8
Fontina (Stella)	1 oz.	113	.6
Frankenmuth, natural (Kraft)	1 oz.	113	.6
Gjetost, natural (Kraft)	1 oz.	135	13.0
Gorgonzola (Foremost Blue Moon)	1 oz.	110	Tr.
Gorgonzola, natural (Kraft)	1 oz.	112	.4
Gouda, baby (Foremost Blue Moon)	1 oz.	120	Tr.
Gouda, natural (Kraft)	1 oz.	108	.5
Gruyère (Gerber)	1 oz.	101	.5
Gruyère, natural (Kraft)	1 oz.	110	.6
Jack-dry, natural (Kraft)	1 oz.	102	.4

(USDA): United States Department of Agriculture
DNA: Data Not Available
*Prepared as Package Directs

Food and Description	Measure or Quantity	Calories	Carbohydrates (grams)
Jack-fresh, natural (Kraft)	1 oz.	95	.4
Lagerkase, natural (Kraft)	1 oz.	108	.3
Leyden, natural (Kraft)	1 oz.	80	.7
Liederkranz (Borden)	1 oz.	86	.4
Limburger, natural (USDA)	1 oz.	98	.6
Limburger, natural (Kraft)	1 oz.	98	.6
MacLaren's, process, cold pack (Kraft)	1 oz.	109	.6
Monterey Jack (Frigo)	1 oz.	103	.4
Monterey Jack, natural (Kraft)	1 oz.	103	.4
Mozzarella:			
(Frigo)	1 oz.	79	.3
Natural, low moisture, part skim (Kraft)	1 oz.	84	.3
Natural, low moisture, part skim, pizza (Kraft)	1 oz.	79	.3
Muenster, natural (Kraft)	1 oz.	100	.3
Muenster, process, slices (Kraft)	1 oz.	102	.6
Neufchâtel:			
(Borden) *Eagle Brand*	1 oz.	73	1.0
Loaf (Kraft)	1 oz.	69	.7
Natural (Kraft) *Calorie-Wise*	1 oz.	70	.7
Swankyswigs (Kraft):			
Olive-pimento	1 oz.	70	1.2
Pimento	1 oz.	67	1.4
Pineapple	1 oz.	70	2.7
Relish	1 oz.	71	3.3
Roka	1 oz.	80	.6
Nippy Whipped (Kraft)	1 oz.	82	.9
Nuworld (Kraft)	1 oz.	104	.7
Old English loaf, process, slices (Kraft)	1 oz.	105	.5
Parmesan:			
Natural:			
(USDA)	1 oz.	111	.8
(Frigo)	1 oz.	107	.8
(Kraft)	1 oz.	107	.8
(Stella)	1 oz.	103	.9
Grated:			
(USDA)	1 cup (3.7 oz.)	416	3.0
(USDA)	1 T.	26	.2
(Borden)	1 T.	26	.2
(Buitoni)	1 T.	22	1.5
(Frigo)	1 T.	27	.2

(USDA): United States Department of Agriculture
DNA: Data Not Available
*Prepared as Package Directs

Food and Description	Measure or Quantity	Calories	Carbo-hydrates (grams)
(Kraft)	1 oz.	127	1.0
Shredded (Kraft)	1 oz.	114	.9
Parmesan & Romano, grated:			
(Borden)	1 oz.	143	.9
(Borden)	1 T.	31	.2
Pepato (Frigo)	1 oz.	110	.8
Pimento American, process:			
(USDA)	1 oz.	105	.5
(Borden)	1 oz.	105	.5
Loaf or slices (Kraft)	1 oz.	104	.4
Pizza:			
(Frigo)	1 oz.	73	.3
(Kraft)	1 oz.	73	.3
Shredded (Kraft)	1 oz.	86	.4
Port du Salut (Foremost Blue Moon)	1 oz.	100	Tr.
Port du Salut, natural (Kraft)	1 oz.	100	.3
Prim-Ost, natural (Kraft)	1 oz.	134	13.0
Provolone (Frigo)	1 oz.	99	.5
Provolone or Provoloncini, natural (Kraft)	1 oz.	99	.5
Ricotta cheese (Sierra)	1 oz.	50	1.3
Romano:			
Natural:			
(Frigo)	1 oz.	110	.8
(Kraft)	1 oz.	110	.8
(Stella)	1 oz.	106	.6
Grated:			
(Buitoni)	1 T.	21	1.5
(Frigo)	1 T.	29	.2
(Kraft)	1 oz.	134	1.0
Shredded (Kraft)	1 oz.	121	.9
Roquefort, natural:			
(USDA)	1 oz.	105	.5
(Borden)	1 oz.	105	.5
(Kraft)	1 oz.	105	.5
Sap Sago, natural (Kraft)	1 oz.	76	1.7
Sardo Romano, natural (Kraft)	1 oz.	110	.8
Scamorze (Frigo)	1 oz.	79	.3
Scamorze, natural (Kraft)	1 oz.	100	.3
Swiss, domestic:			
Natural:			
(USDA)	1 oz.	105	1.0
(Foremost Blue Moon)	1 oz.	105	1.0

(USDA): United States Department of Agriculture
DNA: Data Not Available
*Prepared as Package Directs

Food and Description	Measure or Quantity	Calories	Carbohydrates (grams)
(Kraft)	1 oz.	104	.5
(Sealtest)	1 oz.	105	.5
Process:			
(USDA)	1 oz.	101	.5
(Borden)	1 oz.	101	.5
Loaf (Kraft)	1 oz.	93	.5
Slices (Kraft)	1 oz.	95	.6
With American (Kraft)	1 oz.	99	.5
With Muenster (Kraft)	1 oz.	98	.6
Washed curd, natural (Kraft)	1 oz.	108	.6
CHEESE CAKE, frozen (Mrs. Smith's)	⅙ of 8″ cake	483	38.8
CHEESE CAKE MIX:			
*(Jell-O)	⅙ of cake including crust (4.4 oz.)	349	44.2
*(Royal) *No-Bake*	⅛ of 9″ cake (including crust)	264	31.4
CHEESE DIP (See **DIP**)			
CHEESE FONDUE, home recipe (USDA)	4 oz.	301	11.3
CHEESE FOOD, process:			
American:			
(USDA)	1 oz.	92	2.0
(Borden)	1 oz.	92	2.0
Grated, used in *Kraft Dinner*	1 oz.	129	8.4
Slices (Kraft)	1 oz.	94	2.1
(Foremost Blue Moon)	1 oz.	87	1.5
With bacon (Kraft)	1 oz.	101	.7
Blue, cold pack (Kraft)	1 oz.	89	2.2
Cheddar, cold pack (Kraft)	1 oz.	90	2.4
Links:			
Bacon, garlic or jalapeño (Kraft)	1 oz.	93	2.2
Nippy (Kraft)	1 oz.	93	2.2
Smokelle (Kraft)	1 oz.	93	2.2
Swiss (Kraft)	1 oz.	91	1.4
Loaf:			
Munst-ett (Kraft)	1 oz.	101	1.7
Pimento *Velveeta* (Kraft)	1 oz.	90	2.5
Pizzalone (Kraft)	1 oz.	90	.5
Sharp (Kraft)	1 oz.	97	1.1

(USDA): United States Department of Agriculture
DNA: Data Not Available
*Prepared as Package Directs

Food and Description	Measure or Quantity	Calories	Carbo-hydrates (grams)
Super blend (Kraft)	1 oz.	92	1.6
Super blend with caraway (Kraft)	1 oz.	94	1.6
Velveeta, California only (Kraft)	1 oz.	90	2.5
CHEESE PIE (Tastykake)	4-oz. pie	357	51.2
CHEESE PUFF, hors d'oeuvres, frozen (Durkee)	1 piece (.5 oz.)	74	2.9
CHEESE SAUCE CASSEROLE BASE (Pennsylvania Dutch)	6¾-oz. pkg. (3 cups cooked)	877	107.8
CHEESE SOUFFLE:			
Home recipe (USDA)	4 oz.	247	7.0
Frozen (Stouffer's)	12-oz. pkg.	730	35.0
CHEESE SPREAD:			
American:			
Process (USDA)	1 oz.	82	2.3
Process (Borden)	1 oz.	82	2.3
Process, (Kraft) *Swankyswig*	1 oz.	77	1.7
(Nabisco) *Snack Mate*	1 oz.	83	2.2
(Nabisco) *Snack Mate*	1 tsp.	15	.4
Cheddar (Nabisco) *Snack Mate*	1 tsp.	15	.4
Cheese & bacon (Kraft) *Swankyswig*	1 oz.	92	.6
Cheez Whiz, process (Kraft)	1 oz.	76	1.7
Garlic, process (Kraft) *Swankyswig*	1 oz.	86	2.2
Imitation (Kraft) *Calorie-Wise*	1 oz.	48	3.6
Imitation (Kraft) *Tasty Loaf*	1 oz.	48	3.6
Limburger (Kraft)	1 oz.	70	.3
Neufchâtel:			
Bacon & horseradish (Kraft) *Party Snacks*	1 oz.	74	.7
Chipped beef (Kraft) *Party Snacks*	1 oz.	67	1.2
Chive (Kraft) *Party Snacks*	1 oz.	69	.8
Clam (Kraft) *Party Snacks*	1 oz.	67	.8
Onion soup (Kraft) *Party Snacks*	1 oz.	66	1.6
Pimento (Kraft) *Party Snacks*	1 oz.	67	1.4
Old English (Kraft) *Swankyswig*	1 oz.	97	.6
Onion flavor, French (Nabisco) *Snack Mate*	1 tsp.	15	.4

(USDA): United States Department of Agriculture
DNA: Data Not Available
*Prepared as Package Directs

Food and Description	Measure or Quantity	Calories	Carbo-hydrates (grams)
Phenix or *Phenix Pimento* (Kraft)	1 oz.	80	2.3
Pimento:			
(Sealtest)	1 oz.	77	1.7
(Nabisco) *Snack Mate*	1 tsp.	16	.4
Cheez Whiz (Kraft)	1 oz.	76	1.7
Neufchâtel (Kraft)	1 oz.	67	1.4
Process (Kraft) *Swankyswig*	1 oz.	77	1.7
Velveeta, process (Kraft)	1 oz.	84	2.6
Sharpie, process (Kraft)	1 oz.	90	.5
Smokelle Swankyswig, process			
(Kraft)	1 oz.	90	.5
Velveeta, process (Kraft)	1 oz.	84	2.6
CHEESE STRAW:			
(USDA)	1 oz.	128	9.8
(Durkee)	1 piece (8 grams)	29	1.2
CHELOIS WINE (Great Western)			
12% alcohol	3 fl. oz.	78	2.2
CHENIN BLANC WINE (Louis			
M. Martini) dry, 12½% alcohol	3 fl. oz.	90	.2
CHERIMOYA, raw (USDA):			
Whole	1 lb. (weighed with skin & seeds)	247	63.1
Flesh only	4 oz.	107	27.2
CHERI SUISSE, Swiss liqueur			
(Leroux) 60 proof	1 fl. oz.	90	10.2
CHERRY:			
Sour:			
Fresh (USDA):			
Whole	1 lb. (weighed with stems)	213	52.5
Whole	½ cup (2 oz.)	33	8.2
Pitted	½ cup (2.8 oz.)	45	11.0
Canned, syrup pack, pitted (USDA):			
Light syrup	4 oz. (with liq.)	84	21.2
Heavy syrup	½ cup (with liq.)	116	29.5
Heavy syrup	4 oz. (with liq.)	101	26.0
Extra heavy syrup	4 oz. (with liq.)	127	32.4

(USDA): United States Department of Agriculture
DNA: Data Not Available
*Prepared as Package Directs

Food and Description	Measure or Quantity	Calories	Carbo-hydrates (grams)
Canned, water pack, pitted:			
(USDA)	4 oz. (with liq.)	49	12.2
(USDA)	½ cup (3.8 oz.)	46	11.5
(Musselman's)	4 oz.	55	D.N.A.
(Stokely-Van Camp)	½ cup	49	12.2
Frozen, pitted (USDA):			
Sweetened	½ cup (4.6 oz.)	146	36.1
Unsweetened	4 oz.	62	15.2
Sweet:			
Fresh (USDA):			
Whole	1 lb. (weighed with stems)	286	71.0
Whole	½ cup (2.8 oz.)	50	12.4
Pitted	½ cup (2.8 oz.)	57	14.3
Canned, syrup pack, pitted (USDA):			
Light syrup	4 oz. (with liq.)	74	18.7
Heavy syrup	4 oz. (with liq.)	92	23.2
Heavy syrup	½ cup (with liq.)	96	24.2
Extra heavy syrup	4 oz. (with liq.)	114	29.0
Canned, water or dietetic pack, pitted:			
Solids & liq. (USDA)	4 oz.	55	13.5
Solids & liq. (Blue Boy)	4 oz.	52	10.4
Dark, Bing (Yes Madame)	½ cup	63	11.3
Royal Anne:			
Solids & liq., heavy syrup (USDA)	½ cup (4.6 oz.)	105	26.7
Solids & liq. (Diet Delight)	½ cup (4.3 oz.)	58	11.3
Unsweetened (S and W) Nutradiet	14 whole cherries (3.5 oz.)	47	10.6
(White Rose)	4 oz.	64	15.0
(Yes Madame)	½ cup	61	14.0
Frozen, with syrup, quick thaw (Birds Eye)	½ cup (5 oz.)	170	42.6
CHERRY ALMOND CAKE (Van de Kamp's)	1 cake	1227	D.N.A.
CHERRY, BLACK, SOFT DRINK:			
Sweetened:			
(Canada Dry)	6 fl. oz.	93	24.2
(Dr. Brown's)	6 fl. oz.	81	20.2

Food and Description	Measure or Quantity	Calories	Carbo-hydrates (grams)
(Hoffman)	6 fl. oz.	90	22.5
(Key Food)	6 fl. oz.	81	20.2
(Kirsch)	6 fl. oz.	88	22.1
(Shasta)	6 fl. oz.	88	22.2
(Waldbaum)	6 fl. oz.	81	20.2
Unsweetened or low calorie:			
(Dr. Brown's) *Slim-Ray*	6 fl. oz.	3	.8
(Hoffman)	6 fl. oz.	3	.8
(No-Cal)	6 fl. oz.	2	0.
(Shasta)	6 fl. oz.	<1	<.1
CHERRY CAKE MIX:			
*(Duncan Hines)	1 cake	2222	384.0
Chip (Betty Crocker)	1-lb. 3.5-oz. pkg.	1814	348.8
CHERRY, CANDIED:			
(USDA)	1 oz.	96	24.6
(Liberty)	1 oz.	93	22.6
CHERRY DRINK:			
(Hi-C)	6 fl. oz.	92	22.7
*(Wyler's)	6 fl. oz.	63	15.8
Cherry-apple (BC)	6 fl. oz.	102	D.N.A.
CHERRY EXTRACT, imitation			
(Ehlers)	1 tsp.	8	D.N.A.
CHERRY FRUIT ROLL, frozen			
(Chun King)	1 oz.	64	10.4
CHERRY FRUIT SPREAD (Vita):			
With brandy wine flavor	1 T.	9	D.N.A.
With papaya	1 T.	9	D.N.A.
CHERRY HEERING, Danish liqueur, 49 proof	1 fl. oz.	80	10.0
CHERRY JELLY (Slenderella)	1 T.	24	6.0
CHERRY KARISE, liqueur (Leroux) 49 proof	1 fl. oz.	71	7.6
CHERRY KIJAFA, Danish wine, 17.5% alcohol	3 fl. oz.	148	15.3

(USDA): United States Department of Agriculture
DNA: Data Not Available
*Prepared as Package Directs

Food and Description	Measure or Quantity	Calories	Carbo-hydrates (grams)
CHERRY LIQUEUR:			
(Bols) 60 proof	1 fl. oz.	96	8.9
(Hiram Walker) 60 proof	1 fl. oz.	82	8.0
(Leroux) 60 proof	1 fl. oz.	80	7.6
CHERRY, MARASCHINO:			
(USDA)	1 oz. (with liq.)	33	8.3
(Liberty)	1 average cherry	8	1.9
CHERRY PIE:			
Home recipe (USDA)	⅙ of 9″ pie (5.6 oz.)	412	60.7
Cherry-apple (Tastykake)	4-oz. pie	373	56.8
Frozen:			
Unbaked (USDA)	5 oz.	364	55.4
Baked (USDA)	5 oz.	413	63.0
(Banquet)	5 oz.	352	50.2
(Morton)	⅙ of 20-oz. pie	258	37.0
(Mrs. Smith's)	⅙ of 8″ pie	274	35.4
CHERRY PIE FILLING:			
(Lucky Leaf)	8 oz.	242	58.2
(Musselman's)	1 cup	400	D.N.A.
***CHERRY-PLUM DANISH DESSERT** (Junket)	½ cup	138	33.8
CHERRY PRESERVE, dietetic, morello or cherry-pineapple (Dia-Mel)	1 T.	22	5.4
CHERRY SOFT DRINK, sweetened:			
(Canada Dry)	6 fl. oz.	85	22.2
Fanta	6 fl. oz.	87	21.0
(Hires)	6 fl. oz.	81	20.2
(Nedick's)	6 fl. oz.	81	20.2
(White Rock)	6 fl. oz.	90	D.N.A.
(Yoo-Hoo)	6 fl. oz.	90	18.0
High-protein (Yoo-Hoo)	6 fl. oz.	114	24.6
(Yukon Club)	6 fl. oz.	87	21.8
CHERRY SYRUP, dietetic:			
(Dia-Mel)	1 T.	22	5.5
(No-Cal) black	1 tsp.	<1	Tr.

(USDA): United States Department of Agriculture
DNA: Data Not Available
*Prepared as Package Directs

Food and Description	Measure or Quantity	Calories	Carbohydrates (grams)
CHERRY TURNOVER, frozen (Pepperidge Farm)	1 piece	280	D.N.A.
CHERRY WINE (Mogen David) 12% alcohol	3 fl. oz.	126	16.9
CHERVIL, raw (USDA)	1 oz.	16	3.3
CHESTNUT (USDA):			
Fresh, in shell	1 lb. (weighed in shell)	713	154.7
Fresh, shelled	4 oz.	220	47.8
Dried, in shell	1 lb. (weighed in shell)	1402	292.4
Dried, shelled	4 oz.	428	89.1
CHESTNUT FLOUR (See **FLOUR, CHESTNUT**)			
CHEWING GUM:			
Sweetened:			
(USDA)	1 stick (3 grams)	10	3.0
Bazooka, bubble, 1¢ size	1 piece	18	4.5
Bazooka, bubble, 5¢ size	1 piece	85	21.2
Beechies	1 tablet	6	1.6
Beech-Nut	1 stick	10	2.5
Beemans	1 stick	9	2.3
Black Jack	1 stick	9	2.3
Chiclets	1 piece	6	1.1
Chiclets, tiny size	5¢ pkg.	65	D.N.A.
Cinnamint	1 stick	10	2.3
Clove	1 stick	9	2.3
Dentyne	1 piece	4	1.2
Doublemint	1 stick	8	2.3
Fruit Punch	1 stick	10	2.3
Juicy Fruit	1 stick	9	2.4
Peppermint (Clark)	1 stick	10	2.3
Sour (Warner-Lambert)	1 piece	10	D.N.A.
Sour lemon (Clark)	1 stick	10	2.3
Spearmint (Wrigley's)	1 stick	8	2.2
Teaberry	1 stick	10	2.3
Unsweetened or dietetic:			
All flavors (Clark)	1 stick	7	1.7
All flavors (Estee)	1 stick	6	1.6

Food and Description	Measure or Quantity	Calories	Carbo-hydrates (grams)
Bazooka, bubble, sugarless	1 piece	16	Tr.
Bubble (Estee)	1 piece	4	0.
(Harvey's)	1 stick	4	1.0
Peppermint (Amurol)	1 stick	5	1.8

CHIANTI WINE:
(Antinori):

Classico, 12½% alcohol	3 fl. oz.	87	6.3
1955, 12½% alcohol	3 fl. oz.	87	6.3
Vintage, 12½% alcohol	3 fl. oz.	87	6.3
Brolio Classico, 13% alcohol	3 fl. oz.	66	.3
(Gancia) Classico, 12½% alcohol	3 fl. oz.	75	D.N.A.
(Italian Swiss Colony):			
Gold Medal, 12.1% alcohol	3 fl. oz.	65	1.4
Private Stock, Tipo, 12% alcohol	3 fl. oz.	59	<.1
(Louis M. Martini) 12½% alcohol	3 fl. oz.	90	.2

CHICKEN (See also **CHICKEN, CANNED**) (USDA):

Broiler, cooked, meat only	4 oz.	154	0.
Capon, raw	1 lb. (weighed ready-to-cook)	937	0.
Fryer:			
Raw:			
Ready-to-cook	1 lb. (weighed ready-to-cook)	382	0.
Breast	1 lb. (weighed with bone)	394	0.
Drumstick	1 lb. (weighed with bone)	313	0.
Thigh	1 lb. (weighed with bone)	435	0.
Fried. A 2½-pound chicken (weighed before cooking with bone) will give you:			
Back	1 back (2⅕ oz.)	139	2.7
Breast	½ breast (3⅓ oz.)	154	1.1
Leg or drumstick	1 leg (2 oz.)	87	.4
Neck	1 neck (2.1 oz.)	121	1.9
Rib	1 rib (¾ oz.)	42	.8
Thigh	1 thigh (2¼ oz.)	118	1.2
Wing	1 wing (1¾ oz.)	78	.8
Fried skin	1 oz.	119	2.6

(USDA): United States Department of Agriculture
DNA: Data Not Available
*Prepared as Package Directs

Food and Description	Measure or Quantity	Calories	Carbohydrates (grams)
Hen and cock:			
Raw	1 lb. (weighed ready-to-cook)	987	0.
Stewed:			
Meat only	4 oz.	236	0.
Chopped	½ cup (2.5 oz.)	150	0.
Diced	½ cup (2.4 oz.)	139	0.
Ground	½ cup (2.3 oz.)	137	0.
Roaster:			
Raw	1 lb. (weighed ready-to-cook)	791	0.
Roasted:			
Dark meat without skin	4 oz.	209	0.
Light meat without skin	4 oz.	206	0.
CHICKEN A LA KING:			
Home recipe (USDA)	4 oz.	217	5.7
Canned (College Inn)	4 oz.	107	2.7
Canned (Richardson & Robbins)	½ cup	166	3.0
Frozen (Banquet) cookin' bag	5 oz.	140	9.0
CHICKEN BARONET (Lipton)	1 pkg.	634	90.6
CHICKEN BOUILLON/BROTH, cube or powder (See also **CHICKEN SOUP**):			
(Croyden House)	1 tsp.	12	2.5
(Herb-Ox)	1 cube	6	.6
(Herb-Ox)	1 packet	14	1.0
(Knorr Swiss)	1 cube	13	D.N.A.
(Knorr Swiss)	1 tsp.	11	D.N.A.
(Maggi)	1 cube or 1 tsp.	8	1.1
(Wyler's)	1 cube or 1 tsp.	6	.8
CHICKEN CACCIATORE			
(Hormel)	1-lb. can	386	8.2
CHICKEN, CANNED:			
Boned:			
(USDA)	4 oz.	225	0.
(USDA)	½ cup	200	0.
(College Inn)	4 oz.	299	0.
(Lynden)	5-oz. jar	450	0.
(Richardson & Robbins)	4 oz.	239	.9
Whole (College Inn)	4 oz.	342	0.

(USDA): United States Department of Agriculture
DNA: Data Not Available
*Prepared as Package Directs

Food and Description	Measure or Quantity	Calories	Carbo-hydrates (grams)
CHICKEN, CREAMED, frozen			
(Stouffer's)	11½-oz. pkg.	613	16.2
CHICKEN DINNER:			
Canned:			
Dumpling (Morton House)	12¾-oz. can	545	D.N.A.
Dumpling (Sweet Sue)	24-oz. can	940	D.N.A.
Noodle (Heinz)	8-oz. can	172	15.9
Frozen:			
Cantonese (Chun King)	11-oz. dinner	302	D.N.A.
Chicken & dumplings:			
Buffet (Banquet)	2-lb. pkg.	1306	110.8
(Tom Thumb)	3-lb. 8-oz. tray	1920	112.6
Fried:			
With mashed potato, carrots, peas, corn & beans (USDA)	12 oz.	588	38.4
(Banquet)	11-oz. dinner	542	48.2
(Morton)	11-oz. dinner	435	22.0
(Swanson)	12-oz. dinner	600	46.6
(Swanson) 3-course	16-oz. dinner	652	90.8
CHICKEN & DUMPLINGS (See **CHICKEN DINNER**)			
CHICKEN FRICASSEE:			
Home recipe (USDA)	4 oz.	183	3.6
Canned (College Inn)	4 oz.	108	3.0
Canned (Richardson & Robbins)	½ cup	114	2.6
CHICKEN, FRIED, frozen			
(Swanson)	8.5-oz. pkg.	483	37.8
CHICKEN, GIZZARD (USDA):			
Raw	4 oz.	128	.8
Simmered	4 oz.	168	.8
CHICKEN LIVER (See **LIVER**)			
CHICKEN LIVER, CHOPPED			
(Mrs. Kornberg's)	1 oz.	43	D.N.A.
CHICKEN LIVER PUFF, hors d'oeuvres, frozen (Durkee)	1 piece (.5 oz.)	64	3.1

(USDA): United States Department of Agriculture
DNA: Data Not Available
*Prepared as Package Directs

Food and Description	Measure or Quantity	Calories	Carbohydrates (grams)
CHICKEN & NOODLES:			
Home recipe (USDA)	8 oz.	348	24.2
Frozen, escalloped (Stouffer's)	11½-oz. pkg.	589	35.9
Frozen (Swanson)	8-oz. pkg.	285	17.3
CHICKEN PIE:			
Baked, home recipe (USDA)	8 oz.	532	41.6
Frozen:			
Commercial, unheated (USDA)	8 oz.	496	50.4
(Banquet)	8 oz.	412	37.8
(Morton)	8¼ oz.	460	37.2
(Stouffer's)	10-oz. pie	722	44.2
(Swanson)	8-oz. pie	503	52.9
(Van de Kamp's)	10½-oz. pie	601	D.N.A.
CHICKEN PUFF, hors d'oeuvres, frozen (Durkee)	1 piece (.5 oz.)	42	3.0
CHICKEN RAVIOLI (Lyden)	14½-oz. can	364	53.0
CHICKEN & RICE with VEGETABLES (Morton House)	12¾-oz. can	690	D.N.A.
CHICKEN SOUP, canned:			
*Barley (Manischewitz)	8 oz. (by wt.)	83	12.4
Broth:			
(Campbell)	8 oz. (by wt.)	82	2.7
*Diet, condensed (Claybourne)	1 cup	9	0.
(College Inn)	8 oz.	32	.1
Low calorie (College Inn)	8 oz.	9	.1
(Richardson & Robbins)	1 cup	17	.2
With noodles (College Inn)	8 oz.	20	2.2
With rice (College Inn)	8 oz.	44	7.7
With rice (Richardson & Robbins)	1 cup	45	1.4
Consommé:			
Condensed (USDA)	8 oz. (by wt.)	41	3.4
*Prepared with equal volume water (USDA)	1 cup	22	1.9
Cream of:			
Condensed (USDA)	8 oz. (by wt.)	179	15.2
*Prepared with equal volume milk (USDA)	1 cup (8.4 oz.)	175	14.2

(USDA): United States Department of Agriculture
DNA: Data Not Available
*Prepared as Package Directs

Food and Description	Measure or Quantity	Calories	Carbo-hydrates (grams)
*Prepared with equal volume water (USDA)	1 cup (8.4 oz.)	94	7.9
Condensed (Campbell)	8 oz. (by wt.)	172	14.3
*(Heinz)	1 cup	101	9.2
(Heinz) *Great American*	1 cup	102	8.4
& Dumplings, condensed (Campbell)	8 oz. (by wt.)	188	9.5
Egg drop, frozen (Temple)	8 oz.	49	D.N.A.
Gumbo:			
Condensed (USDA)	8 oz. (by wt.)	104	13.8
*Prepared with equal volume water (USDA)	1 cup (8.8 oz.)	55	7.4
Condensed (Campbell)	8 oz. (by wt.)	111	17.0
& Noodle:			
Condensed (USDA)	8 oz. (by wt.)	120	15.0
*Prepared with equal volume water (USDA)	1 cup (8.8 oz.)	65	8.2
Condensed (Campbell)	8 oz. (by wt.)	123	16.3
Noodle-O's (Campbell)	8 oz. (by wt.)	134	17.9
*(Heinz)	1 cup	68	7.9
*(Manischewitz)	8 oz. (by wt.)	46	4.2
(Tillie Lewis) dietetic	1 cup	54	4.5
With dumplings (Heinz) *Great American*	1 cup (by wt.)	84	8.4
With stars, condensed (Campbell)	8 oz. (by wt.)	113	13.8
*With stars (Heinz)	1 cup	67	7.6
& Rice:			
Condensed (USDA)	8 oz. (by wt.)	89	10.7
*Prepared with equal volume water (USDA)	1 cup (8.8 oz.)	50	6.0
Condensed (Campbell)	8 oz. (by wt.)	98	11.1
*(Heinz)	1 cup	58	6.9
*(Manischewitz)	8 oz. (by wt.)	48	5.4
With mushrooms (Heinz), *Great American*	1 cup	91	10.9
Vegetable:			
Condensed (USDA)	8 oz. (by wt.)	141	17.5
*Prepared with equal volume water (USDA)	1 cup (8.8 oz.)	79	9.9
Condensed (Campbell)	8 oz. (by wt.)	136	17.2
*(Manischewitz)	8 oz. (by wt.)	55	7.7
*(Heinz)	1 cup	77	10.1
*With Kasha (Manischewitz)	8 oz. (by wt.)	41	5.4

(USDA): United States Department of Agriculture
DNA: Data Not Available
*Prepared as Package Directs

Food and Description	Measure or Quantity	Calories	Carbohydrates (grams)
CHICKEN SOUP MIX:			
& Noodle:			
(USDA)	1 oz.	109	16.5
*(USDA)	1 cup (8.1 oz.)	50	7.4
*(Golden Grain)	1 cup	58	8.8
(Lipton)	1 pkg. (2 oz.)	217	29.2
With diced chicken (Lipton)	1 pkg. (1.75 oz.)	206	26.8
*(Wyler's)	6 fl. oz.	33	4.0
& Rice:			
(USDA)	1 oz.	100	17.8
*(USDA)	1 cup (8 oz.)	46	8.0
(Lipton)	1 pkg. (1.5 oz.)	186	23.8
*Rice-A-Roni	1 cup	63	10.9
*(Wyler's)	6 fl. oz.	37	6.0
Vegetable (Lipton)	1 pkg. (2 oz.)	210	29.8
*Vegetable (Wyler's)	6 fl. oz.	28	4.0
CHICKEN SPREAD (Underwood)	1 T.	31	3.3
CHICKEN STEW:			
Canned:			
(B&M)	1 cup (8.8 oz.)	168	14.2
(Bounty)	8 oz. (by wt.)	186	15.4
With dumplings (Heinz)	8-oz. can	188	17.0
Frozen, in white wine cream sauce			
(Swanson)	6-oz. pkg.	243	3.7
CHICK-PEAS or GARBANZOS (USDA):			
Dry	1 lb.	1633	276.7
Dry	1 cup (7 oz.)	720	122.0
CHICORY GREENS, raw (USDA):			
Untrimmed	½ lb. (weighed untrimmed)	37	7.1
Trimmed	4 oz.	23	2.0
CHICORY, WITLOOF, Belgian or French endive, raw, bleached head (USDA):			
Untrimmed	½ lb. (weighed untrimmed)	31	6.5
Trimmed, cut	½ cup (.9 oz.)	4	.8

Food and Description	Measure or Quantity	Calories	Carbo-hydrates (grams)
CHILI or CHILI CON CARNE:			
Canned, beans only, Western-style sauce (Morton House)	15-oz. can	545	D.N.A.
Canned, with beans:			
(USDA)	1 cup (8.8 oz.)	332	30.5
(Armour Star)	15½-oz. can	682	59.3
(Austex)	15½-oz. can (1¾ cups)	584	53.6
(Bounty)	8 oz.	270	21.8
(Chef Boy-Ar-Dee)	7½ oz. (¼ of 30-oz. can)	259	24.1
(College Inn)	8 oz.	465	18.6
(Heinz)	8-oz. can	286	23.8
(Hormel)	2-lb. 8-oz. can	1400	106.6
(Hormel)	1-lb. 8-oz. can	811	44.2
(Hormel)	15-oz. can	626	41.6
(Hormel)	8-oz. can	274	17.5
(Morton House)	15-oz. can	925	D.N.A.
(Rosarita)	8 oz.	376	27.2
(Rutherford)	8 oz.	379	D.N.A.
(Silver Skillet)	8 oz.	334	19.6
(Stokely-Van Camp)	1 cup	332	30.5
(Wilson)	5 oz.	204	13.7
Canned, without beans:			
(USDA)	1 cup (9 oz.)	510	14.8
(Armour Star)	15½-oz. can	837	25.5
(Austex)	15-oz. can (1¾ cups)	851	24.7
(Bunker Hill)	10¼-oz. can	657	D.N.A.
(Chef Boy-Ar-Dee)	7⅝ oz. (½ of 15¼-oz. can)	331	14.0
(Hormel)	15-oz. can	770	15.7
(Morton House)	15-oz. can	1065	D.N.A.
(Nalley's)	8 oz.	352	12.8
(Rutherford)	6 oz.	335	D.N.A.
(Stokely-Van Camp)	1 cup	510	14.8
(Wilson)	8 oz.	434	13.1
Frozen, with beans:			
Cookin' bag (Banquet)	8 oz.	310	21.5
Dinner (Swanson)	11¼-oz. dinner	459	58.6
CHILI BEEF SOUP:			
Condensed (Campbell)	8 oz. (by wt.)	297	41.5
*(Heinz)	1 cup	174	19.8

(USDA): United States Department of Agriculture
DNA: Data Not Available
*Prepared as Package Directs

Food and Description	Measure or Quantity	Calories	Carbo-hydrates (grams)
(Heinz) *Great American*	1 cup	163	20.1
CHILI CON CARNE MIX:			
With added seasonings (USDA)	1 oz.	96	16.0
With added seasonings (USDA)	1 T.	50	8.0
*With meat and beans (Durkee)	2½ cups (2¼-oz. dry pkg.)	800	80.0
*Without meat and beans (Durkee)	1¼ cups (2¼-oz. dry pkg.)	160	35.0
(Chili Products)	1 oz.	94	15.6
(Mexene)	1 oz.	97	16.1
CHILI DOG SAUCE MIX			
(McCormick)	1 oz.	21	4.5
CHILI SAUCE:			
(USDA)	1 T.	16	3.8
(Heinz)	1 T.	20	4.6
(Hunt's)	1 oz.	29	7.0
CHILI SEASONING MIX:			
Chili-O (French's)	1¾-oz. pkg.	125	24.0
(Lawry's)	1.6-oz. pkg.	137	23.6
(Wyler's)	1⅝-oz. pkg.	D.N.A.	22.0
CHINESE DATE (See **JUJUBE**)			
CHINESE DINNER, frozen			
(Swanson)	11-oz. dinner	356	40.9
CHIPS (See **CRACKERS** for corn chips and **POTATO CHIPS**)			
CHITTERLINGS, canned (Hormel)	1-lb. 2-oz. can	832	.5
CHIVES, raw (USDA)	½ lb.	64	13.1
CHOCO FIZZ (Dia-Mel)	1 tsp.	7	.7
CHOCOLATE, BAKING:			
Bitter or unsweetened:			
(USDA)	1 oz.	143	8.2
(Baker's)	1 oz. (1 sq.)	136	7.7

(USDA): United States Department of Agriculture
DNA: Data Not Available
*Prepared as Package Directs

Food and Description	Measure or Quantity	Calories	Carbo-hydrates (grams)
Pre-melted, *Choco-Bake*	1-oz. packet	172	10.2
(Hershey's)	1 oz.	169	6.6
Sweetened:			
German's sweet (Baker's)	1 oz. (4½ sq.)	144	15.6
Semisweet (Baker's)	1 oz. (1 sq.)	133	18.1
Chips, semisweet (Baker's)	1 oz. (⅙ cup)	133	18.1
Chips, semisweet (Ghirardelli)	⅓ cup	299	35.6
Chips, milk (Hershey's)	1 oz.	152	15.9
Chips, semisweet (Hershey's)	1 oz.	145	17.2
Morsels, milk (Nestlé's)	1 oz.	143	17.2
Morsels, semisweet (Nestlé's)	1 oz.	137	18.1
Morsels, semisweet mint (Nestlé's)	1 oz.	136	18.0
CHOCOLATE CAKE:			
Home recipe (USDA):			
Without icing	2 oz.	208	29.5
With chocolate icing	⅟₁₆ of 10″ cake	443	67.0
With uncooked, white icing	⅟₁₆ of 10″ cake	443	71.0
Almond (Van de Kamp's)	2 layer cake	3377	D.N.A.
Frozen (Pepperidge Farm)	1″ x 3″ piece	175	D.N.A.
Fudge layer, frozen (Pepperidge Farm)	1″ x 3″ piece	174	D.N.A.
Milk (Van de Kamp's)	2 layer cake	2825	D.N.A.
Pecan (Van de Kamp's)	2 layer cake	3366	D.N.A.
CHOCOLATE CAKE MIX (See also **FUDGE CAKE MIX**):			
Chocolate pudding (Betty Crocker)	11-oz. pkg.	1254	265.1
Chocolate loaf (Pillsbury)	1 oz.	120	21.8
Chocolate malt (USDA)	1 oz.	116	22.4
Chocolate malt (Betty Crocker)	1-lb. 2.5-oz. pkg.	2183	418.1
*Chocolate malt, uncooked white icing (USDA)	4 oz.	392	75.5
*Deep chocolate (Duncan Hines)	1 cake	2334	384.0
*Deep chocolate (Duncan Hines)	⅟₁₂ of cake (2.5 oz.)	194	32.0
German chocolate (Pillsbury)	1 oz.	121	22.0
*German chocolate (Swans Down)	⅟₁₂ of cake	187	35.8
German chocolate (Betty Crocker)	1-lb. 2.5-oz. pkg.	2183	418.1
Milk chocolate (Betty Crocker)	1-lb. 2.5-oz. pkg.	2164	408.8
*Swiss chocolate (Duncan Hines)	1 cake	2374	384.0
*Swiss chocolate (Duncan Hines)	⅟₁₂ of cake (2.5 oz.)	194	32.0
CHOCOLATE CANDY (See **CANDY**)			

(USDA): United States Department of Agriculture
DNA: Data Not Available
*Prepared as Package Directs

Food and Description	Measure or Quantity	Calories	Carbo-hydrates (grams)
CHOCOLATE DRINK (Borden):			
Dutch	1 qt.	724	106.8
Dutch, canned	9½-oz. can	232	32.1
CHOCOLATE DRINK MIX:			
Dutch, instant (Borden):			
*With water	6 fl. oz.	87	18.8
*With skim milk	6 fl. oz.	188	27.6
*With whole milk	6 fl. oz.	207	27.4
Hot (USDA)	1 cup (4.9 oz.)	545	102.7
Hot (USDA)	1 oz.	111	21.0
Hot (Hershey's)	1 oz.	116	20.6
Quik (Nestlé's) regular or fudge	2 heaping tsp.	56	14.4
CHOCOLATE, GROUND			
(Ghirardelli)	¼ cup	163	30.4
CHOCOLATE, HOT, home			
recipe (USDA)	1 cup	238	26.0
CHOCOLATE ICE CREAM (See also individual brands):			
(Sealtest)	⅙ qt.	191	23.6
French (Prestige)	⅙ qt.	250	24.1
CHOCOLATE ICE CREAM MIX			
(Junket)	6 serving pkg. (4 oz.)	380	94.4
CHOCOLATE PIE:			
Chiffon, home recipe (USDA)	⅙ of 9″ pie (4.9 oz.)	459	61.2
Meringue, home recipe (USDA)	⅙ of 9″ pie (4.9 oz.)	353	46.9
Nut (Tastykake)	4½-oz. pie	451	64.3
Frozen, cream:			
(Banquet)	2½-oz. serving	202	28.5
(Morton)	¼ of 14.5-oz. pie	290	40.6
(Mrs. Smith's)	⅙ of 8″ pie	214	25.5
CHOCOLATE PIE FILLING:			
*Regular, fudge (Jell-O)	½ cup (5.3 oz.)	179	31.0
*Cream (Jell-O)	⅛ of 8″ pie (including crust)	336	42.4
(My-T-Fine)	1 oz.	123	25.6
Almond (My-T-Fine)	1 oz.	124	25.5
Fudge (My-T-Fine)	1 oz.	122	25.5

(USDA): United States Department of Agriculture
DNA: Data Not Available
*Prepared as Package Directs

Food and Description	Measure or Quantity	Calories	Carbo-hydrates (grams)
*Dutch (Royal) *No-Bake*	⅛ of 9″ pie including crust)	255	31.3
Low calorie (D-Zerta):			
*With whole milk	½ cup (4.5 oz.)	97	9.3
*With nonfat milk	½ cup (4.5 oz.)	58	9.5
CHOCOLATE PUDDING, sweetened:			
Home recipe with starch base, (USDA)	4 oz.	168	29.1
Canned:			
(Betty Crocker)	1-lb. 2-oz. can	684	117.0
Dutch (Bounty)	4 oz.	173	31.8
Fudge (Betty Crocker)	1-lb. 2-oz. can	684	118.8
CHOCOLATE PUDDING MIX:			
Sweetened:			
Regular:			
Dry (USDA)	1 oz.	102	26.0
*Prepared with milk (USDA)	4 oz.	141	25.9
*(Jell-O)	½ cup (5.3 oz.)	179	31.0
(My-T-Fine)	1 oz.	123	25.6
*(Royal)	½ cup (5.1 oz.)	190	30.7
*(Royal) *Dark 'N' Sweet*	½ cup (5.1 oz.)	195	30.7
*(Thank You)	½ cup	175	29.2
Almond (My-T-Fine)	1 oz.	124	25.5
*Fudge (Jell-O)	½ cup (5.3 oz.)	179	31.0
Fudge (My-T-Fine)	1 oz.	122	25.5
*Tapioca (Royal)	½ cup (5.1 oz.)	185	29.2
Instant:			
Dry (USDA)	1 oz.	101	25.7
*Prepared with milk, without cooking (USDA)	4 oz.	142	27.7
*(Jell-O)	½ cup (5.3 oz.)	177	30.5
(My-T-Fine)	1 oz.	107	23.3
*(Royal)	½ cup (5.2 oz.)	200	32.8
*(Royal) *Dark 'N' Sweet*	½ cup (5.2 oz.)	200	32.8
*(Royal) *Shake-A-Pudd'N*	½ cup (6.1 oz.)	200	40.7
*Fudge (Jell-O)	½ cup (5.3 oz.)	177	30.5
*Malt (Royal) *Shake-A-Pudd'N*	½ cup (6.1 oz.)	200	40.7
Nut (My-T-Fine)	1 oz.	110	22.9
Low calorie or dietetic:			
*With nonfat milk (Dia-Mel)	4 oz.	53	8.2
*With whole milk (Dia-Mel)	4 oz.	90	8.1

(USDA): United States Department of Agriculture
DNA: Data Not Available
*Prepared as Package Directs

Food and Description	Measure or Quantity	Calories	Carbo-hydrates (grams)
*With nonfat milk (D-Zerta)	½ cup (4.5 oz.)	66	12.0
*With whole milk (D-Zerta)	½ cup (4.5 oz.)	102	12.0
CHOCOLATE RENNET CUSTARD MIX (Junket):			
Powder:			
Dry	1 oz.	116	25.2
*Prepared with whole milk	4 oz.	113	14.9
Tablet:			
Dry	1 tablet	1	.2
*Prepared with whole milk & sugar	4 oz.	101	13.4
CHOCOLATE SOFT DRINK:			
(Devil Shake)	6 fl. oz.	90	D.N.A.
(Yoo-Hoo)	6 fl. oz.	90	18.0
High protein (Yoo-Hoo)	6 fl. oz.	114	24.6
CHOCOLATE SYRUP:			
Sweetened:			
Fudge (USDA)	1 oz.	94	15.3
Thin type (USDA)	1 oz.	70	17.8
(Cocoa Marsh)	1 T.	50	D.N.A.
(Hershey's)	1 oz.	69	16.5
Low calorie, *Choco Sip* (Dia-Mel)	1 T.	14	3.5
CHOP SUEY:			
Home recipe, with meat (USDA)	4 oz.	136	5.8
Canned:			
With meat (USDA)	4 oz.	70	4.8
Beef (Chun King)	4 oz.	61	D.N.A.
Chicken (Hung's)	¾ cup	90	9.2
Meatless (Hung's)	¾ cup	84	8.2
Vegetable (Hung's)	¾ cup	30	4.6
Frozen, beef (Chun King)	4 oz.	63	D.N.A.
CHOP SUEY VEGETABLES, canned, drained (Chun King)	4 oz.	22	3.2
CHOW CHOW:			
Sour (USDA)	1 oz.	8	1.2
Sweet (USDA)	1 oz.	33	7.7
(Crosse & Blackwell)	1 T.	9	1.0

(USDA): United States Department of Agriculture
DNA: Data Not Available
*Prepared as Package Directs

Food and Description	Measure or Quantity	Calories	Carbo-hydrates (grams)
CHOW MEIN:			
Home recipe, chicken, without noodles (USDA)	4 oz.	116	4.5
Canned:			
Without noodles (USDA)	4 oz.	43	8.1
Chicken:			
(Chun King)	8 oz.	82	12.2
(Hung's)	¾ cup	76	7.6
& noodles (Chun King)	8 oz.	111	D.N.A.
Subgum (Chun King)	8 oz.	78	D.N.A.
Meatless:			
(Chun King)	8 oz.	62	11.8
(Hung's)	¾ cup	72	6.5
& noodles (Chun King)	8 oz.	74	D.N.A.
Frozen:			
Chicken (Chun King)	8 oz.	112	10.6
Chicken (Temple)	11-oz. pkg.	178	D.N.A.
Meatless (Chun King)	8 oz.	94	15.4
Shrimp (Chun King)	8 oz.	88	13.2
Shrimp (Temple)	12-oz. pkg.	199	D.N.A.
CHOW MEIN NOODLES (See **NOODLES, CHOW MEIN**)			
CHUB, raw (USDA):			
Whole	1 lb. (weighed whole)	217	0.
Meat only	4 oz.	165	0.
CHUTNEY, *Major Grey's* (Crosse & Blackwell)	1 T.	53	13.1
CIDER (See **APPLE CIDER**)			
CINNAMON, GROUND (Information supplied by General Mills Laboratory)	1 oz.	114	25.1
CINNAMON STICKS, frozen (Aunt Jemima)	3 pieces (1.8 oz.)	148	22.0
CITRON, CANDIED:			
(USDA)	1 oz.	89	22.7
(Liberty)	1 oz.	93	22.6

(USDA): United States Department of Agriculture
DNA: Data Not Available
*Prepared as Package Directs

Food and Description	Measure or Quantity	Calories	Carbo-hydrates (grams)
CITRUS COOLER (Hi-C)	6 fl. oz.	92	22.7
CITRUS SALAD, canned (See **GRAPEFRUIT & ORANGE SECTIONS**)			
CITRUS SOFT DRINK, low calorie (No-Cal)	6 fl. oz.	2	0.
CLACKERS, cereal (General Mills)	1 cup (1 oz.)	111	22.1
CLAM:			
Raw, meat only (USDA)	4 med. clams	65	1.7
Raw, hard or round, meat & liq. (USDA)	1 lb. (weighed in shell)	71	6.1
Raw, soft, meat & liq. (USDA)	1 lb. (weighed in shell)	142	5.3
Raw, soft, meat only (USDA)	4 oz.	93	1.5
Canned:			
Solids & liq. (USDA)	4 oz.	59	3.2
Solids & liq. (USDA)	3 med. clams (3 oz.)	45	2.0
Meat only (USDA)	4 oz.	111	2.1
Chopped & minced, solids & liq. (Doxsee)	4 oz.	59	3.2
Chopped, solids & liq. (Doxsee)	4 oz.	66	D.N.A.
Chopped, meat only (Doxsee)	4 oz.	111	2.1
Steamed, meat & broth (Doxsee)	1 pt. 8 fl. oz.	152	D.N.A.
Steamed, meat only (Doxsee)	1 pt. 8 fl. oz.	66	D.N.A.
Whole (Doxsee)	4 oz.	62	D.N.A.
CLAM CHOWDER:			
Manhattan, canned:			
Condensed (USDA)	8 oz. (by wt.)	150	22.7
*Prepared with equal volume water (USDA)	1 cup (9 oz.)	84	12.8
Condensed (Campbell)	8 oz. (by wt.)	143	20.9
(Crosse & Blackwell)	6½ oz. (½ can)	61	12.9
Condensed (Doxsee)	10.5 oz. (by wt.)	155	D.N.A.
*(Doxsee)	1 cup	62	D.N.A.
New England:			
Canned:			
(Crosse & Blackwell)	6½ oz. (½ can)	101	10.3
Condensed (Doxsee)	10.5 oz. (by wt.)	155	D.N.A.

(USDA): United States Department of Agriculture
DNA: Data Not Available
*Prepared as Package Directs

Food and Description	Measure or Quantity	Calories	Carbo-hydrates (grams)
*(Doxsee)	1 cup	139	D.N.A.
Frozen:			
Condensed (USDA)	8 oz. (by wt.)	243	19.5
*Prepared with equal volume water (USDA)	8 oz. (by wt.)	123	10.0
*Prepared with equal volume milk (USDA)	8 oz. (by wt.)	195	15.2
Condensed (Campbell)	8 oz. (by wt.)	245	20.2
CLAM COCKTAIL (Sau-Sea)	4 oz.	80	19.1
CLAM FRITTERS, home recipe (USDA)	4 oz.	353	35.0
CLAM JUICE/LIQUOR, canned:			
(USDA)	1 cup (8.4 oz.)	45	5.0
(Doxsee)	8 oz.	43	D.N.A.
CLAM STEW, frozen (Mrs. Paul's)	8 oz.	244	20.0
CLAM STICKS, frozen (Mrs. Paul's)	4 oz.	286	D.N.A.
CLARET WINE:			
(Gold Seal) 12% alcohol	3 fl. oz.	82	.4
(Italian Swiss Colony-Gold Medal) 12.3% alcohol	3 fl. oz.	63	.7
(Louis M. Martini) 12.5% alcohol	3 fl. oz.	90	.2
(Taylor) 12.5% alcohol	3 fl. oz.	72	D.N.A.
CLARISTINE LIQUEUR (Leroux) 86 proof	1 fl. oz.	114	10.8
CLORETS:			
Chewing gum	1 piece	6	1.3
Mint	1 piece	6	1.6
CLUB SODA SOFT DRINK, any brand:			
Regular	6 fl. oz.	0	0.
Dietetic	6 fl. oz.	0	0.
COCOA, dry:			
Low fat (USDA)	1 T.	10	3.1

(USDA): United States Department of Agriculture
DNA: Data Not Available
*Prepared as Package Directs

Food and Description	Measure or Quantity	Calories	Carbohydrates (grams)
Medium low fat (USDA)	1 T.	12	2.9
Medium high fat (USDA)	1 T.	14	2.8
High fat (USDA)	1 T.	16	2.8
Unsweetened (Droste)	1 T.	21	2.9
(Hershey's)	1 cup	337	11.8
(Hershey's)	1 oz.	111	4.0
(Hershey's)	1 T.	27	2.5
COCOA-CREAM SOFT DRINK:			
(Hoffman)	6 fl. oz.	88	21.9
(Yukon Club)	6 fl. oz.	88	21.9
COCOA, HOME RECIPE (USDA)	1 cup	242	27.2
COCOA KRISPIES, cereal			
(Kellogg's)	1 cup (1 oz.)	113	23.8
COCOA MIX:			
With nonfat dry milk (USDA)	1 oz.	102	20.1
Without milk (USDA)	1 oz.	98	25.3
Sweet milk cocoa (Hershey's)	1 oz.	116	20.6
(Nestlé's) *Ever Ready*	3 heaping tsp.	102	19.2
Instant (Hershey's)	1 oz.	105	25.0
Instant (Swiss Miss)	1 oz.	106	20.4
COCOA PUFFS, cereal			
(General Mills)	1 cup (1 oz.)	107	25.0
COCONUT:			
Fresh (USDA):			
Whole	1 lb. (weighed in shell)	816	22.2
Meat only	4 oz.	392	21.0
Meat only	2″ x 2″ x ½″ piece (1.6 oz.)	161	6.3
Grated	½ cup (1.4 oz.)	138	3.8
Dried, canned:			
Unsweetened (USDA)	4 oz.	751	26.1
Shredded, sweetened (USDA)	½ cup (1.6 oz.)	252	24.5
Angel Flake (Baker's)	½ cup (2 oz.)	270	22.4
Shred & cookie (Baker's)	½ cup (2 oz.)	280	23.2
COCONUT CAKE, frozen			
(Pepperidge Farm)	1″ x 3″ piece	175	D.N.A.

(USDA): United States Department of Agriculture
DNA: Data Not Available
*Prepared as Package Directs

Food and Description	Measure or Quantity	Calories	Carbo-hydrates (grams)
COCONUT CAKE MIX:			
Toasted (Betty Crocker)	1-lb. 3.5-oz. pkg.	2360	436.8
*(Duncan Hines)	1 cake	2367	384.0
COCONUT PIE:			
Cream:			
(Tastykake)	4-oz. pie	467	48.4
Frozen:			
(Banquet)	2½ oz.	209	24.2
(Mrs. Smith's)	⅙ of 8″ pie	204	24.5
Custard:			
Home recipe (USDA)	⅙ of 9″ pie (5.4 oz.)	357	37.8
Frozen:			
Baked, home recipe (USDA)	5 oz.	354	41.9
Unbaked, home recipe (USDA)	5 oz.	291	38.5
(Banquet)	5 oz.	294	39.8
(Mrs. Smith's)	⅙ of 8″ pie	273	31.7
COCONUT PIE FILLING MIX:			
Custard, dry (USDA)	1 oz.	133	20.0
*Custard, prepared with egg yolk & milk (USDA)	4 oz. (including crust)	228	32.7
*Cream (Jell-O)	½ cup (5.3 oz.)	179	31.0
*Cream (Jell-O)	⅛ of 8″ pie (including crust)	345	42.3
COCONUT PUDDING MIX:			
*Cream (Jell-O)	½ cup (5.3 oz.)	179	31.0
*Cream, instant (Jell-O)	½ cup (5.3 oz.)	177	30.5
*Toasted, instant (Royal)	½ cup (5 oz.)	185	28.2
COCONUT SOFT DRINK (Yoo-Hoo):			
Regular	6 fl. oz.	90	18.0
High protein	6 fl. oz.	114	24.6
***COCO WHEATS**, cereal*	2 T.	82	16.8
COD:			
Raw, whole (USDA)	1 lb. (weighed whole)	110	0.
Raw, meat only (USDA)	4 oz.	89	0.
Broiled (USDA)	4 oz.	193	0.

(USDA): United States Department of Agriculture
DNA: Data Not Available
*Prepared as Package Directs

Food and Description	Measure or Quantity	Calories	Carbo-hydrates (grams)
Canned (USDA)	4 oz.	97	0.
Dehydrated, lightly salted (USDA)	4 oz.	425	0.
Dried, salted (USDA)	4 oz.	148	0.
Frozen, fillets (Taste O'Sea)	4 oz.	80	0.
Frozen, Alaska (Van de Kamp's)	1 pkg.	473	0.
COFFEE:			
*Regular (Maxwell House)	1 cup	2	.4
*Regular (Yuban)	1 cup	2	.4
Instant:			
Dry (USDA)	1 oz.	37	Tr.
*(USDA)	1 cup	2	Tr.
*(Chase & Sanborn)	5 fl. oz.	3	<.1
*(Maxwell House)	1 cup	3	.7
Nescafé	1 slightly rounded tsp.	4	.7
*(Yuban)	1 cup	3	.7
Decaffeinated:			
Decaf	1 tsp.	4	.6
Sanka	1 cup	3	.7
Siesta	5 fl. oz.	3	.1
*Freeze-dried:			
Maxim	1 cup	3	.8
Taster's Choice	1 slightly rounded tsp.	4	.7
COFFEE BREAK, cream substitute (Seneca)	1 oz.	20	3.9
COFFEE CAKE:			
(Drake's)	1 small cake pkg.	357	52.8
Almond brittle (Van de Kamp's)	9½-oz. cake	1449	D.N.A.
Almond crispy (Van de Kamp's)	1 piece (3 oz.)	449	D.N.A.
Apple (Van de Kamp's)	9-oz. cake	977	D.N.A.
Bear claw (Van de Kamp's)	1 piece (2.2 oz.)	127	D.N.A.
Butterfly (Van de Kamp's)	1 piece (2.3 oz.)	187	D.N.A.
Butter horn (Van de Kamp's)	1 piece (2.2 oz.)	287	D.N.A.
Cinnamon, 1-lb. loaf (Van de Kamp's)	1 slice (.8 oz.)	85	D.N.A.
Danish cluster (Van de Kamp's)	1 piece (1 oz.)	150	D.N.A.
Danish pastry (USDA)	2 oz.	239	25.9
Dutch ring (Van de Kamp's)	10-oz. cake	1107	D.N.A.
French pecan (Van de Kamp's)	12-oz. cake	1458	D.N.A.

(USDA): United States Department of Agriculture
DNA: Data Not Available
*Prepared as Package Directs

Food and Description	Measure or Quantity	Calories	Carbo-hydrates (grams)
Rosette (Van de Kamp's)	1 piece (2.5 oz.)	349	D.N.A.
Swedish twist (Van de Kamp's)	12-oz. cake	1356	D.N.A.
Walnut swirl (Van de Kamp's)	1 piece (1.5 oz.)	266	D.N.A.

COFFEE CAKE MIX:
Dry (USDA)	4 oz.	489	87.5
*Prepared with egg & milk (USDA)	2 oz.	183	29.7
*(Aunt Jemima)	⅛ of cake (1.8 oz.)	181	30.0

COFFEE FLAVORING, low
calorie (Coffee Time)	1 fl. oz.	<1	.1

COFFEE-MATE, cream substitute
	1 tsp.	11	1.0

COFFEE-RICH, cream substitute
	1 oz.	44	3.5

COFFEE SOFT DRINK, low
calorie (No-Cal)	6 fl. oz.	2	<.1

COFFEE SOUTHERN, liqueur
	1 fl. oz.	85	7.0

COGNAC (See **DISTILLED LIQUOR**)

COLA SOFT DRINK:
Sweetened:
(Canada Dry)	6 fl. oz.	77	19.8
(Clicquot Club)	6 fl. oz.	82	20.5
Coca-Cola	6 fl. oz.	72	18.0
(Cott)	6 fl. oz.	82	20.5
(Dr. Brown's)	6 fl. oz.	81	20.2
(Hoffman)	6 fl. oz.	81	20.2
(Key Food)	6 fl. oz.	81	20.2
(Kirsch)	6 fl. oz.	80	20.1
(Mission)	6 fl. oz.	82	20.5
Mr. Cola	6 fl. oz.	79	20.3
Pepsi-Cola	6 fl. oz.	78	19.5
(Shasta)	6 fl. oz.	76	19.4
(Waldbaum)	6 fl. oz.	81	20.2
(White Rock)	6 fl. oz.	78	D.N.A.
Cherry (Shasta)	6 fl. oz.	76	19.4
Low calorie:			
(Dia-Mel)	6 fl. oz.	1	D.N.A.
Diet Pepsi-Cola	6 fl. oz.	35	8.8

(USDA): United States Department of Agriculture
DNA: Data Not Available
*Prepared as Package Directs

Food and Description	Measure or Quantity	Calories	Carbo-hydrates (grams)
(Dr. Brown's) *Slim-Ray*	6 fl. oz.	3	.8
(Hoffman)	6 fl. oz.	3	.8
(No-Cal)	6 fl. oz.	<1	<.1
(Shasta)	6 fl. oz.	<1	<.1
Cherry (Shasta)	6 fl. oz.	<1	<.1
Tab	6 fl. oz.	1	.1
COLA SYRUP, dietetic (No-Cal)	1 tsp.	<1	Tr.
COLD DUCK WINE, (Italian Swiss Colony-Private Stock) 12% alcohol	3 fl. oz.	75	4.3
COLESLAW, home recipe (USDA):			
Prepared with commercial French dressing	4 oz.	108	8.6
Prepared with homemade French dressing	4 oz.	146	5.8
Prepared with mayonnaise	4 oz.	163	5.4
Prepared with mayonnaise-type salad dressing	4 oz.	112	8.1
Prepared with mayonnaise-type salad dressing	1 cup (4.2 oz.)	118	8.5
COLLARDS:			
Raw (USDA):			
Leaves including stems	1 lb.	181	32.7
Leaves only	½ lb.	70	11.6
Boiled, drained (USDA):			
Leaves, cooked in large amount water	4 oz.	35	5.4
Leaves & stems, cooked in small amount water	4 oz.	33	5.6
Leaves & stems, cooked in small amount of water	1 cup (6.7 oz.)	55	9.0
Frozen:			
(USDA)	1 lb.	145	26.3
Boiled, drained solids (USDA)	½ cup (3 oz.)	26	4.8
Chopped (Birds Eye)	⅓ pkg. (3.3 oz.)	29	4.5
COLLINS MIX (Bar-Tender's)	1 serving (⅝ oz.)	70	17.4
COLLINS MIXER, SOFT DRINK (See **TOM COLLINS SOFT DRINK**)			
CONCENTRATE, cereal (Kellogg's)	⅓ cup (1 oz.)	106	15.5

Food and Description	Measure or Quantity	Calories	Carbo-hydrates (grams)
CONCORD WINE:			
(Gold Seal) 13-14% alcohol	3 fl. oz.	125	9.8
(Mogen David) 12% alcohol	3 fl. oz.	120	16.0
(Mogen David) dry, 12% alcohol	3 fl. oz.	24	1.8
CONSOMME MADRILENE, canned, clear or red (Crosse & Blackwell)	6½ oz. (½ can)	33	2.4
COOK-IN-A-BOWL, cereal (Ralston Purina):			
Apple-cinnamon	1 packet (1.1 oz.)	125	D.N.A.
Whole wheat	1 packet (1 oz.)	112	D.N.A.
COOKIE COMMERCIAL. The following are listed by type or brand name:			
Almond toast, Mandel (Stella D'oro)	1 piece	58	D.N.A.
Angelica Goodies (Stella D'oro)	1 piece	100	14.6
Angel puffs, dietetic (Stella D'oro)	1 piece	17	1.4
Anginetti (Stella D'oro)	1 piece	19	1.6
Animal cracker:			
(USDA)	1 oz.	122	22.7
(Nabisco) *Barnum's*	1 piece (3 grams)	12	2.0
(Sunshine)	1 piece (2 grams)	10	1.8
Anisette sponge (Stella D'oro)	1 piece	50	8.4
Anisette toast (Stella D'oro)	1 piece	34	6.8
Applesauce (Sunshine)	1 piece (7 grams)	33	4.4
Applesauce, iced (Sunshine)	1 piece (¾ oz.)	104	14.1
Apple strudel (Nabisco)	1 piece (.4 oz.)	48	6.8
Assortments:			
(USDA)	1 oz.	136	20.1
(Nabisco) *Famous*	1 piece (.5 oz.)	71	9.1
(Nabisco), *Pride* sandwich	1 piece (.4 oz.)	54	7.3
(Stella D'oro) *Lady Stella Assortment*	1 piece	45	D.N.A.
(Sunshine) *Lady Joan Party Assortment*	1 piece (8 grams)	42	5.9
Bordeaux (Pepperidge Farm)	1 piece (8 grams)	38	5.4
Breakfast Treats (Stella D'oro)	1 piece	99	15.0
Brown edge wafers (Nabisco)	1 piece (6 grams)	28	4.1
Brownie:			
(Tastykake)	1 pkg. (2¼ oz.)	242	34.0

(USDA): United States Department of Agriculture
DNA: Data Not Available
*Prepared as Package Directs

COOKIE (Continued)

Food and Description	Measure or Quantity	Calories	Carbo-hydrates (grams)
Chocolate nut, old fashioned			
(Pepperidge Farm)	1 piece (.4 oz.)	59	6.4
Nut fudge (Nab) *Bake Shop*	1 pkg. (2 oz.)	265	33.6
Peanut butter (Tastykake)	1 pkg. (1¾ oz.)	239	32.0
Pecan fudge (Keebler)	1 pkg. (1⅞ oz.)	245	27.9
Frozen, with nuts & chocolate			
icing (USDA)	1 oz.	119	17.2
Brown sugar (Nabisco) *Family*			
Favorites	1 piece (5 grams)	25	3.0
Brussels (Pepperidge Farm)	1 piece (8 grams)	42	4.7
Butter:			
Thin, rich (USDA)	1 oz.	130	20.1
(Burry's)	1 piece	23	D.N.A.
(Nabisco)	1 piece (8 grams)	37	5.7
(Sunshine)	1 piece (5 grams)	24	3.5
Buttercup (Keebler)	1 piece (5 grams)	24	3.7
Butterscotch Fudgies (Tastykake)	1 pkg. (1¾ oz.)	251	35.0
Capri (Pepperidge Farm)	1 piece (.6 oz.)	70	6.5
Caramel peanut logs (Nabisco)			
Hey Days	1 piece (.8 oz.)	122	13.4
Chocolate & chocolate-covered:			
(USDA)	1 oz.	126	20.3
(Van de Kamp's)	1 piece (.7 oz.)	79	D.N.A.
Kings (Sunshine)	1 piece (1.1 oz.)	135	19.6
Melody (Nabisco)	1 piece (7 grams)	31	5.1
Nuggets (Sunshine)	1 piece (4 grams)	23	3.3
Peanut bars (Nabisco) *Ideal*	1 piece (.6 oz.)	94	10.3
Pin Wheel cakes (Nabisco)	1 piece (1.1 oz.)	139	20.9
Puffs (Sunshine)	1 piece (.5 oz.)	63	10.6
Snaps (Nabisco)	1 piece (4 grams)	18	2.7
Wafers (Nabisco) *Famous*	1 piece (6 grams)	28	4.7
Wafers (Sunshine)	1 piece (3 grams)	13	2.6
Wafers (Sunshine) Ice Box	1 piece (7 grams)	30	4.8
Chocolate chip:			
(USDA)	1 oz.	134	19.8
(Nab)	1.2-oz. pkg. (6 pieces)	176	23.6
(Nabisco)	1 piece (.4 oz.)	51	7.5
(Nabisco) *Chips Ahoy*	1 piece (.4 oz.)	51	7.5
(Nabisco) *Family Favorites*	1 piece (7 grams)	33	4.5
Snaps (Nabisco)	1 piece (5 grams)	21	3.4
Old fashioned (Pepperidge			
Farm)	1 piece (.4 oz.)	54	6.4
(Sunshine)	1 piece (7 grams)	37	4.8

(USDA): United States Department of Agriculture
DNA: Data Not Available
*Prepared as Package Directs

Food and Description	Measure or Quantity	Calories	Carbo-hydrates (grams)
Coconut (Sunshine)	1 piece (.5 oz.)	76	9.9
Choc-O-Chip (Tastykake)	1¾-oz. pkg. (4 pieces)	283	34.8
(Van de Kamp's)	1 piece (.5 oz.)	66	D.N.A.
Cinnamon, old fashioned (Pepperidge Farm)	1 piece (.4 oz.)	59	8.2
Cinnamon wafers (Sunshine)	1 piece (4 grams)	20	3.2
Clover Leaves (Sunshine)	1 piece (5 grams)	25	3.7
Coco Creme (Wise)	1 piece (9 grams)	39	6.5
Coconut:			
Bars (USDA)	1 oz.	140	18.1
Bars (Nabisco)	1 piece (⅓ oz.)	45	6.3
Bars (Sunshine)	1 piece (.4 oz.)	47	7.6
Chocolate chip (Nabisco)	1 piece (.5 oz.)	76	9.0
Chocolate drop (Keebler)	1 piece (.5 oz.)	75	8.5
Coconut Kiss (Tastykake)	1¾-oz. pkg. (4 pieces)	318	33.2
Family Favorites (Nabisco)	1 piece (3 grams)	16	2.2
Como Delight (Stella D'oro)	1 piece	153	18.3
Cowboys and Indians (Nabisco)	1 piece (2 grams)	10	1.8
Creme Wafer Stick (Dutch Twin)	1 piece	36	5.9
Creme Wafer Stick (Nabisco)	1 piece (9 grams)	50	5.9
Crests Cakes (Nabisco)	1 piece (.5 oz.)	54	10.4
Cup Custard (Sunshine)	1 piece (.6 oz.)	79	10.3
Danish Swirls (Nabisco)	1 piece (.4 oz.)	49	7.0
Danish Wedding (Keebler)	1 piece (6 grams)	33	5.0
Date and nut (Sunshine)	1 piece (¾ oz.)	82	14.7
Devil's food cake:			
(Nab)	1¾ oz. (4 pieces)	192	38.2
(Nabisco)	1 piece (.5 oz.)	58	11.4
(Sunshine)	1 piece (.5 oz.)	55	10.9
Dresden (Pepperidge Farm)	1 piece (4 grams)	18	2.5
Dutch Apple (Keebler)	1 piece (6 grams)	34	4.7
Dutch Crunch (Keebler)	1 piece (10 grams)	44	6.7
Dutch Girl (Van de Kamp's)	1 piece (.3 oz.)	53	D.N.A.
Egg Jumbo (Stella D'oro)	1 piece	37	D.N.A.
Fig bar:			
(USDA)	1 oz.	101	21.4
(Keebler)	1 piece (.6 oz.)	71	14.4
(Nab) *Fig Newton*	2½-oz. pkg. (2 pieces)	269	70.1
(Nabisco) *Fig Newton*	1 piece (.6 oz.)	59	10.9
(Sunshine)	1 piece (.4 oz.)	42	8.8
Fortune (Chun King)	1 oz.	125	D.N.A.

(USDA): United States Department of Agriculture
DNA: Data Not Available
*Prepared as Package Directs

Food and Description	Measure or Quantity	Calories	Carbo-hydrates (grams)
Frosted cake (Sunshine)	1 piece (.6 oz.)	68	14.8
Fruit:			
California fruit bar (Stella D'oro)	1 piece	72	11.6
Golden fruit (Sunshine)	1 piece (⅔ oz.)	73	16.2
Iced fruit (Nabisco)	1 piece (.6 oz.)	70	14.0
Fudge:			
Chip, old fashioned (Pepperidge Farm)	1 piece (.4 oz.)	52	7.0
Eton Fudge Stick (Keebler)	1 piece (.4 oz.)	55	6.3
Fudge Stripes (Keebler)	1 piece (.4 oz.)	57	7.5
Fudgetown, chocolate or vanilla base (Burry's)	1 piece	67	D.N.A.
Penguin Fudge (Keebler)	1 piece (.8 oz.)	111	14.0
Gaucho (Burry's)	1 piece	72	D.N.A.
Gingersnap:			
(USDA)	1 oz.	119	22.6
Crumbs (USDA)	1 cup (4 oz.)	483	91.8
Large (Sunshine)	1 piece (7 grams)	32	5.7
Old fashioned (Nabisco)	1 piece (7 grams)	30	5.5
Small (Sunshine)	1 piece (3 grams)	14	2.5
Zu Zu (Nabisco)	1 piece (4 grams)	16	3.1
Graham Cracker (See CRACKER, Graham)			
Hermit bar, frosted (Tastykake)	1 pkg. (2 oz.)	321	60.8
Hydrox (Sunshine)	1 piece (.4 oz.)	46	6.7
Jumble (Drake's)	1 piece	78	11.8
Kreemlined wafers (Sunshine)	1 piece (8 grams)	45	6.2
Ladyfingers (USDA)	1 oz.	102	18.3
Lemon:			
Creme sandwich (Keebler)	1 piece	85	12.0
Jumble rings (Nabisco)	1 piece (.5 oz.)	70	11.3
Nut crunch, old fashioned (Pepperidge Farm)	1 piece (.4 oz.)	58	6.6
Punch (Burry's)	1 piece	62	D.N.A.
Snaps (Nabisco)	1 piece (4 grams)	16	3.1
Lickety Splits, chocolate or vanilla base (Burry's)	1 piece	57	D.N.A.
Lido (Pepperidge Farm)	1 piece (.6 oz.)	90	10.3
Lisbon (Pepperidge Farm)	1 oz.	151	18.1
Macaroon:			
(USDA)	1 oz.	135	18.7
(Sunshine)	1 piece (.6 oz.)	85	12.1
Almond (Tastykake)	2-oz. pkg. (2 pieces)	336	35.1

Food and Description	Measure or Quantity	Calories	Carbo-hydrates (grams)
Butter flavored (Sunshine)	1 piece (8 grams)	39	4.9
Coconut (Nabisco) *Bake Shop*	1 piece (.7 oz.)	87	12.1
Coconut (Sunshine)	1 piece (.7 oz.)	81	12.8
Coconut (Van de Kamp's)	1 piece (.7 oz.)	89	D.N.A.
Sandwich (Nabisco)	1 piece (.5 oz.)	71	9.5
Marshmallow:			
(USDA)	1 oz.	116	20.5
Mallomar (Nabisco)	1 piece (.5 oz.)	60	8.7
Mallo Puff (Sunshine)	1 piece (.6 oz.)	70	13.1
Puffs (Nabisco)	1 piece (.7 oz.)	94	12.7
Sandwich (Nabisco)	1 piece (8 grams)	32	5.7
Twirls (Nabisco)	1 piece (1.1 oz.)	133	21.8
Marble sponge (Stella D'oro)	1 piece	50	D.N.A.
Margherite, chocolate (Stella D'oro)	1 piece	73	10.6
Margherite, white (Stella D'oro)	1 piece	73	10.5
Marquisette (Pepperidge Farm)	1 oz.	149	17.3
Milano (Pepperidge Farm)	1 piece (.4 oz.)	61	7.2
Milco, dandies (Sunshine)	1 piece (.6 oz.)	91	12.3
Milco, sugar wafers (Sunshine)	1 piece (.5 oz.)	80	10.1
Minarets (Nabisco)	1 piece (10 grams)	46	5.6
Minarets cakes (Nab)	1-oz. pkg. (3 pieces)	144	17.9
Mint sandwich, cocoa-covered (Nabisco)	1 piece (.6 oz.)	88	10.6
Molasses (USDA)	1 oz.	120	21.5
Mr. Chips (Burry's), coconut, mint, oatmeal or regular	1 piece	42	D.N.A.
Naples, plain (Pepperidge Farm)	1 oz.	149	18.4
Naples, enriched (Pepperidge Farm)	1 oz.	151	17.6
Nassau (Pepperidge Farm)	1 piece (.6 oz.)	82	9.2
Nut Sundae (Sunshine)	1 piece (.6 oz.)	74	12.0
Oatmeal:			
(Drake's)	1 piece	83	12.5
(Nabisco) *Family Favorites*	1 piece (5 grams)	24	3.8
(Nabisco) home style	1 piece (.5 oz.)	61	9.0
(Sunshine)	1 piece (.4 oz.)	60	8.9
(Van de Kamp's)	1 piece (.6 oz.)	59	D.N.A.
Iced (Keebler)	1 piece (.6 oz.)	82	12.8
Irish, old fashioned (Pepperidge Farm)	1 piece (.4 oz.)	51	7.2
Old fashioned (Keebler)	1 piece (.6 oz.)	79	11.7
Raisin (USDA)	1 oz.	128	20.8
Raisin (Nabisco) *Bake Shop*	1 piece	76	11.4
Raisin bar (Tastykake)	1 pkg. (2¼ oz.)	298	47.6
Raisin, iced (Nabisco)	1 piece (.4 oz.)	57	8.2

(USDA): United States Department of Agriculture
DNA: Data Not Available
*Prepared as Package Directs

Food and Description	Measure or Quantity	Calories	Carbo-hydrates (grams)
Raisin, old fashioned (Pepperidge Farm)	1 piece (.4 oz.)	54	7.3
Old Country Treats (Stella D'oro)	1 piece	55	D.N.A.
Orleans (Pepperidge Farm)	1 piece (6 grams)	30	3.8
Peanut & peanut butter:			
(USDA)	1 oz.	134	19.0
(Sunshine)	1 piece (6 grams)	33	3.8
Bars, cocoa-covered (Nabisco)			
Crowns	1 piece (.6 oz.)	94	10.3
Crunch (Sunshine)	1 piece (.5 oz.)	68	8.1
Creme patties (Nab)	1.8-oz. pkg. (8 pieces)	272	31.0
Creme patties (Nabisco)	1 piece (7 grams)	34	3.9
Creme patties cocoa-covered (Nabisco) fancy	1 piece (.4 oz.)	198	6.4
Creme sticks, cocoa-covered (Nabisco)	1 piece (9 grams)	48	5.8
Patties (Sunshine)	1 piece (6 grams)	30	4.2
Pecan Krunch (Sunshine)	1 piece (.5 oz.)	78	8.4
Pecan Sandies (Keebler)	1 piece (.6 oz.)	85	9.2
Pfefferneuse (Stella D'oro)	1 piece	40	D.N.A.
Pirouettes, vanilla (Pepperidge Farm)	1 piece (7 grams)	38	4.6
Pitter Patter (Keebler)	1 piece (.6 oz.)	84	10.9
Pizzelle (Stella D'oro)	1 piece	56	D.N.A.
Raisin:			
(USDA)	1 oz.	107	22.9
Bar, iced (Keebler)	1 piece (.6 oz.)	81	11.0
Fruit biscuit (Nabisco)	1 piece (.5 oz.)	56	11.8
Rich 'n' Chips (Keebler)	1 piece (.5 oz.)	73	8.9
Sandwich, creme:			
(USDA)	1 oz.	140	19.6
Cameo (Nabisco)	1 piece (.5 oz.)	68	10.5
Chocolate fudge:			
(Keebler)	1 piece	99	13.0
(Nabisco) *Cookie Break*	1 piece (.4 oz.)	52	7.0
(Sunshine)	1 piece (.5 oz.)	74	9.3
Empire (Keebler)	1 piece (.6 oz.)	80	11.3
Lemon (Keebler)	1 piece	85	12.0
Orbit (Sunshine)	1 piece (.4 oz.)	51	7.4
Oreo (Nab)	1.7-oz. pkg. (6 pieces)	239	34.1
Oreo (Nabisco)	1 piece (.4 oz.)	50	7.1

(USDA): United States Department of Agriculture
DNA: Data Not Available
*Prepared as Package Directs

Food and Description	Measure or Quantity	Calories	Carbo-hydrates (grams)
Oreo & Swiss (Nab)	1.7-oz. pkg. (6 pieces)	246	33.4
Oreo & Swiss creme (Nabisco)	1 piece (10 grams)	50	6.8
Social Tea (Nabisco)	1 piece (.4 oz.)	51	7.2
Swiss (Nab)	1.8-oz. pkg. (6 pieces)	260	32.9
Vanilla (Nabisco) *Cookie Break*	1 piece (.4 oz.)	52	7.0
Vanilla, French (Keebler)	1 piece (.6 oz.)	95	13.3
Vienna Finger (Sunshine)	1 piece (.5 oz.)	69	11.1
Scooter Pies (Burry's) any flavor	1 piece	162	D.N.A.
Scooter Puffs (Burry's) any flavor	1 piece	62	D.N.A.
Sesame, Regina (Stella D'oro)	1 piece	48	5.8
Shortbread or shortcake:			
(USDA)	1 oz.	141	18.5
(Nabisco) *Dandy*	1 piece (.4 oz.)	46	7.7
Cherry nut (Van de Kamp's)	1 piece (.4 oz.)	59	D.N.A.
Lorna Doone (Nab)	1.7-oz. pkg. (6 pieces)	242	29.6
Lorna Doone (Nabisco)	1 piece (7 grams)	38	4.4
Pecan (Nabisco)	1 piece (.5 oz.)	77	8.7
Scottie (Sunshine)	1 piece (8 grams)	39	4.9
Striped (Nabisco)	1 piece (10 grams)	50	6.8
Vanilla (Tastykake)	2¼-oz. pkg. (6 pieces)	352	43.8
Sierra Eclairs, (Burry's) any flavor	1 piece	62	D.N.A.
Smack Wafers (Sunshine)	1 piece (2 grams)	10	1.2
Social Tea Biscuit (Nabisco)	1 piece (5 grams)	21	3.6
Spiced wafers (Nabisco)	1 piece (8 grams)	33	6.0
Sprinkles (Sunshine)	1 piece (.6 oz.)	71	13.6
Sugar cookie:			
(Van de Kamp's)	1 piece (.6 oz.)	79	D.N.A.
Brown, old fashioned (Pepperidge Farm)	1 piece (.4 oz.)	50	6.8
Old fashioned (Keebler)	1 piece (.6 oz.)	78	12.4
Old fashioned (Pepperidge Farm)	1 piece (.4 oz.)	52	7.2
Rings (Nabisco)	1 piece (.5 oz.)	68	10.6
Sugar wafer:			
(USDA)	1 oz.	137	20.8
(Nab)	1½-oz. pkg. (6 pieces)	220	30.0
(Nabisco) *Biscos*	1 piece (4 grams)	18	2.5
(Sunshine)	1 piece (.4 oz.)	47	6.8

(USDA): United States Department of Agriculture
DNA: Data Not Available
*Prepared as Package Directs

Food and Description	Measure or Quantity	Calories	Carbohydrates (grams)
Assorted (Dutch Twin)	1 piece	34	4.7
Chocolate (Keebler)	1 piece (6 grams)	31	3.5
Krisp Kreem (Keebler)	1 piece (6 grams)	31	3.7
Regent (Sunshine)	1 piece (5 grams)	23	3.4
Strawberry (Keebler)	1 piece (6 grams)	31	3.7
Vanilla (Keebler)	1 piece (6 grams)	31	3.7
Swedish Kreme (Keebler)	1 piece (.6 oz.)	98	12.2
Tahiti (Pepperidge Farm)	1 piece (.5 oz.)	77	7.9
Toy (Sunshine)	1 piece (3 grams)	13	2.1
Vanilla creme (Wise)	1 piece (9 grams)	38	6.4
Vanilla snap (Nabisco)	1 piece (3 grams)	12	2.3
Vanilla wafer:			
(USDA)	1 oz.	131	21.1
(Keebler)	1 piece (4 grams)	19	2.6
Nilla (Nabisco)	1 piece (4 grams)	18	2.9
(Sunshine)	1 piece (3 grams)	14	2.1
Venice (Pepperidge Farm)	1 piece (.4 oz.)	57	6.4
Waffle creme (Dutch Twin)	1 piece	44	6.1
Waffle creme (Nabisco) *Biscos*	1 piece (8 grams)	46	5.6
Yum Yums (Sunshine)	1 piece (.5 oz.)	83	10.4

COOKIE DIETETIC:

Food and Description	Measure or Quantity	Calories	Carbohydrates (grams)
Almond chocolate wafer (Estee)	1 wafer	27	2.6
Apple pastry (Stella D'oro)	1 piece	93	15.0
Assorted (Estee)	1 piece	28	3.4
Assorted filled wafers (Estee)	1 piece	25	3.0
Belgian Treats (Estee)	1 piece	32	3.0
Chocolate chip (Dia-Mel)	1 piece (9 grams)	40	3.7
Chocolate chip (Estee)	1 piece	34	4.1
Chocolate continental (Stella D'oro)	1 piece	21	D.N.A.
Chocolate Holland-filled wafer (Estee)	1 piece	21	2.0
Chocolate mint wafer (Dia-Mel)	1 piece (9 grams)	43	3.2
Chocolate & vanilla wafer (Estee)	1 piece	27	3.6
Coconut bar continental (Stella D'oro)	1 piece	34	D.N.A.
Coconut tea (Dia-Mel)	1 piece (7 grams)	32	2.8
Expresso Wafers (Estee)	1 piece	22	1.9
Fig pastry (Stella D'oro)	1 piece	95	15.8
French continental (Stella D'oro)	1 piece	36	D.N.A.
Fruit flavored wafer (Estee)	1 piece	21	2.0
Fudge nut (Estee)	1 piece	12	1.6

(USDA): United States Department of Agriculture
DNA: Data Not Available
*Prepared as Package Directs

Food and Description	Measure or Quantity	Calories	Carbo-hydrates (grams)
Half moon continental (Stella D'oro)	1 piece	28	D.N.A.
Kichel (Stella D'oro)	1 piece	8	.6
Metrecal (Drackett) any flavor	1 piece (6 grams)	25	3.0
Monties (Estee)	1 piece	37	3.2
Oatmeal raisin (Estee)	1 piece	28	3.8
Oatmeal raisin (Dia-Mel)	1 piece (7 grams)	29	2.7
Peach-apricot pastry (Stella D'oro)	1 piece	94	15.0
Prune pastry (Stella D'oro)	1 piece	90	15.0
Ripple Supreme (Dia-Mel)	1 piece (12 grams)	54	4.4
Royal Nuggets (Stella D'oro)	1 piece	1	.1
Sandwich (Estee)	1 piece	37	4.5
Sandwich (Dia-Mel)	1 piece (9 grams)	44	3.2
Vanilla continental (Stella D'oro)	1 piece	24	D.N.A.
Vanilla filled wafer (Estee)	1 piece	28	3.1
Vanilla Holland-filled wafer (Estee)	1 piece	21	2.0
COOKIE DOUGH, refrigerated:			
Unbaked, plain (USDA)	1 oz.	127	16.7
(Pillsbury):			
Brownie	1 oz.	110	17.3
Butterscotch nut	1 oz.	128	15.2
Chocolate chip	1 oz.	116	17.0
Fudge nut	1 oz.	119	15.9
Oatmeal raisin	1 oz.	116	16.8
Peanut butter	1 oz.	129	16.0
Sugar	1 oz.	125	16.1
COOKIE, HOME RECIPE:			
Brownie with nuts (USDA)	1 oz.	137	14.4
Chocolate chip (USDA)	1 oz.	146	17.0
Sugar, soft, thick (USDA)	1 oz.	126	19.3
COOKIE MIX:			
Plain, dry (USDA)	1 oz.	140	18.9
*Plain, prepared with egg & water (USDA)	1 oz.	140	18.4
*Plain, prepared with milk (USDA)	1 oz.	139	18.9
Brownie:			
Dry, without egg (USDA)	1 oz.	125	21.6
Dry, with egg (USDA)	1 oz.	119	22.3
*Dry, with egg, prepared with water & nuts (USDA)	1 oz.	114	17.0

(USDA): United States Department of Agriculture
DNA: Data Not Available
*Prepared as Package Directs

Food and Description	Measure or Quantity	Calories	Carbohydrates (grams)
*Dry, without egg, prepared with egg, water & nuts (USDA)	1 oz.	121	17.9
*Family size (Duncan Hines)	1/24 of cake	141	20.0
*Regular size (Duncan Hines)	1/16 of cake	143	20.0
Butterscotch (Betty Crocker)	1-lb. pkg.	2032	342.4
Butterscotch, chocolate chip (Betty Crocker)	1-lb. pkg.	2096	332.8
Fudge (Betty Crocker)	1-lb. pkg.	1968	340.8
Fudge (Betty Crocker)	1 oz.	123	21.3
Fudge (Pillsbury)	1 oz.	125	21.7
Fudge, with chocolate chip (Betty Crocker)	1-lb. pkg.	2048	334.4
German chocolate (Betty Crocker)	1-lb. 3-oz. pkg.	2375	419.9
Walnut (Betty Crocker)	1-lb. 5-oz. pkg.	2730	420.0
Walnut (Betty Crocker)	1 oz.	130	20.0
Walnut (Pillsbury)	1 oz.	125	21.7
Date bar (Betty Crocker)	14-oz. pkg.	1974	250.6
Macaroon, coconut (Betty Crocker)	13-oz. pkg.	1755	243.1
Vienna Dream bar (Betty Crocker)	12.5-oz. pkg.	1725	238.8
*With morsels (Nestlé's)	1 piece (.4 oz.)	52	7.2
*Without morsels (Nestlé's)	1 piece (8 grams)	42	5.7

COOKING FATS (See **FATS**)

CORDIAL (See individual kinds of liqueur by flavor or brand name)

CORDON D'ALSACE, Alsatian wine, 12% alcohol (Willm)	3 fl. oz.	66	3.6
CORDON DE BORDEAUX, French Bordeaux, red or white (Chanson) 11½% alcohol	3 fl. oz.	60	6.3
CORDON DE BOURGOGNE, French white Burgundy, (Chanson) 11½% alcohol	3 fl. oz.	81	6.3
CORDON DU RHONE, French red Rhone wine, (Chanson) 12% alcohol	3 fl. oz.	84	6.3

(USDA): United States Department of Agriculture
DNA: Data Not Available
*Prepared as Package Directs

Food and Description	Measure or Quantity	Calories	Carbo-hydrates (grams)
CORN:			
Fresh, white or yellow (USDA):			
Raw, untrimmed, on cob	1 lb. (weighed in husk)	157	36.1
Raw, trimmed on cob	1 lb. (husk removed)	240	55.1
Boiled, kernels, cut from cob, drained	1 cup (5.9 oz.)	114	26.3
Boiled, whole	4.9-oz. ear (5″ x 1¾″)	70	16.0
Canned, regular pack:			
Golden or yellow, whole kernel:			
Solids & liq., vacuum pack (USDA)	4 oz.	94	23.2
Solids & liq., wet pack (USDA)	½ cup (3 oz.)	84	20.1
Drained solids, wet pack (USDA)	½ cup (3 oz.)	72	17.0
Drained solids (Butter Kernel)	½ cup	75	18.0
Drained solids (Cannon)	4 oz.	95	22.5
(Fall River)	½ cup	75	18.0
(Green Giant)	½ cup	75	18.0
(Stokely-Van Camp)	½ cup	75	18.0
With red & green sweet pepper (Green Giant)	4 oz.	82	D.N.A.
White, whole kernel:			
Solids & liq., wet pack (USDA)	½ cup (2.8 oz.)	52	12.5
Drained solids, wet pack (USDA)	4 oz.	95	22.5
Drained liq., wet pack (USDA)	4 oz.	29	7.8
(Fall River)	½ cup	70	16.4
(Green Giant)	4 oz.	77	D.N.A.
Canned, white or yellow, dietetic pack:			
Solids & liq., wet pack (USDA)	4 oz.	65	15.4
Drained solids (USDA)	4 oz.	86	20.4
Drained liq. (USDA)	4 oz. (by wt.)	19	4.9
Solids & liq. (Blue Boy)	4 oz.	78	16.0
Solids & liq. (Diet Delight)	½ cup (4.4 oz.)	69	16.6
(S and W) *Nutradiet*	4 oz.	58	11.8
(Tillie Lewis)	½ cup (4.5 oz.)	73	14.8
Canned, cream style, white or yellow, regular pack:			
Solids & liq. (USDA)	½ cup (4.4 oz.)	102	25.0

(USDA): United States Department of Agriculture
DNA: Data Not Available
*Prepared as Package Directs

Food and Description	Measure or Quantity	Calories	Carbo-hydrates (grams)
(Butter Kernel)	½ cup	92	22.5
Golden (Fall River)	½ cup	92	22.5
Golden (Green Giant)	4 oz.	105	D.N.A.
White (Fall River)	½ cup	91	21.9
White (Green Giant)	4 oz.	103	D.N.A.
White or golden (Stokely-Van Camp)	½ cup	102	25.0
Canned, cream style, dietetic pack:			
Solids & liq. (USDA)	4 oz.	93	21.0
Solids & liq. (Blue Boy)	4 oz.	105	20.6
(S and W) *Nutradiet*	4 oz.	95	19.6
Frozen:			
On the cob:			
(USDA)	4 oz.	111	25.6
Boiled, drained (USDA)	4 oz.	107	24.5
(Birds Eye)	1 ear (3.5 oz.)	98	21.9
Kernel:			
Not thawed (USDA)	4 oz.	93	22.3
Boiled, drained solids (USDA)	½ cup (3.2 oz.)	72	17.1
(Birds Eye)	½ cup (3.3 oz.)	77	18.0
(Blue Goose)	4 oz.	102	20.6
(Stokely-Van Camp)	4 oz.	93	22.3
In butter sauce:			
(Birds Eye)	½ cup (3.3 oz.)	101	15.6
Niblets (Green Giant) boil-in-the-bag	4 oz.	133	18.6
White Shoe Peg (Green Giant) boil-in-the-bag	4 oz.	137	17.7
Mexicorn (Green Giant) boil-in-the-bag	4 oz.	128	16.6
Cream style:			
(Birds Eye)	½ cup (3.3 oz.)	79	19.2
(Green Giant) boil-in-the-bag	4 oz.	108	24.3
With peas & tomatoes (Birds Eye)	½ cup (3.3 oz.)	68	14.8

CORNBREAD:

Food and Description	Measure or Quantity	Calories	Carbo-hydrates (grams)
Corn pone, home recipe, prepared with white, whole-ground cornmeal (USDA)	4 oz.	231	41.1
Corn sticks, frozen (Aunt Jemima)	3 pieces (2 oz.)	171	27.0
Johnnycake, home recipe prepared with yellow degermed cornmeal (USDA)	4 oz.	303	51.6

Food and Description	Measure or Quantity	Calories	Carbo-hydrates (grams)
Southern-style, home recipe, prepared with degermed cornmeal (USDA)	4 oz.	254	39.3
Southern-style, home recipe, prepared with whole-ground cornmeal (USDA)	4 oz.	235	33.0
Spoonbread, home recipe, prepared with white whole-ground cornmeal (USDA)	4 oz.	221	19.2
CORNBREAD MIX:			
Dry (USDA)	1 oz.	122	20.1
*Prepared with egg & milk (USDA)	4 oz.	264	37.3
*(Aunt Jemima)	⅙ of cornbread (2.4 oz.)	225	35.0
(Pillsbury) *Ballard*	1 oz.	103	19.2
CORN BURSTS, cereal	1 cup (1 oz.)	110	25.6
CORN CHEX, cereal	1¼ cups (1 oz.)	111	24.7
CORN CHIPS (See **CRACKERS**)			
CORNED BEEF:			
Uncooked, boneless, medium fat (USDA)	1 lb.	1329	0.
Cooked, boneless, medium fat (USDA)	4 oz.	422	0.
Canned:			
Lean (USDA)	4 oz.	210	0.
Medium fat (USDA)	4 oz.	245	0.
Fat (USDA)	4 oz.	298	0.
(Vienna)	4 oz.	272	.4
CORNED BEEF HASH, canned:			
With potato (USDA)	4 oz.	205	12.1
(Armour Star)	15½-oz. can	837	36.0
(Austex)	15-oz. can	769	45.5
(Bounty)	4 oz.	209	12.1
(Hormel)	15-oz. can	570	30.6
(Morton House)	15-oz. can	890	D.N.A.
(Nalley's)	4 oz.	209	9.1
(Silver Skillet)	4 oz.	217	10.9
(Wilson)	4 oz.	205	8.2

(USDA): United States Department of Agriculture
DNA: Data Not Available
*Prepared as Package Directs

Food and Description	Measure or Quantity	Calories	Carbohydrates (grams)
CORNED BEEF HASH DINNER, frozen (Swanson)	12½-oz. dinner	511	55.0
CORNED BEEF SPREAD (Underwood)	1 T.	27	Tr.
CORN FLAKES, cereal:			
(USDA)	1 cup (1 oz.)	112	24.7
Crushed (USDA)	1 cup (2.4 oz.)	270	59.7
Frosted (USDA)	1 cup (1.5 oz.)	166	39.2
Country (General Mills)	1 cup (¾ oz.)	83	18.3
(Kellogg's)	1 cup (¾ oz.)	79	18.3
(Ralston Purina)	1 cup (1 oz.)	111	24.0
(Van Brode)	1 oz.	106	24.2
Dietetic (Van Brode)	1 oz.	109	24.9
CORN FRITTER:			
Home recipe (USDA)	4 oz.	428	45.0
Frozen (Mrs. Paul's)	4 oz.	432	45.6
CORN GRITS (See **HOMINY**)			
CORNMEAL, WHITE or YELLOW:			
Bolted (USDA)	1 oz.	103	21.1
Degermed:			
Dry (USDA)	1 cup (4.6 oz.)	470	101.1
Dry (USDA)	1 oz.	103	22.2
Cooked (USDA)	4 oz.	57	12.1
Self-rising, degermed (USDA)	1 cup (5 oz.)	491	105.9
Self-rising, whole-ground (USDA)	1 oz.	98	20.4
Whole-ground, unbolted (USDA)	1 cup (4.2 oz.)	419	87.0
Whole-ground, unbolted (USDA)	1 oz.	101	20.9
Cooked:			
(Albers)	½ cup	60	12.8
Enriched (Aunt Jemima)	½ cup	63	14.2
Enriched (Quaker)	½ cup	63	14.2
CORN PUDDING, home recipe (USDA)	4 oz.	118	14.7
CORN SALAD, raw (USDA):			
Untrimmed	1 lb. (weighed untrimmed)	91	15.7
Trimmed	4 oz.	24	4.1

(USDA): United States Department of Agriculture
DNA: Data Not Available
*Prepared as Package Directs

Food and Description	Measure or Quantity	Calories	Carbo-hydrates (grams)
CORN SOUFFLE, frozen			
(Stouffer's)	12-oz. pkg.	492	57.0
CORNSTARCH:			
(USDA)	1 cup (4.5 oz.)	465	112.0
(USDA)	1 T.	30	7.0
(Argo)	1 T.	30	7.0
(Kingford's)	1 T.	30	7.0
(Duryea's)	1 T.	30	7.0
CORN STICK (See **CORNBREAD**)			
CORN SYRUP, light & dark			
blend (USDA)	1 T.	58	15.0
CORN TOTAL, cereal	1 oz.	111	24.3
COTTAGE PUDDING, home			
recipe (USDA):			
Without sauce	2 oz.	195	30.8
With chocolate sauce	2 oz.	180	32.1
With strawberry sauce	2 oz.	166	27.4
COUGH DROP:			
(Beech-Nut)	1 drop	10	2.4
(F & F)	1 drop	11	D.N.A.
(H-B)	1 drop	8	1.9
(Luden's):			
Honey lemon	1 drop	8	D.N.A.
Honey licorice	1 drop	8	D.N.A.
Menthol	1 drop	9	2.1
Wild cherry	1 drop	9	D.N.A.
(Pine Bros.)	1 drop	10	2.5
(Smith Brothers)	1 drop	7	2.1
COUNTRY-STYLE SAUSAGE,			
smoked links (USDA)	1 oz.	98	0.
COWPEA (USDA):			
Immature seeds:			
Raw, whole	1 lb. (weighed in pods)	317	54.4
Raw, shelled	1 lb.	576	98.9
Boiled, drained solids	½ cup (2.8 oz.)	88	14.5

(USDA): United States Department of Agriculture
DNA: Data Not Available
*Prepared as Package Directs

Food and Description	Measure or Quantity	Calories	Carbo-hydrates (grams)
Canned, solids & liq.	4 oz.	79	14.1
Frozen (See **BLACK-EYED PEAS,** frozen)			
Young pods with seeds:			
Raw, whole	1 lb. (weighed untrimmed)	182	39.2
Boiled, drained solids	4 oz.	39	7.9
Mature seeds, dry:			
Raw	1 lb.	1556	279.9
Raw	½ cup (3.5 oz.)	343	61.7
Cooked	½ cup (4.4 oz.)	95	17.1
CRAB, all species:			
Fresh:			
Steamed, whole (USDA)	1 lb. (weighed in shell)	202	1.1
Steamed, meat only (USDA)	4 oz.	106	.6
(Epicure)	½ cup	50	.6
Canned:			
Drained solids (USDA)	4 oz.	115	1.3
(Del Monte)	7½-oz. can	215	D.N.A.
(Harris Atlantic)	4 oz.	115	1.3
Alaska King, drained solids (Icy Point)	7½-oz. can	215	2.3
Alaska King, drained solids (Pillar Rock)	7½-oz. can	215	2.3
Frozen, Alaska King, thawed & drained (Wakefield's)	4 oz.	95	.6
CRAB COCKTAIL, King crab (Sau-Sea)	4-oz. jar	80	18.4
CRAB, DEVILED:			
Home recipe (USDA)	4 oz.	213	15.1
Frozen (Mrs. Paul's)	4 oz.	214	15.2
CRAB IMPERIAL, home recipe (USDA)	4 oz.	167	4.4
CRAB NEWBURG, Alaska King, frozen (Stouffer's)	12-oz. pkg.	562	13.6
CRAB SOUP (Crosse & Blackwell)	6½ oz. (½ can)	59	8.3

(USDA): United States Department of Agriculture
DNA: Data Not Available
*Prepared as Package Directs

Food and Description	Measure or Quantity	Calories	Carbo-hydrates (grams)
CRAB APPLE, fresh (USDA):			
Whole	1 lb. (weighed whole)	284	74.3
Flesh only	4 oz.	77	20.2
CRACKER, PUFFS and CHIPS:			
Appeteasers (Nabisco):			
Crescent roll shaped	1 piece (<1 gram)	3	.5
Ham tasting, shaped	1 piece (<1 gram)	2	.4
Onion shaped	1 piece (<1 gram)	2	.3
Arrowroot biscuit (Nabisco)	1 piece (5 grams)	22	3.5
Arrowroot biscuit (Sunshine)	1 piece (4 grams)	15	2.9
Bacon flavored thins (Nabisco)	1 piece (2 grams)	10	1.2
Bacon toast (Keebler)	1 piece (3 grams)	15	2.0
Barbecue snack wafer (Sunshine)	1 piece (3 grams)	17	2.0
Barbecue Vittles (General Mills)	32 pieces (½ oz.)	67	9.1
Bows (General Mills)	22 pieces (½ oz.)	81	7.5
Bugles (General Mills)	15 pieces (½ oz.)	81	7.5
Butter (USDA)	1 oz.	130	19.1
Butter thins (Keebler)	1 piece	16	D.N.A.
Butter thins (Nabisco)	1 piece (3 grams)	14	1.5
Buttons (General Mills)	48 pieces (½ oz.)	73	7.8
Cheese flavored (See also individual brand names in this grouping):			
(USDA)	1 oz.	136	17.1
Cheese 'n Bacon flavored sandwich (Nab)	1.4-oz. pkg. (6 pieces)	196	18.0
Cheese-N-Cheese (Wise)	1 piece (6 grams)	32	3.8
Cheese-Nips (Nab)	1½-oz. pkg. (39 pieces)	195	28.5
Cheese-Nips (Nabisco)	1 piece (<1 gram)	5	.7
Cheese on Rye sandwich (Nab)	1.4-oz. pkg. (6 pieces)	209	19.3
Chee-Tos, cheese-flavored puffs	1 oz.	159	15.0
Cheez Doodles (Old London)	1 oz.	133	17.3
Cheez It (Sunshine)	1 piece (1 gram)	6	.6
Che-zo (Keebler)	1 piece (<1 gram)	5	.6
Combo Cheez sandwich (Austin's)	1 piece	26	D.N.A.
Cheese Pixies (Wise)	1 oz.	158	14.5
Cheez Waffles (Austin's)	1 piece	26	D.N.A.
Ritz cheese (Nabisco)	1 piece (3 grams)	18	1.9

(USDA): United States Department of Agriculture
DNA: Data Not Available
*Prepared as Package Directs

Food and Description	Measure or Quantity	Calories	Carbohydrates (grams)
Sesame cheese snack (Sunshine)	1 cracker (3 grams)	16	2.2
Shapies, dip delights (Nabisco)	1 piece (2 grams)	8	.8
Shapies, shells (Nabisco)	1 piece (2 grams)	9	.8
Skinny Dips (Keebler)	1 piece (1 gram)	5	.7
Thins (Pepperidge Farm)	1 piece (3 grams)	10	1.6
Thins, dietetic (Estee)	1 thin	6	.8
Tid Bit (Nab)	1½-oz. pkg. (113 pieces)	192	28.9
Tid Bit (Nabisco)	1 piece (<1 gram)	4	.6
Toast (Keebler)	1 piece (3 grams)	16	1.9
Twists (Nalley's)	1 oz.	137	14.1
Waffies (Old London)	1 oz.	147	13.0
Cheese & peanut butter sandwich:			
(USDA)	1 oz.	139	15.9
(Austin's)	1 piece	43	4.5
(Nab) *O-So-Gud*	1 oz. (4 pieces)	145	16.8
(Nab) *Squares*	1 ⅔-oz. pkg. (6 pieces)	230	47.0
(Nab) *Variety Pack*	1 ⅔-oz. pkg. (6 pieces)	229	24.8
(Wise)	1 piece (7 grams)	34	3.5
Chicken in a Biskit (Nabisco)	1 piece (2 grams)	10	1.2
Chippers (Nabisco)	1 piece (3 grams)	14	1.8
Chipsters (Nabisco)	1 piece (<1 gram)	2	.3
Cinnamon Crisp (Keebler)	1 section (4 grams)	17	2.7
Club, with or without salt (Keebler)	1 section (3 grams)	15	2.0
Corn Chips:			
(Fritos)	1 oz.	164	15.2
(Old London)	1 oz.	150	14.6
(Wise)	1 oz.	166	14.8
Barbecue flavored (Wise)	1 oz.	160	15.3
Crown Pilot (Nabisco)	1 piece (.6 oz.)	72	12.4
Dipsy Doodles (Old London)	1 oz.	150	14.6
Doo Dads (Nabisco)	1 oz.	143	18.1
Duet (Nabisco)	1 piece (4 grams)	17	2.3
Euphrates (Burry's), original, onion or rye	1 cracker	22	D.N.A.
Flings, cheese-flavored curls (Nabisco)	1 piece (2 grams)	10	.6
Flings, Swiss- & ham-flavored curls (Nabisco)	1 piece (2 grams)	9	1.0
French Fried Potato Crisps (General Mills)	16 pieces (½ oz.)	78	7.5

(USDA): United States Department of Agriculture
DNA: Data Not Available
*Prepared as Package Directs

Food and Description	Measure or Quantity	Calories	Carbo-hydrates (grams)
Goldfish (Pepperidge Farm):			
Cheese	1 oz.	142	18.1
Cheese	1 piece (<1 gram)	2	.4
Lightly salted	1 oz.	136	19.0
Lightly salted	1 piece (<1 gram)	2	.4
Graham:			
(USDA)	1 oz.	109	20.8
(USDA)	2 small or 1 med. (7 grams)	28	5.2
(Nabisco)	1 piece (7 grams)	30	5.4
(Sunshine)	1 piece (4 grams)	17	3.0
Chocolate or cocoa-covered:			
(USDA)	1 oz.	135	19.2
(Burry's) Crunchy	1 piece	46	D.N.A.
(Keebler) *Deluxe*	1 piece (8 grams)	42	5.6
(Nabisco)	1 piece (.4 oz.)	55	7.0
(Nabisco) *Fancy*	1 piece (.5 oz.)	68	8.9
(Nabisco) *Pantry*	1 piece (.4 oz.)	62	8.5
(Sunshine) *Delito*	1 piece (8 grams)	41	5.5
Sugar honey-coated:			
(USDA)	1 oz.	29	5.4
(Keebler)	1 section (4 grams)	17	2.8
(Nabisco) *Honey Maid*	1 piece (7 grams)	30	5.5
(Sunshine)	1 piece (7 grams)	30	5.2
Hi-Ho (Sunshine)	1 piece (3 grams)	17	2.0
Krispy, salted tops (Sunshine)	1 piece (3 grams)	12	2.1
Krispy, unsalted tops (Sunshine)	1 piece (3 grams)	12	2.0
Matzo (See **MATZO**)			
Melba toast (See **MELBA**)			
Milk lunch (Burry's)	1 piece	36	D.N.A.
Milk lunch (Nabisco) *Royal Lunch*	1 piece (.4 oz.)	54	7.8
New Daisys (General Mills)	28 pieces (½ oz.)	68	8.8
Onion flavored:			
French (Nabisco)	1 piece (2 grams)	11	1.6
Rings (Old London)	1 oz.	136	21.2
Rings (Wise)	1 oz.	126	22.2
Skinny Dips (Keebler)	1 piece (1 gram)	5	.7
Tam (Manischewitz)	1 piece	14	D.N.A.
Toast (Keebler)	1 piece (3 grams)	18	2.1
Onion Waffies (Old London)	1 oz.	138	13.4
OTC (Original Trenton Cracker) regular or wine	1 piece	23	4.4
Oyster:			
(USDA)	1 cup (1 oz.)	119	20.6

(USDA): United States Department of Agriculture
DNA: Data Not Available
*Prepared as Package Directs

CRACKER, PUFFS AND CHIPS (Continued)

Food and Description	Measure or Quantity	Calories	Carbohydrates (grams)
(Keebler)	1 piece (<1 gram)	2	.2
Oysterettes (Nabisco)	1 piece (<1 gram)	3	.6
Soup & oyster (Nabisco) *Dandy*	1 piece (<1 gram)	3	.5
(Sunshine)	1 piece (<1 gram)	4	.7
Party Toast (Keebler)	1 piece (3 grams)	15	1.9
Peanut butter sandwich:			
& jelly flavored (Nabisco)	1.3-oz. pkg. (6 pieces)	180	23.9
Malted milk (Nab)	1½-oz. pkg. (6 pieces)	224	24.0
Toast (Wise)	1 piece (7 grams)	33	3.7
Toasty (Austin's)	1 piece	37	D.N.A.
Peanut butter & cheese (See Cheese & Peanut Butter Sandwich)			
Pizza Spins (General Mills)	½ oz. (32 pieces)	72	8.0
Ritz (Nabisco)	1 piece (3 grams)	18	2.0
Ry Brot (Burry's)	1 piece	67	D.N.A.
Rye thins (Pepperidge Farm)	1 piece	10	1.8
Rye toast (Keebler)	1 section (4 grams)	17	2.2
Saltine:			
(USDA)	1 oz.	123	20.3
(USDA)	2″ sq. (4 grams)	17	2.8
Regular (Flavor Kist)	1 piece	12	2.2
Premium (Nab)	.9-oz. pkg. (8 pieces)	114	18.9
Premium (Nabisco)	1 piece (3 grams)	12	2.0
Premium (Nabisco), unsalted tops	1 piece (3 grams)	12	2.0
Rye (Flavor Kist)	1 piece	13	2.2
Sesame (Flavor Kist)	1 piece	13	2.2
Zesta (Keebler)	1 section (2 grams)	12	2.0
Sea Toast(Keebler)	1 piece (.5 oz.)	62	11.1
Sesa Wheat (Austin's)	1 piece	34	3.7
Sesame bread wafer (Keebler)	1 piece (3 grams)	16	2.0
Sesame bread wafer (Nabisco)			
Meal Mates	1 piece (4 grams)	22	2.9
Sip 'N Chips snacks (Nabisco)	1 piece (2 grams)	8	1.0
Sociables (Nabisco)	1 piece (2 grams)	10	1.3
Soda (USDA)	1 oz.	124	20.0
Soda (USDA)	2½″ sq. (6 grams)	24	4.0
Souperfish (Burry's)	1 piece	9	D.N.A.
Swedish rye wafers (Keebler)	1 piece (5 grams)	5	3.8
Tam Tam (Manischewitz)	1 piece	13	1.7
Toasted wafers (Sunshine)	1 wafer (2 grams)	10	1.2
Tomato onion (Sunshine)	1 piece (3 grams)	15	2.5
Tortilla chips (Frito-Lay) *Doritos*	1 oz.	149	16.7

(USDA): United States Department of Agriculture
DNA: Data Not Available
*Prepared as Package Directs

Food and Description	Measure or Quantity	Calories	Carbo-hydrates (grams)
Tortilla chips (Old London)	1 oz.	129	16.3
Town House (Keebler)	1 piece (4 grams)	18	2.2
Triangle Thins (Nabisco)	1 piece (2 grams)	8	1.1
Triscuit wafers (Nabisco)	1 piece (4 grams)	22	2.9
Uneeda Biscuit, unsalted tops (Nabisco)	1 piece (5 grams)	22	3.7
Wafer-ets (Hol-Grain):			
Rice, salted or unsalted	1 piece	12	2.5
Wheat, salted or unsalted	1 piece	6	1.4
Waldorf salt-free (Keebler)	1 section (3 grams)	14	2.4
Waverly wafers (Nabisco)	1 piece (4 grams)	18	2.6
Wheat *Skinny Dips* (Keebler)	1 piece (1 gram)	5	.7
Wheat thins (Nabisco)	1 piece (2 grams)	9	1.1
Wheat toast (Keebler)	1 piece (3 grams)	16	1.9
Whistles (General Mills)	17 pieces (½ oz.)	71	8.0
White thins (Pepperidge Farm)	1 piece	10	1.9
Whole-wheat (USDA)	1 oz.	114	19.3
CRACKER CRUMBS:			
Graham (USDA)	1 cup (3 oz.)	330	63.0
Graham (Keebler)	3 oz.	368	64.1
Graham (Nabisco)	1 cup (3.7 oz.)	432	76.6
CRACKER JACK (See **POPCORN**)			
CRACKER MEAL:			
(USDA)	3 oz.	373	60.0
(USDA)	1 T.	43	7.3
Salted (Nabisco)	1 cup (3 oz.)	318	67.8
Unsalted (Nabisco)	1 cup (3 oz.)	318	67.7
Crax (Keebler):			
Fine, medium or coarse	3 oz.	316	68.5
Zesty	3 oz.	363	61.5
CRACKER PIE CRUST MIX (See **PIECRUST MIX**)			
CRANBERRY:			
Fresh:			
Untrimmed (USDA)	1 lb. (weighed with stems)	200	47.0
Stems removed (USDA)	1 cup (4 oz.)	52	12.2
(Ocean Spray)	1 oz.	14.7	2.7
Dehydrated (USDA)	1 oz.	104	23.8

(USDA): United States Department of Agriculture
DNA: Data Not Available
*Prepared as Package Directs

Food and Description	Measure or Quantity	Calories	Carbo-hydrates (grams)
CRANBERRY JUICE COCKTAIL:			
(USDA)	½ cup (4.4 oz.)	82	20.8
(Ocean Spray)	½ cup	83	19.7
CRANBERRY JUICE DRINK			
(Ocean Spray)	½ cup	94	23.0
CRANBERRY-ORANGE RELISH:			
Uncooked (USDA)	4 oz.	202	51.5
(Ocean Spray)	4 oz.	209	51.8
CRANBERRY-PAPAYA FRUIT SPREAD (Vita)	1 T.	9	D.N.A.
CRANBERRY PIE (Tastykake)	4-oz. pie	376	57.7
CRANBERRY SAUCE:			
Home recipe, sweetened, unstrained (USDA)	4 oz.	202	51.6
Canned:			
Sweetened, strained (USDA)	½ cup (4.8 oz.)	199	51.0
Sweetened, strained (USDA)	4 oz.	166	42.5
Jellied (Ocean Spray)	4 oz.	184	42.8
Whole berry (Ocean Spray)	4 oz.	192	44.4
CRANBREAKER MIX (Bar-Tender's)	1 serving (⅝ oz.)	70	17.4
CRANPRUNE JUICE DRINK (Ocean Spray)	½ cup	82	20.1
CRAPPIE, white, raw, meat only (USDA)	4 oz.	90	0.
CRAYFISH, freshwater (USDA):			
Raw, in shell	1 lb. (weighed in shell)	39	.7
Raw, meat only	4 oz.	82	1.4
CREAM:			
Half and half:			
(USDA)	½ cup (4.2 oz.)	162	5.5
(USDA)	1 T.	20	1.0

(USDA): United States Department of Agriculture
DNA: Data Not Available
*Prepared as Package Directs

Food and Description	Measure or Quantity	Calories	Carbo-hydrates (grams)
10.5% fat (Sealtest)	½ cup	150	5.0
12.0% fat (Sealtest)	½ cup	164	4.9
Light, table, or coffee:			
(USDA)	1 cup (8.5 oz.)	505	10.0
(USDA)	1 T.	30	1.0
18% fat (Sealtest)	1 T.	28	.6
25% fat (Sealtest)	1 T.	37	.5
Light whipping:			
(USDA)	1 cup (8.4 oz.)	717	8.6
(USDA)	1 T.	45	.5
(Sealtest)	1 T.	44	.5
Heavy whipping:			
(USDA)	1 cup (8.4 oz.)	840	7.0
(USDA)	1 T.	55	Tr.
(Sealtest)	1 T.	52	.5
Sour:			
(USDA)	1 cup	506	10.3
(USDA)	2 T.	63	1.3
(Borden)	1 cup	454	7.7
(Borden)	2 T.	57	1.0
(Breakstone)	2 T.	56	1.0
(Sealtest)	2 T.	57	1.0
Imitation:			
(Borden) *Zest*, 13.5% vegetable fat	1 pt.	776	28.0
(Borden) *Zest*, 13.5% vegetable fat	2 T.	97	3.5
(Breakstone)	2 T	60	2.2
Sour cream, dried (Information supplied by General Mills Laboratory)	1 oz.	188	8.1
Sour dressing, cultured (Breakstone)	2 T.	56	1.6
CREAMIES (Tastykake):			
Banana cake	1 pkg. (1⅞ oz.)	238	34.5
Chocolate	1 pkg. (1⅞ oz.)	290	29.3
Koffee Kake	1 pkg. (1⅞ oz.)	303	47.2
Vanilla	1 pkg. (1⅞ oz.)	292	32.3
***CREAM OF RICE,** cereal	4 oz.	82	17.9
CREAM PUFF, home recipe, with custard filling (USDA)	2 oz.	133	11.7

(USDA): United States Department of Agriculture
DNA: Data Not Available
*Prepared as Package Directs

Food and Description	Measure or Quantity	Calories	Carbo-hydrates (grams)
CREAMSICLE (Popsicle Industries)	3 fl. oz.	96	20.0
CREAM or CREME SOFT DRINK:			
Sweetened:			
(Canada Dry)	6 fl. oz.	93	24.2
(Dr. Brown's)	6 fl. oz.	81	20.4
Fanta	6 fl. oz.	96	24.0
(Hoffman)	6 fl. oz.	87	21.6
(Key Food)	6 fl. oz.	81	20.4
(Kirsch)	6 fl. oz.	77	19.6
(Shasta)	6 fl. oz.	84	21.3
(Waldbaum)	6 fl. oz.	81	20.4
(Yukon Club)	6 fl. oz.	84	21.0
Low calorie:			
(Dr. Brown's)	6 fl. oz.	3	.8
(Hoffman)	6 fl. oz.	3	.8
(No-Cal)	6 fl. oz.	2	<.1
(Shasta)	6 fl. oz.	<1	<.1
CREAM SUBSTITUTE (See individual brand names)			
CREAM OF WHEAT, cereal:			
Instant or quick, dry	1⅓ oz. (1 cup cooked)	133	28.5
Mix'n Eat	1-oz. pkg.	101	21.2
Regular, dry	1⅓ oz. (1 cup cooked)	133	28.8
CREME D'AMANDE LIQUEUR (Garnier) 60 proof	1 fl. oz.	111	15.6
CREME D'APRICOT LIQUEUR (Old Mr. Boston) 42 proof	1 fl. oz.	66	6.0
CREME DE BANANE LIQUEUR:			
(Garnier) 60 proof	1 fl. oz.	96	11.5
(Old Mr. Boston) 42 proof	1 fl. oz.	66	6.0
CREME DE BLACKBERRY LIQUEUR (Old Mr. Boston) 42 proof	1 fl. oz.	66	6.0

(USDA): United States Department of Agriculture
DNA: Data Not Available
*Prepared as Package Directs

Food and Description	Measure or Quantity	Calories	Carbo-hydrates (grams)
CREME DE CACAO LIQUEUR:			
Brown or white:			
(Bols) 54 proof	1 fl. oz.	101	11.8
(Garnier) 54 proof	1 fl. oz.	97	13.1
(Hiram Walker) 54 proof	1 fl. oz.	104	15.0
(Leroux) brown, 54 proof	1 fl. oz.	101	14.3
(Leroux) white, 54 proof	1 fl. oz.	98	13.3
(Old Mr. Boston) 42 proof	1 fl. oz.	84	7.0
(Old Mr. Boston) 54 proof	1 fl. oz.	95	7.0
CREME DE CAFE LIQUEUR			
(Leroux) 60 proof	1 fl. oz.	104	13.6
CREME DE CASSIS LIQUEUR:			
(Garnier) 36 proof	1 fl. oz.	83	13.5
(Leroux) 35 proof	1 fl. oz.	88	14.9
CREME DE CHERRY LIQUEUR:			
black cherry (Old Mr. Boston) 42 proof	1 fl. oz.	66	6.0
CREME DE COFFEE LIQUEUR,			
(Old Mr. Boston) 42 proof	1 fl. oz.	66	6.0
CREME DE MENTHE LIQUEUR,			
green or white:			
(Bols) 60 proof	1 fl. oz.	112	13.0
(Garnier) 60 proof	1 fl. oz.	110	15.3
(Hiram Walker) 60 proof	1 fl. oz.	94	11.2
(Leroux) green, 60 proof	1 fl. oz.	110	15.2
(Leroux) white, 60 proof	1 fl. oz.	101	12.8
(Old Mr. Boston) 42 proof	1 fl. oz.	66	6.0
(Old Mr. Boston) 60 proof	1 fl. oz.	94	8.5
CREME DE NOYAUX LIQUEUR:			
(Bols) 60 proof	1 fl. oz.	115	13.7
(Leroux) 60 proof	1 fl. oz.	108	14.6
CREME DE PEACH LIQUEUR			
(Old Mr. Boston) 42 proof	1 fl. oz.	66	6.0
CREME SOFT DRINK (See **CREAM SOFT DRINK**)			
CREMORA, non-dairy (Borden)	1 tsp.	11	1.1

(USDA): United States Department of Agriculture
DNA: Data Not Available
*Prepared as Package Directs

Food and Description	Measure or Quantity	Calories	Carbohydrates (grams)
CRESS, GARDEN (USDA):			
Raw, whole	1 lb. (weighed untrimmed)	103	17.7
Boiled, drained solids	4 oz.	26	4.3
Boiled in small amount of water, drained solids (USDA)	1 cup (6.3 oz.)	41	6.8
CRISP RICE (Van Brode):			
Regular	1 oz.	106	24.7
Dietetic	1 oz.	109	25.5
CRISPY CRITTERS, cereal	1 cup (1 oz.)	110	23.0
CROAKER (USDA):			
Atlantic:			
Raw, meat only	4 oz.	109	0.
Baked	4 oz.	151	0.
White, raw, meat only	4 oz.	95	0.
Yellowfin, raw, meat only	4 oz.	101	0.
CRULLER (See **DOUGHNUT**)			
CUCUMBER, fresh (USDA):			
Eaten with skin	½ lb. (weighed whole)	33	7.4
Eaten without skin	½ lb. (weighed with skin)	23	5.3
Unpared, 10-oz. cucumber	7½″ x 2″ pared cucumber (7.3 oz.)	28	6.6
Pared	6 slices (2″ x ⅛″)	7	1.6
Pared & diced	½ cup (2.5 oz.)	10	2.3
CUPCAKE:			
Home recipe (USDA):			
Without icing	1.4-oz. cupcake (2¾″)	146	22.4
With chocolate icing	1.8-oz. cupcake (2¾″)	184	29.7
With boiled white icing	1.8-oz. cupcake (2¾″)	176	30.9
With uncooked white icing	1.8-oz. cupcake (2¾″)	184	31.6
Commercial:			
Chocolate (Hostess)	1 cupcake	205	29.4

(USDA): United States Department of Agriculture
DNA: Data Not Available
*Prepared as Package Directs

Food and Description	Measure or Quantity	Calories	Carbo-hydrates (grams)
Chocolate (Tastykake)	1 cupcake (1 oz.)	192	33.0
Chocolate, chocolate creme filled (Tastykake)	1 cupcake (1¼ oz.)	128	23.2
Coconut (Tastykake)	1 cupcake (¾ oz.)	92	16.7
Creme filled, chocolate butter cream (Tastykake)	1 cupcake (1⅛ oz.)	161	23.1
Lemon creme filled (Tastykake)	1 cupcake (⅞ oz.)	124	17.1
Orange (Hostess)	1 cupcake	185	26.7
Orange creme filled (Tastykake)	1 cupcake (⅞ oz.)	133	17.1
Vanilla creme filled (Tastykake)	1 cupcake (⅞ oz.)	123	16.4
Vanilla *Triplets* (Tastykake)	1 cupcake (.8 oz.)	101	16.1
CUPCAKE MIX:			
(USDA)	4 oz.	497	86.0
*Prepared with eggs, milk, without icing (USDA)	2 oz.	198	31.6
*Prepared with eggs, milk, with chocolate icing (USDA)	2 oz.	203	33.6
(Flako)	.8-oz. cupcake (1/16 of pkg.)	101	16.0
CURACAO LIQUEUR:			
Curaçao-Blue (Bols) 64 proof	1 fl. oz.	105	10.3
Curaçao-Orange (Bols) 64 proof	1 fl. oz.	100	8.8
(Garnier) 60 proof	1 fl. oz.	100	12.7
(Hiram Walker) 60 proof	1 fl. oz.	96	11.8
(Leroux) 60 proof	1 fl. oz.	84	9.5
CURRANT, fresh (USDA):			
Black European:			
Whole	1 lb. (weighed with stems)	240	58.2
Stems removed	4 oz.	61	14.9
Red & white:			
Whole	1 lb. (weighed with stems)	220	53.2
Stems removed	4 oz.	57	13.7
Stems removed	1 cup (3.8 oz.)	55	13.3
*CURRANT-RASPBERRY DANISH DESSERT (Junket)	½ cup	138	33.8
CURRY POWDER (Crosse & Blackwell)	1 T.	26	4.9

(USDA): United States Department of Agriculture
DNA: Data Not Available
*Prepared as Package Directs

Food and Description	Measure or Quantity	Calories	Carbo-hydrates (grams)
CUSK, (USDA):			
Raw, drawn	1 lb. (weighed drawn, head & tail on)	197	0.
Raw, meat only	1 lb.	340	0.
Steamed	4 oz.	120	0.
CUSTARD, home recipe, baked (USDA)	½ cup (4.4 oz.)	142	13.8
CUSTARD APPLE, bullock's-heart, raw (USDA):			
Whole	1 lb. (weighed with skin & seeds)	266	66.3
Flesh only	4 oz.	302	75.2
CUSTARD PUDDING MIX:			
Dry, with vegetable gum base (USDA)	1 oz.	109	28.0
*Prepared with whole milk (USDA)	4 oz.	149	25.6
*Prepared with whole milk (Jell-O)	½ cup (5 oz.)	165	22.5
*Prepared with nonfat milk (Jell-O)	½ cup (5.1 oz.)	130	22.0
Real egg (Lynden)	4-oz. pkg.	441	71.0
*(Royal)	½ cup (4.8 oz.)	145	21.4
CUSTARD PIE:			
Home recipe (USDA)	⅙ of 9″ pie (5.4 oz.)	331	35.6
Frozen (Banquet)	5 oz.	274	41.2
Frozen egg custard (Mrs. Smith's)	⅙ of 8″ pie	248	28.8

D

Food and Description	Measure or Quantity	Calories	Carbo-hydrates (grams)
DAIQUIRI COCKTAIL:			
(Calvert) 60 proof	3 fl. oz.	190	9.5
(Hiram Walker) 52.5 proof	3 fl. oz.	177	12.0
DAIQUIRI MIX (Bar-Tender's)	1 serving (⅝ oz.)	70	17.2
DAMSON PLUM (See **PLUM**)			

(USDA): United States Department of Agriculture
DNA: Data Not Available
*Prepared as Package Directs

Food and Description	Measure or Quantity	Calories	Carbo- hydrates (grams)
DANDELION GREENS, raw (USDA):			
Trimmed	1 lb.	204	41.7
Boiled, drained solids	½ cup (3.2 oz.)	30	6.0
DANISH PASTRY (See **COFFEE CAKE**)			
DANISH-STYLE VEGETABLES, frozen (Birds Eye)	⅓ pkg. (3⅓ oz.)	96	7.6
DATE, dry: Domestic:			
With pits (USDA)	1 lb. (weighed with pits)	1081	287.7
Without pits (USDA)	4 oz.	311	83.0
Without pits, chopped (USDA)	1 cup (6.3 oz.)	488	129.8
California (Cal-Date)	2 oz.	153	42.8
California (Cal-Date)	1 date	35	5.8
California (Garden of the Setting Sun)	5 dates	150	40.5
Chopped (Dromedary)	1 cup (5 oz.)	493	115.2
Pitted (Dromedary)	1 cup (5 oz.)	470	112.6
Imported (Bordo):			
Iraq	4 oz.	359	91.4
Iraq	4 average dates	76	19.3
Dehydrated (Vacu-Dry)	1 oz.	98	26.1
DELAWARE WINE:			
(Gold Seal) 12% alcohol	3 fl. oz.	87	2.4
(Great Western) 12% alcohol	3 fl. oz.	82	3.0
DEVIL DOGS (Drake's)	1 cake	171	24.1
DEVIL'S FOOD CAKE: Home recipe (USDA):			
Without icing	1⁄16 of 10″ layer cake	439	62.4
With chocolate icing	1⁄16 of 10″ layer cake	443	67.0
With uncooked white icing	1⁄16 of 10″ layer cake	442	71.0
Commercial, frozen:			
With chocolate icing (USDA)	2 oz.	215	31.5

(USDA): United States Department of Agriculture
DNA: Data Not Available
*Prepared as Package Directs

Food and Description	Measure or Quantity	Calories	Carbohydrates (grams)
With whipped cream filling & chocolate icing (USDA)	2 oz.	210	24.8
(Pepperidge Farm)	1″ x 3″ piece	174	D.N.A.
DEVIL'S FOOD CAKE MIX:			
Dry (USDA)	4 oz.	460	87.3
*With chocolate icing (USDA)	⅟₁₆ of 9″ cake	234	40.2
(Betty Crocker)	1-lb. 2.5-oz. pkg.	2164	416.2
Butter recipe (Betty Crocker)	1-lb. 2.5-oz. pkg.	2109	431.0
*(Duncan Hines)	1 cake	2337	384.0
*(Duncan Hines)	⅟₁₂ of cake	194	32.0
Red Devil (Pillsbury)	1 oz.	119	21.5
*(Swans Down)	⅟₁₂ of cake	106	36.4
DEWBERRY, fresh (See **BLACKBERRY,** fresh)			
DIAMOND WINE (Great Western) 12% alcohol	3 fl. oz.	76	1.7
DING DONG (Hostess)	1 cake	173	20.8
DINKEY TWINKY (Hostess)	1 cake	152	22.4
DINNER, frozen (See individual listings such as **BEEF DINNER, CHICKEN DINNER, CHINESE DINNER, ENCHILADA DINNER,** etc.)			
DIP:			
Bacon-horseradish, neufchâtel cheese (Kraft) *Ready Dip*	1 oz.	71	.8
Bacon-horseradish, sour cream (Kraft) *Teez*	1 oz.	55	1.4
Blue cheese, neufchâtel cheese (Kraft) *Ready Dip*	1 oz.	69	1.6
Blue cheese, sour cream (Kraft) *Teez*	1 oz.	49	1.4
Clam, neufchâtel cheese (Kraft) *Ready Dip*	1 oz.	66	1.8
Clam, sour cream (Kraft) *Teez*	1 oz.	45	1.5
Dill pickle & neufchâtel cheese (Kraft) *Ready Dip*	1 oz.	67	2.4

(USDA): United States Department of Agriculture
DNA: Data Not Available
*Prepared as Package Directs

Food and Description	Measure or Quantity	Calories	Carbo-hydrates (grams)
Onion:			
(Borden)	1 oz.	48	1.8
Neufchâtel cheese (Kraft) *Ready Dip*	1 oz.	68	2.0
Sour cream (Kraft) *Teez*	1 oz.	46	2.1
(Sealtest)	1 oz.	46	1.5
Tasty Tartar (Borden)	1 oz.	48	1.8
Western Bar B-Q (Borden)	1 oz.	48	1.8
DIP MIX (Lawry's):			
Caesar	1 pkg. (.6 oz.)	53	7.8
Fiesta	1 pkg. (.6 oz.)	49	10.5
Garlic Sociable	1 pkg. (.6 oz.)	56	11.4
Green onion	1 pkg. (.6 oz.)	57	8.3
Guacamole	1 pkg. (.6 oz.)	60	5.5
Toasted onion	1 pkg. (.6 oz.)	46	8.6

DISTILLED LIQUOR. The values below apply to unflavored bourbon whiskey, brandy, Canadian whisky, gin, Irish whiskey, rum, rye whiskey, Scotch whisky, tequila, and vodka. The caloric content of distilled liquors depends on the percentage of alcohol. The proof is twice the alcohol percent and the following values apply to all brands. (USDA):

80 proof	1 fl. oz.	65	Tr.
86 proof	1 fl. oz.	70	Tr.
90 proof	1 fl. oz.	73	Tr.
94 proof	1 fl. oz.	76	Tr.
100 proof	1 fl. oz.	82	Tr.

DOCK, including **SHEEP SORREL:**			
Raw, whole (USDA)	1 lb. (weighed untrimmed)	89	17.8
Boiled, drained solids (USDA)	4 oz.	22	4.4
DOGFISH, spiny, raw, meat only (USDA)	4 oz.	177	0.
DOLLY VARDEN, raw, flesh & skin (USDA)	4 oz.	163	0.

(USDA): United States Department of Agriculture
DNA: Data Not Available
*Prepared as Package Directs

Food and Description	Measure or Quantity	Calories	Carbo-hydrates (grams)
DOUGHNUT:			
Cake type:			
(USDA)	4 oz.	443	58.2
(USDA)	1 piece (1.1 oz.)	125	16.0
(Van de Kamp's)	1 piece (1½ oz.)	174	D.N.A.
Yeast-leavened (USDA)	4 oz.	469	42.3
Chocolate:			
(Hostess)	1 piece (2.1 oz.)	280	D.N.A.
Coated gem (Hostess)	1 piece (.6 oz.)	110	D.N.A.
Long John (Van de Kamp's)	1 piece (2.1 oz.)	179	D.N.A.
Cruller (Van de Kamp's)	1 piece (1½ oz.)	161	D.N.A.
Cruller, old-fashioned (Hostess)	1 piece	100	D.N.A.
Powdered (Morton)	1 piece	75	6.7
Sugared (Hostess):			
Regular	1 piece (1.8 oz.)	233	D.N.A.
Gem, mini	1 piece (½ oz.)	95	D.N.A.
Gem, chocolate inside	1 piece (½ oz.)	100	D.N.A.
Sugar & spice (Morton)	1 piece	76	6.9
DRAMBUIE LIQUEUR, 80 proof (Hiram Walker)	1 fl. oz.	110	11.0
DR. BROWN'S CEL-RAY TONIC, soft drink	6 fl. oz.	66	16.5
DREAMSICLE (Popsicle Industries)	3 fl. oz.	87	D.N.A.
DR. PEPPER, soft drink:			
Regular	6 fl. oz.	71	17.4
Sugar free	6 fl. oz.	2	.4
DRUM, raw (USDA):			
Freshwater:			
Whole	1 lb. (weighed whole)	143	0.
Meat only	4 oz.	137	0.
Red:			
Whole	1 lb. (weighed whole)	149	0.
Meat only	4 oz.	91	0.
DUCK, raw (USDA):			
Domesticated:			
Ready-to-cook	1 lb. (weighed ready-to-cook)	1213	0.

(USDA): United States Department of Agriculture
DNA: Data Not Available
*Prepared as Package Directs

Food and Description	Measure or Quantity	Calories	Carbo-hydrates (grams)
Flesh only	4 oz.	187	0.
Wild:			
Dressed	1 lb. (weighed dressed)	613	0.
Flesh only	4 oz.	156	0.
DUTCH CAKE MIX, Double			
Dutch (Pillsbury)	1 oz.	117	21.5

E

ECLAIR, home recipe, with custard filling & chocolate icing (USDA)	4 oz.	271	26.3
EEL (USDA):			
Raw, meat only	4 oz.	264	0.
Smoked, meat only	4 oz.	374	0.
EGG, CHICKEN (USDA):			
Raw:			
White only	1 large egg	15	Tr.
White only, large	1 cup (9 oz.)	130	2.0
Yolk only	1 large egg	60	Tr.
Yolk only, large	1 cup (8.4 oz.)	835	1.4
Whole, small	1 egg	60	.3
Whole, medium	1 egg	71	.4
Whole, large	1 egg	81	.4
Whole, large	1 cup (8.9 oz.)	409	2.2
Whole, extra large	1 egg	94	.5
Whole, jumbo	1 egg	105	.6
Cooked:			
Boiled	1 large egg	80	Tr.
Fried in fat	1 large egg	100	Tr.
Omelet, mixed with milk & cooked in fat	1 large egg	110	1.5
Poached	1 large egg	80	Tr.
Scrambled, mixed with milk & cooked in fat	1 large egg	110	1.5
Scrambled, mixed with milk & cooked in fat	1 cup (7.8 oz.)	376	4.8
Dried:			
Whole	1 oz.	168	1.2
Whole	1 cup (3.8 oz.)	639	4.4
Yolk	1 cup (3.4 oz.)	637	2.4

(USDA): United States Department of Agriculture
DNA: Data Not Available
*Prepared as Package Directs

Food and Description	Measure or Quantity	Calories	Carbo-hydrates (grams)
EGG, DUCK, raw (USDA)	1 egg	135	.5
EGG, GOOSE, raw (USDA)	1 egg	264	1.9
EGG, TURKEY, raw (USDA)	1 egg	132	1.9
EGG FOO YOUNG, frozen (Chun King)	6 oz. (½ pkg.)	126	D.N.A.
EGG NOG:			
Dairy:			
(Borden) 4.69% fat	½ cup	132	16.3
(Borden) 6.0% fat	½ cup	151	16.3
(Borden) 8.0% fat	½ cup	171	16.3
(Sealtest) 6.8% fat	½ cup	177	17.8
(Sealtest) 8.8% fat	½ cup	195	17.2
With alcohol (Old Mr. Boston) 30 proof	1 fl. oz.	83	4.5
EGGPLANT:			
Raw, whole (USDA)	1 lb. (weighed untrimmed)	92	20.6
Boiled, drained solids (USDA)	4 oz.	22	4.6
Boiled, drained solids, diced (USDA)	1 cup (7 oz.)	38	8.2
Frozen, sticks (Mrs. Paul's)	1 oz.	38	D.N.A.
EGG ROLL, frozen:			
Meat (Chun King)	1 oz.	64	7.8
Shrimp (Chun King)	1 oz.	58	7.6
Shrimp & meat (Chun King)	1 oz.	46	5.7
Shrimp (Hung's)	1 piece	131	15.6
***EGGSTRA** (Tillie Lewis)	½ of 7-oz. dry pkg. (1 large egg)	43	2.2
ELDERBERRY, fresh (USDA):			
Whole	1 lb. (weighed with stems)	307	67.9
Stems removed	4 oz.	82	18.6
ENCHILADA, frozen:			
Beef:			
(Banquet)	5 pieces	936	91.8

(USDA): United States Department of Agriculture
DNA: Data Not Available
*Prepared as Package Directs

Food and Description	Measure or Quantity	Calories	Carbo-hydrates (grams)
With sauce (Banquet) cookin' bag	1 piece (3 oz.)	130	14.5
(Patio)	1 piece (2 in pkg.)	280	D.N.A.
(Patio)	1 piece (8 in pkg.)	150	D.N.A.
Cheese:			
(Patio)	1 piece (2 in pkg.)	166	D.N.A.
(Van de Kamp's)	1 pkg.	387	D.N.A.
Chicken (Van de Kamp's)	1 pkg.	365	D.N.A.
ENCHILADA DINNER, frozen:			
Beef:			
(Banquet)	12-oz. dinner	467	61.0
(Patio)	1 dinner	682	D.N.A.
(Rosarita)	12-oz. dinner	511	D.N.A.
Cheese:			
(Banquet)	12-oz. dinner	482	58.2
(Patio)	1 dinner	418	D.N.A.
(Rosarita)	12-oz. dinner	436	D.N.A.
ENDIVE, BELGIAN or FRENCH (See **CHICORY, WITLOOF**)			
ENDIVE, CURLY, raw (USDA):			
Untrimmed	1 lb. (weighed un-trimmed)	80	16.4
Trimmed	½ lb.	46	9.2
Cut up or shredded	1 cup (2.5 oz.)	14	2.9
ESCAROLE, raw (USDA):			
Untrimmed	1 lb. (weighed un-trimmed)	80	16.4
Trimmed	½ lb.	46	9.2
Cut up or shredded	1 cup (2.5 oz.)	14	2.9
EULACHON or SMELT, raw, flesh only (USDA)	4 oz.	134	0.
EXTRACT (See individual listings)			

F

FARINA (See also *CREAM OF WHEAT*):			
Regular:			
Dry:			
(USDA)	1 oz.	105	21.8
Cream, enriched (H-O)	1 cup	635	135.3

(USDA): United States Department of Agriculture
DNA: Data Not Available
*Prepared as Package Directs

Food and Description	Measure or Quantity	Calories	Carbo-hydrates (grams)
Cream, enriched (H-O)	1 T.	40	8.5
(Pearls of Wheat)	1 cup	608	128.6
Cooked:			
*(USDA)	1 cup (8.4 oz.)	100	21.0
*(USDA)	4 oz.	48	9.9
*(Quaker)	1 cup (1 oz. dry)	100	22.0
Quick-cooking (USDA):			
Dry	1 oz.	103	21.2
Cooked	4 oz.	49	10.1
Instant-cooking (USDA):			
Dry	1 oz.	103	21.2
Cooked	4 oz.	62	12.9
FAT, COOKING, vegetable:			
(USDA)	1 cup	1768	0.
(USDA)	1 T.	110	0.
Snowdrift	1 T.	110	0.
Spry	1 cup	1530	0.
Spry	1 T.	96	0.
FENNEL LEAVES, raw (USDA):			
Untrimmed	1 lb. (weighed un-trimmed)	118	21.5
Trimmed	4 oz.	32	5.8
FESTIVAL MAIN MEAL MEAT, canned (Wilson Sinclair):			
Beef roast	3 oz.	100	0.
Corned beef brisket	3 oz.	135	0.
Ham	3 oz.	129	.8
Picnic	3 oz.	137	.8
Pork loin, smoked	3 oz.	114	.8
Pork roast	3 oz.	133	0.
Turkey & dressing	3 oz.	159	8.5
Turkey roast	3 oz.	87	0.
FIG:			
Fresh:			
(USDA)	1 lb.	363	92.1
Small (USDA)	1.3-oz. fig (1½″ dia.)	30	7.6
Candied (USDA)	1 oz.	85	21.0
Canned, regular pack (USDA):			
Light syrup, solids & liq.	4 oz.	74	19.0

(USDA): United States Department of Agriculture
DNA: Data Not Available
*Prepared as Package Directs

Food and Description	Measure or Quantity	Calories	Carbo- hydrates (grams)
Heavy syrup, solids & liq.	4 oz.	95	24.7
Heavy syrup, solids & liq.	½ cup (4.4 oz.)	106	27.6
Extra heavy syrup, solids & liq.	4 oz.	117	30.3
Canned, unsweetened or dietetic pack:			
Water pack, solids & liq. (USDA)	4 oz.	55	14.0
Kadota, solids & liq. (Diet De- light)	½ cup (4.3 oz.)	58	11.1
Whole, unsweetened (S and W) *Nudradiet*	6 figs (3.5 oz.)	52	12.2
Dehydrated, white, slices (Vacu- Dry)	1 oz.	98	24.4
Dried:			
(USDA)	1 cup (5.9 oz.)	453	114.9
(USDA)	4 oz.	311	78.0
(USDA)	.7-oz. fig (2″ x 1″)	60	15.0
FIG JUICE *Real Fig*	½ cup	61	15.8
FILBERT or HAZELNUT (USDA):			
Whole	1 lb. (weighed in shell)	1323	34.9
Shelled	1 oz.	180	4.8
FINNAN HADDIE (See **HADDOCK,** Smoked)	4 oz.	117	0.
FISH (See individual listings)			
FISH, BREADED, frozen:			
Raw (Sea Pass)	4 oz.	129	D.N.A.
Precooked (Sea Pass)	4 oz.	150	D.N.A.
FISH CAKE:			
Home recipe, fried (USDA)	2 oz.	98	5.2
Frozen:			
Fried, reheated (USDA)	2 oz.	153	9.8
(Commodore)	2 oz.	102	9.8
(Mrs. Paul's)	2 oz.	156	10.0
FISH CRISPS, frozen (Commodore)	1 oz.	64	D.N.A.

(USDA): United States Department of Agriculture
DNA: Data Not Available
*Prepared as Package Directs

Food and Description	Measure or Quantity	Calories	Carbohydrates (grams)
FISH DINNER, frozen:			
(Morton)	8¾-oz. dinner	335	28.2
With French fries (Swanson)	9¾-oz. dinner	429	41.4
FISH FILLETS (Mrs. Paul's)	2 oz.	102	3.8
FISH FLAKES, canned (USDA)	4 oz.	126	0.
FISH LOAF, home recipe, cooked (USDA)	4 oz.	141	8.3
FISH STICK, frozen:			
Cooked, commercial, 3.8″ x 1″ x ½″ sticks (USDA)	10 sticks (8-oz. pkg.)	400	14.8
Cooked (Booth)	1 oz.	50	1.8
(Commodore)	1 oz.	50	1.9
(Mrs. Paul's)	1 oz.	51	1.9
Precooked, breaded (Sea Pass)	1 oz.	41	D.N.A.
FLICK, instant (Ghirardelli)	1 T.	47	10.8
FLIP, soft drink (Dad's)	6 fl. oz.	75	18.4
FLORIDA PUNCH, fruit drink (Hi-C)	6 fl. oz.	98	24.1
FLOUNDER:			
Raw:			
Whole (USDA)	1 lb. (weighed whole)	118	0.
Meat only (USDA)	4 oz.	90	0.
Meat only (Booth)	4 oz.	90	0.
Baked (USDA)	4 oz.	229	0.
Frozen, dinner, low calorie (Taste O'Sea)	1 dinner	200	D.N.A.
FLOUR:			
Buckwheat, dark (USDA)	1 oz.	94	20.4
Buckwheat, light (USDA)	1 oz.	96	22.6
Carob or St. John's-bread (USDA)	1 oz.	51	22.9
Chestnut (USDA)	1 oz.	103	21.6
Corn (USDA)	1 oz.	104	21.8

(USDA): United States Department of Agriculture
DNA: Data Not Available
*Prepared as Package Directs

Food and Description	Measure or Quantity	Calories	Carbo-hydrates (grams)
Cottonseed (Information supplied by General Mills Laboratory)	1 oz.	101	7.7
Fish, from whole fish (USDA)	1 oz.	95	0.
Lima bean (USDA)	1 oz.	97	17.9
Potato (USDA)	1 oz.	100	22.7
Rye:			
Light:			
(USDA)	1 oz.	101	22.1
Unsifted, spooned (USDA)	1 cup (3.6 oz.)	360	78.6
Sifted, spooned (USDA)	1 cup (3.1 oz.)	314	68.6
Medium (USDA)	1 oz.	99	21.2
Dark:			
(USDA)	1 oz.	93	19.3
Unstirred (USDA)	1 cup (4.5 oz.)	418	87.2
Stirred (USDA)	1 cup (4.4 oz.)	415	86.4
Soybean, defatted (USDA)	1 oz.	92	10.8
Soybean, high fat (USDA)	1 oz.	108	9.4
Sunflower seed (USDA)	1 oz.	96	10.7
Wheat:			
All-purpose:			
(USDA)	1 oz.	103	21.6
Unsifted, dipped (USDA)	1 cup (5 oz.)	520	108.8
Unsifted, spooned (USDA)	1 cup (4.4 oz.)	458	95.8
Sifted, spooned (USDA)	1 cup (4 oz.)	422	88.2
Bread:			
(USDA)	1 oz.	104	21.2
Unsifted, dipped (USDA)	1 cup (4.8 oz.)	496	101.6
Unsifted, spooned (USDA)	1 cup (4.3 oz.)	448	91.8
Sifted, spooned (USDA)	1 cup (4.1 oz.)	427	86.6
Cake:			
(USDA)	1 oz.	103	22.5
Unsifted, dipped (USDA)	1 cup (4.2 oz.)	433	94.4
Unsifted, spooned, (USDA)	1 cup (3.9 oz.)	404	88.1
Sifted, spooned (USDA)	1 cup (3.4 oz.)	360	78.6
Gluten:			
(USDA)	1 oz.	107	13.4
Unsifted, dipped (USDA)	1 cup (5 oz.)	536	67.0
Unsifted, spooned (USDA)	1 cup (4.8 oz.)	510	63.7
Sifted, spooned (USDA)	1 cup (4.8 oz.)	514	64.2
Self-rising:			
(USDA)	1 oz.	100	21.0
Unsifted, dipped (USDA)	1 cup (4.6 oz.)	458	96.4
Unsifted, spooned (USDA)	1 cup (4.4 oz.)	447	94.2
Sifted, spooned (USDA)	1 cup (3.7 oz.)	373	78.6

(USDA): United States Department of Agriculture
DNA: Data Not Available
*Prepared as Package Directs

FLOUR (Continued)

Food and Description	Measure or Quantity	Calories	Carbo-hydrates (grams)
Whole (USDA)	1 oz.	94	20.1
Whole, stirred, spooned (USDA)	1 cup (4.8 oz.)	456	97.2
Gold Medal, regular (Betty Crocker)	1 oz.	101	21.2
Gold Medal, self-rising (Betty Crocker)	1 oz.	96	20.7
Red Band, enriched (Betty Crocker)	1 oz.	103	22.0
Red Band, self-rising (Betty Crocker)	1 oz.	98	21.5
Softasilk (Betty Crocker)	1 oz.	102	22.2
Wondra, enriched (Betty Crocker)	1 oz.	101	21.0
FOLLE BLANCHE WINE (Louis M. Martini) 12.5% alcohol	3 fl. oz.	90	.2
FOURNIER NATURE (Gold Seal) 12% alcohol	3 fl. oz.	82	.4

FRANKFURTER:
Raw:

Food and Description	Measure or Quantity	Calories	Carbo-hydrates (grams)
All kinds (USDA)	1 frankfurter (10 per lb.)	140	.8
All meat (USDA)	1 frankfurter (10 per lb.)	133	1.1
With cereal (USDA)	1 frankfurter (10 per lb.)	112	.1
(American Kosher)	1 frankfurter	125	D.N.A.
All meat (Armour Star)	1 frankfurter (10 per lb.)	155	D.N.A.
All beef (Eckrich)	1 frankfurter (1.6 oz.)	152	D.N.A.
All meat (Eckrich)	1 frankfurter (1.6 oz.)	152	D.N.A.
Pure beef (Oscar Mayer)	1 frankfurter	145	D.N.A.
(Vienna)	1 frankfurter	121	1.0
All beef (Wilson)	3 oz.	258	1.5
Skinless (Wilson)	3 oz.	262	1.5
Cooked, all kinds (USDA)	1 frankfurter (10 per lb.)	133	.7
Canned (USDA)	2 oz.	125	.1
Canned (Hormel)	2 oz.	162	.4

FRANKS & BEANS (See **BEANS & FRANKS**)

(USDA): United States Department of Agriculture
DNA: Data Not Available
*Prepared as Package Directs

[150]

Food and Description	Measure or Quantity	Calories	Carbo-hydrates (grams)
FRANKS-N-BLANKETS, frozen (Durkee)	1 piece (.4 oz.)	45	1.0
FRENCH TOAST, frozen (Cardinal)	1 slice (1.5 oz.)	165	D.N.A.
FRESCA, soft drink	6 fl. oz.	<1	<.1
FROG LEGS, raw (USDA):			
Bone in	1 lb. (weighed with bone)	215	0.
Meat only	4 oz.	83	0.
FROOT LOOPS, cereal (Kellogg's)	1 cup (1 oz.)	114	24.1
FROSTED SHAKE, any flavor (Borden)	9¼-oz. can	327	45.0
FROSTING (See **CAKE ICING**)			
FROSTY O's, cereal	¾ cup (1 oz.)	111	23.9
FROZEN CUSTARD (See **ICE CREAM**)			
FROZEN DESSERT, vegetable fat product (Sealtest)	⅙ qt.	180	20.7
FRUIT BOWL SOFT DRINK:			
(Hires)	6 fl. oz.	90	22.5
(Nedick's)	6 fl. oz.	90	22.5
FRUIT CAKE (USDA):			
Dark, home recipe	1.1-oz. piece (2″ x 2″ x ½″)	114	17.9
Light, home recipe	1.1-oz. piece (2″ x 2″ x ½″)	116	17.2
FRUIT COCKTAIL:			
Canned, regular pack, solids & liq.:			
Light syrup (USDA)	4 oz.	68	17.8
Heavy syrup (USDA)	4 oz.	86	22.3
Heavy syrup (USDA)	½ cup (4.5 oz.)	98	25.0
Extra heavy syrup (USDA)	4 oz.	104	26.9
With 2 tablespoons liq. (Dole)	½ cup	72	D.N.A.
(Hunt's)	4 oz.	86	22.3

(USDA): United States Department of Agriculture
DNA: Data Not Available
*Prepared as Package Directs

Food and Description	Measure or Quantity	Calories	Carbo-hydrates (grams)
Canned, unsweetened or dietetic pack:			
Water pack, solids & liq. (USDA)	4 oz.	42	11.0
Solids & liq. (Diet Delight)	½ cup (4.3 oz.)	39	8.1
With 2 tablespoons liq. (Dole)	½ cup	36	D.N.A.
(Libby's)	4 oz.	36	11.0
Unsweetened (S and W) *Nutradiet*	4 oz.	39	12.0
Dehydrated, *Fruit Galaxy* (Vacu-Dry)	1 oz.	96	25.2
FRUITFORT, cereal	1 oz.	112	D.N.A.
FRUIT ICE MIX (See individual sherbet flavors)			
FRUIT, MIXED, frozen, quick thaw (Birds Eye)	½ cup (5 oz.)	141	36.1
FRUIT PIE (Hostess)	4¾-oz. pie	453	57.2
***FRUIT PUNCH MIX** (Wyler's)	6 fl. oz.	63	15.7
FRUIT SALAD:			
Bottled chilled (Kraft)	4 oz.	58	12.6
Canned, regular pack, solids & liq. (USDA):			
Light syrup	4 oz.	67	17.6
Heavy syrup	1 cup (8.6 oz.)	184	47.7
Heavy syrup	4 oz.	85	22.0
Extra heavy syrup	4 oz.	102	26.5
Canned, unsweetened or dietetic pack:			
Water pack, solids & liq. (USDA)	4 oz.	40	10.3
Solids & liq. (Diet Delight)	½ cup (4.4 oz.)	31	6.9
(White Rose)	4 oz.	42	10.1
FRUIT-SICLE (Popsicle Industries)	2½ fl. oz.	59	D.N.A.
FUDGE CAKE MIX:			
*Butter recipe (Duncan Hines)	1 cake	3248	432.0
Cherry (Betty Crocker)	1-lb. 2.5-oz. pkg.	2164	410.7

(USDA): United States Department of Agriculture
DNA: Data Not Available
*Prepared as Package Directs

Food and Description	Measure or Quantity	Calories	Carbo-hydrates (grams)
Cherry (Betty Crocker)	1 oz.	117	22.5
Chocolate (Pillsbury)	1 oz.	120	22.1
Dark chocolate (Betty Crocker)	1-lb. 2.5-oz. pkg.	2164	410.7
Dark chocolate (Betty Crocker)	1 oz.	117	22.2
Macaroon (Pillsbury)	1 oz.	124	21.2
*Marble (Duncan Hines)	1 cake	2313	384.0
Sour cream, chocolate flavor (Betty Crocker)	1-lb. 2.5-oz. pkg.	2109	412.6
Sour cream, chocolate flavor (Betty Crocker)	1 oz.	114	22.3
Sour cream flavor (Pillsbury)	1 oz.	118	21.2
Toffee, batter cake (Pillsbury)	1 oz.	119	21.7
FUDGE PUDDING MIX (Thank You)	½ cup	202	25.7
FUDGSICLE, chocolate (Popsicle Industries)	2½ fl. oz.	110	22.4

G

GARBANZO, dry (See **CHICK-PEA,** dry)			
GARBANZO SOUP, canned (Hormel)	15-oz. can	461	30.6
GARLIC, raw (USDA):			
Whole	2 oz. (weighed with skin)	68	15.4
Peeled	1 oz.	38	8.7
GARLIC SPREAD (Lawry's):	1 T.	80	1.2
GAZPACHO SOUP, canned (Crosse & Blackwell)	½ can (6½ oz.)	61	6.8
GEFILTE FISH, canned:			
(Horowitz-Margareten)	1 piece	75	D.N.A.
(Manischewitz)	1 piece (4 oz.)	110	4.2
Jumbo (Manischewitz)	1 piece (2.4 oz.)	64	2.5
Whitefish & pike (Manischewitz)	1 piece (1.8 oz.)	40	1.6

(USDA): United States Department of Agriculture
DNA: Data Not Available
*Prepared as Package Directs

Food and Description	Measure or Quantity	Calories	Carbohydrates (grams)
GELATIN, unflavored, dry:			
(USDA)	1 oz.	95	0.
(USDA)	1 T.	34	0.
(Knox)	1 envelope	28	0.
GELATIN DESSERT POWDER:			
Regular:			
(USDA)	1 oz.	105	24.9
(USDA)	½ cup (3.3 oz.)	347	82.3
*Prepared (USDA)	4 oz.	67	16.0
*Prepared (USDA)	½ cup (4.2 oz.)	70	16.8
*Prepared with fruit added (USDA)	4 oz.	76	18.6
*Prepared with fruit added (USDA)	½ cup (4.2 oz.)	80	19.8
*All fruit flavors (Jell-O)	½ cup (4.9 oz.)	81	18.6
*All flavors (Jells Best)	½ cup	80	18.7
*All flavors (Royal)	½ cup (4.6 oz.)	80	17.7
Dietetic or low calorie:			
*All flavors (D-Zerta)	½ cup (4.3 oz.)	10	0.
*All flavors (Dia-Mel)	4 oz.	11	0.
GELATIN DRINK, any flavor (Knox)	1 envelope	79	14.0
GERMAN DINNER, frozen (Swanson)	11-oz. pkg.	405	42.2
GEVREY-CHAMBERTIN, French red Burgundy (Cruse) 12% alcohol	3 fl. oz.	72	D.N.A.
GEWURZTRAMINER WINE:			
(Louis M. Martini) 12.5% alcohol	3 fl. oz.	90	.2
(Willm) Alsatian, 11-14% alcohol	3 fl. oz.	66	3.6
(Willm) *Clos Gaensbronnel*, 11-14% alcohol	3 fl. oz.	66	3.6
GIN, Unflavored (See **DISTILLED LIQUOR**)			
GIN, FLAVORED:			
Lemon (Old Mr. Boston) 70 proof	1 fl. oz.	76	1.4
Mint (Leroux) 70 proof	1 fl. oz.	70	2.8
Mint (Old Mr. Boston) 70 proof	1 fl. oz.	100	8.0

(USDA): United States Department of Agriculture
DNA: Data Not Available
*Prepared as Package Directs

Food and Description	Measure or Quantity	Calories	Carbo-hydrates (grams)
Orange (Leroux) 70 proof	1 fl. oz.	70	2.8
Orange (Old Mr. Boston) 70 proof	1 fl. oz.	76	1.4
GIN, SLOE:			
(Bols) 66 proof	1 fl. oz.	85	4.7
(Garnier) 60 proof	1 fl. oz.	83	8.5
(Hiram Walker) 60 proof	1 fl. oz.	68	4.8
(Leroux) 60 proof	1 fl. oz.	74	6.0
(Old Mr. Boston) 42 proof	1 fl. oz.	50	2.0
(Old Mr. Boston) 70 proof	1 fl. oz.	76	1.4
GINGER ALE, soft drink:			
Sweetened:			
(Canada Dry)	6 fl. oz.	64	16.5
(Clicquot Club)	6 fl. oz.	65	15.3
(Cott)	6 fl. oz.	65	15.3
(Dr. Brown's)	6 fl. oz.	60	15.0
Fanta	6 fl. oz.	63	15.0
(Hoffman)	6 fl. oz.	60	15.0
(Key Food)	6 fl. oz.	60	15.0
(Kirsch)	6 fl. oz.	59	14.8
(Mission)	6 fl. oz.	65	15.3
(Schweppes)	6 fl. oz.	66	16.2
(Shasta)	6 fl. oz.	65	16.5
(Vernors)	6 fl. oz.	70	17.4
(Waldbaum)	6 fl. oz.	60	15.0
(White Rock)	6 fl. oz.	60	D.N.A.
(Yukon Club)	6 fl. oz.	62	15.3
Low calorie:			
(Dr. Brown's) *Slim Ray*	6 fl. oz.	3	.8
(Hoffman)	6 fl. oz.	3	.8
(No-Cal)	6 fl. oz.	2	<.1
(Shasta)	6 fl. oz.	<1	<.1
(Vernors)	6 fl. oz.	1	0.
GINGER BEER, soft drink:			
(Canada Dry)	6 fl. oz.	71	18.4
(Schweppes)	6 fl. oz.	72	17.6
GINGERBREAD, home recipe			
(USDA)	1.9-oz. piece (2″ x 2″ x 2″)	174	28.6

(USDA): United States Department of Agriculture
DNA: Data Not Available
*Prepared as Package Directs

Food and Description	Measure or Quantity	Calories	Carbo-hydrates (grams)
GINGERBREAD MIX:			
Dry (USDA)	4 oz.	482	88.7
*Prepared (USDA)	2 oz.	156	29.0
(Betty Crocker)	14.5-oz. pkg.	1696	323.4
(Betty Crocker)	1 oz.	117	22.3
*(Dromedary)	1.2-oz. piece (1″ x 4″)	100	18.9
(Pillsbury)	1 oz.	110	22.1
GINGER, CANDIED, (USDA)	1 oz.	96	24.7
GINGER ROOT, fresh (USDA):			
With skin	1 oz.	13	2.5
Without skin	1 oz.	14	2.7
GIN SOUR COCKTAIL (Calvert)			
60 proof	3 fl. oz.	195	10.4
GOLD-O-MINT LIQUEUR			
(Leroux) 25 proof	1 fl. oz.	110	15.2
GOOD HUMOR:			
Bar, ice cream:			
Chocolate chip	1 piece (3 fl. oz.)	239	D.N.A.
Chocolate chip candy, *Super Humor*	1 piece	383	D.N.A.
Chocolate eclair	1 piece (3 fl. oz.)	217	D.N.A.
Choclate fudge cake, *Super Humor*	1 piece	345	D.N.A.
Chocolate malt	1 piece	205	13.6
Toasted almond	1 piece (3 fl. oz.)	234	D.N.A.
Vanilla	1 piece	202	13.2
Cone:			
Ice cream, chocolate burst	1 piece	165	D.N.A.
Ice milk, chocolate	1 piece	88	D.N.A.
Ice milk, vanilla	1 piece	85	D.N.A.
Cup:			
Ice:			
Bon Joy Swirl	1 piece	138	D.N.A.
Italian	1 piece	232	D.N.A.
Venetian	1 piece	115	D.N.A.
Ice cream:			
Chocolate	3 oz.	113	D.N.A.
Chocolate	5 oz.	189	D.N.A.
Vanilla	3 oz.	110	11.6

(USDA): United States Department of Agriculture
DNA: Data Not Available
*Prepared as Package Directs

Food and Description	Measure or Quantity	Calories	Carbo- hydrates (grams)
Vanilla	5 oz.	183	D.N.A.
Frostee Humor bar	1 piece	150	D.N.A.
Frostee shake	1 piece	287	D.N.A.
Humorette	1 piece	103	D.N.A.
Ice Stix:			
Chocolate	1 piece	119	D.N.A.
Chocolate, double	1 piece	151	D.N.A.
Fruit	1 piece	89	D.N.A.
Fruit, double	1 piece	138	D.N.A.
Lollie Jets	1 piece	109	D.N.A.
Wahoos	1 piece	52	D.N.A.
X-5 Jetstars	1 piece	57	D.N.A.
Pint, deluxe French	1 oz.	50	D.N.A.
Sandwich, without crackers:			
Ice cream, grocery pack:			
Chocolate	1 piece	53	D.N.A.
Vanilla	1 piece	51	D.N.A.
Ice milk	1 piece	88	D.N.A.
Sundae:			
Bittersweet	1 piece	282	D.N.A.
Chocolate nut fudge supreme	1 piece	448	D.N.A.
Strawberry	1 piece	221	D.N.A.
Whammy:			
Fruit ice	1 piece (1¾ fl. oz.)	40	D.N.A.
Ice cream	1 piece (1¾ fl. oz.)	140	D.N.A.
Ice milk	1 piece (1¾ fl. oz.)	128	D.N.A.
GOOSE, domesticated (USDA):			
Raw	1 lb. (weighed ready-to-cook)	1172	0.
Roasted, flesh & skin	4 oz.	500	0.
Roasted, flesh only	4 oz.	264	0.
GOOSEBERRY (USDA):			
Fresh	1 lb.	177	44.0
Fresh	1 cup (5.2 oz.)	58	14.6
Canned, water pack, solids & liq.	4 oz.	30	7.5
GOOSE GIZZARD, raw (USDA)	4 oz.	158	0.
GOULASH DINNER (Chef Boy-Ar-Dee)	7⅛-oz. pkg.	263	32.4
GRAACHER HIMMELREICH, German Moselle (Julius Kayser) 10% alcohol	3 fl. oz.	60	2.5

(USDA): United States Department of Agriculture
DNA: Data Not Available
*Prepared as Package Directs

Food and Description	Measure or Quantity	Calories	Carbo-hydrates (grams)
GRAHAM CRACKER (See **CRACKER**)			
GRANADILLA (See **PASSION FRUIT**)			
GRAPE:			
Fresh:			
American type (slip skin), Concord, Delaware, Niagara, Catawba & Scuppernong:			
(USDA)	½ lb. (weighed with stem, skin & seeds)	99	22.5
(USDA)	½ cup (2.7 oz.)	33	7.5
(USDA)	3½″ x 3″ bunch (3.5 oz.)	69	15.7
European type (adherent skin), Malaga, Muscat, Thompson seedless, Emperor & Flame Tokay:			
(USDA)	½ lb. (weighed with stem & seeds)	135	34.9
Whole (USDA)	20 grapes (¾″ dia.)	54	13.8
Whole (USDA)	½ cup (3 oz.)	58	15.0
Halves (USDA)	½ cup (3 oz.)	57	14.8
Canned, solids & liq. (USDA):			
Thompson seedless, heavy syrup	4 oz.	87	22.7
Thompson seedless, water pack	4 oz.	58	15.4
GRAPEADE (Sealtest)	6 fl. oz.	94	24.3
GRAPE DRINK (Hi-C)	6 fl. oz.	88	21.8
***GRAPE DRINK MIX:**			
(Salada)	6 fl. oz.	80	19.4
(Wyler's)	6 fl. oz.	63	15.8
GRAPE JAM, dietetic (Dia-Mel)	1 T.	22	5.4
GRAPE JELLY, dietetic or low calorie:			
(Dia-Mel)	1 T.	22	5.4
Concord (Diet Delight)	1 T.	6	.6
(Kraft)	1 oz.	14	3.3

(USDA): United States Department of Agriculture
DNA: Data Not Available
*Prepared as Package Directs

Food and Description	Measure or Quantity	Calories	Carbohydrates (grams)
(Slenderella)	1 T.	21	5.4
(Tillie Lewis)	1 T.	9	2.1
GRAPE JUICE:			
Canned:			
(USDA)	½ cup (4.5 oz.)	84	21.1
(Heinz)	5½-oz. can	112	27.0
(Seneca)	½ cup	76	18.8
Sweetened (Seneca)	½ cup	104	26.0
Unsweetened (S and W)			
Nutradiet	4 oz.	68	17.4
Frozen, concentrate, sweetened:			
(USDA)	6-fl.-oz. can	395	100.0
*Diluted (USDA)	½ cup	66	16.6
*(Minute Maid)	½ cup	66	16.7
*(Seneca)	½ cup	60	15.6
*(Snow Crop)	½ cup	66	16.7
GRAPE JUICE DRINK, canned:			
(USDA)	6 fl. oz.	101	25.9
Grape-apple (BC)	6 fl. oz.	108	D.N.A.
GRAPE-NUTS, cereal	¼ cup (1 oz.)	100	23.0
GRAPE-NUTS FLAKES, cereal	⅔ cup (1 oz.)	100	23.0
GRAPE PIE (Tastykake)	4-oz. pie	369	51.8
GRAPE SOFT DRINK:			
Sweetened:			
(Canada Dry)	6 fl. oz.	93	24.2
(Clicquot Club)	6 fl. oz.	105	25.1
(Cott)	6 fl. oz.	105	25.1
(Dr. Brown's)	6 fl. oz.	88	21.9
(Dr. Pepper)	6 fl. oz.	102	25.8
Fanta	6 fl. oz.	96	24.0
Grapette	6 fl. oz.	91	23.0
(Hires)	6 fl. oz.	96	24.0
(Hoffman)	6 fl. oz.	96	24.0
(Key Food)	6 fl. oz.	88	21.9
(Mission)	6 fl. oz.	105	25.1
(Nedick's)	6 fl. oz.	96	24.0
(Shasta)	6 fl. oz.	88	22.2
(Waldbaum)	6 fl. oz.	88	21.9

(USDA): United States Department of Agriculture
DNA: Data Not Available
*Prepared as Package Directs

Food and Description	Measure or Quantity	Calories	Carbo-hydrates (grams)
(White Rock)	6 fl. oz.	90	D.N.A.
(Yoo-Hoo)	6 fl. oz.	90	18.0
High-protein (Yoo-Hoo)	6 fl. oz.	114	24.6
(Yukon Club)	6 fl. oz.	96	24.0
Low calorie:			
(Hoffman)	6 fl. oz.	3	.8
(No-Cal)	6 fl. oz.	2	0.
(Shasta)	6 fl. oz.	<1	<.1
GRAPE SYRUP, dietetic (No-Cal)	1 tsp.	<1	Tr.
GRAPEFRUIT:			
Fresh:			
White:			
(USDA)	1 lb. (weighed with seeds & skin)	84	22.0
Seedless type (USDA)	1 lb. (weighed with skin)	87	22.4
(USDA)	½ med. grape-fruit (4¼″ dia.)	55	14.0
(Sunkist)	½ grapefruit	44	11.0
Sections (USDA)	1 cup (7 oz.)	78	20.2
Pink and red:			
(USDA)	1 lb. (weighed with seeds & skin)	87	22.6
Seedless type (USDA)	1 lb. (weighed with skin)	93	24.1
(USDA)	½ med. grapefruit (4¼″ dia.)	60	15.0
Chilled sections (Kraft)	4 oz.	58	12.6
Canned, regular pack, solids & liq. (USDA)	½ cup (4.5 oz.)	90	22.8
Canned, unsweetened or dietetic pack:			
Water pack, solids & liq. (USDA)	½ cup (4.2 oz.)	35	9.0
Solids & liq. (Diet Delight)	½ cup (4.3 oz.)	37	7.3
(Tillie Lewis)	½ cup (4 oz.)	42	10.4
GRAPEFRUIT DRINK (Sealtest)	6 fl. oz.	80	20.0
GRAPEFRUIT JUICE:			
Fresh, pink, red or white, all varieties (USDA)	½ cup (4.3 oz.)	48	11.3

(USDA): United States Department of Agriculture
DNA: Data Not Available
*Prepared as Package Directs

Food and Description	Measure or Quantity	Calories	Carbo-hydrates (grams)
Chilled (Kraft)	½ cup	48	11.1
Canned:			
Sweetened:			
(USDA)	½ cup	65	16.0
(Heinz)	5½-oz. can	62	14.4
(Stokely-Van Camp)	½ cup	65	16.0
(Treesweet)	½ cup	62	D.N.A.
Unsweetened:			
(USDA)	½ cup	50	12.0
(Diet Delight)	½ cup (4.3 oz.)	50	9.7
(Stokely-Van Camp)	½ cup	50	12.0
Pink (Texsun)	½ cup	52	16.1
Frozen, concentrate:			
Sweetened:			
(USDA)	6-oz. can	350	85.0
*Diluted with 3 parts water			
(USDA)	½ cup	58	14.0
*(Minute Maid)	½ cup	58	14.0
*(Snow Crop)	½ cup	58	14.0
*(Treesweet)	½ cup	62	D.N.A.
Unsweetened:			
(USDA)	6-oz. can	300	72.0
*Diluted with 3 parts water			
(USDA)	½ cup	50	12.0
*(Birds Eye)	½ cup (4.2 oz.)	48	12.9
*(Florida Diet)	½ cup	50	10.8
*(Minute Maid)	½ cup	50	12.2
*(7L)	½ cup	50	12.0
*(Snow Crop)	½ cup	50	12.2
Dehydrated, crystals:			
(USDA)	4-oz. can	431	102.9
*Reconstituted (USDA)	½ cup (4.4 oz.)	50	13.0

GRAPEFRUIT-ORANGE JUICE
(USDA):

Canned, unsweetened	½ cup	54	12.5
Canned, sweetened	½ cup	62	15.2
Frozen, concentrate, unsweetened	6-oz. can	327	77.2
*Frozen, concentrate, unsweetened	½ cup	55	13.1

GRAPEFRUIT PEEL, CANDIED:

(USDA)	1 oz.	89	22.9
(Liberty)	1 oz.	93	22.6

(USDA): United States Department of Agriculture
DNA: Data Not Available
*Prepared as Package Directs

Food and Description	Measure or Quantity	Calories	Carbo-hydrates (grams)
GRAPEFRUIT SOFT DRINK:			
Sweetened, golden (Canada Dry)	6 fl. oz.	82	21.3
Sweetened, *Fanta*	6 fl. oz.	87	21.0
Low calorie, pink:			
(Hoffman)	6 fl. oz.	3	.8
(No-Cal)	6 fl. oz.	2	<.1
(Royal Crown)	6 fl. oz.	2	.5
GRAVES WINE (See also individual regional, vineyard or brand names)			
(Barton & Guestier) 12.5% alcohol	3 fl. oz.	65	.6
(Cruse) 11.5% alcohol	3 fl. oz.	69	D.N.A.
GRAVY, canned:			
Beef (Franco-American)	4 oz.	89	7.2
Chicken (Franco-American)	4 oz.	100	6.2
Chicken giblet (Franco-American)	4 oz.	54	5.6
Giblet (Lynden)	7¾-oz. can	264	16.0
Mushroom (B in B)	½ cup	88	D.N.A.
Mushroom (Franco-American)	4 oz.	57	5.7
Mushroom, brown (Green Giant)	4 oz.	37	D.N.A.
GRAVY MASTER	1 fl. oz.	50	8.5
GRAVY with MEAT or TURKEY, canned or frozen:			
Beef chunks (Bunker Hill)	15-oz. can	788	16.0
Chopped beef (Bunker Hill)	10½-oz. can	516	10.0
Sliced beef (Bunker Hill)	15-oz. can	716	16.0
Sliced beef, buffet, frozen (Banquet)	2 lb.	956	21.2
Sliced beef, cookin' bag, frozen (Banquet)	5 oz.	158	4.2
Sliced beef liver (Bunker Hill)	15-oz. can	398	30.0
Sliced turkey, buffet, frozen (Banquet)	2 lb.	677	22.0
GRAVY MIX:			
Beef:			
(Swiss)	1¼-oz. pkg.	107	22.6
(Swiss)	⅞-oz. pkg.	75	15.8
(Wyler's)	1-oz. pkg.	D.N.A.	16.0
Brown:			
*(Durkee)	1 cup (1-oz. dry pkg.)	79	11.2

(USDA): United States Department of Agriculture
DNA: Data Not Available
*Prepared as Package Directs

Food and Description	Measure or Quantity	Calories	Carbo-hydrates (grams)
(French's)	¾-oz. pkg.	72	9.6
*(Kraft)	1 oz.	11	1.4
(Lawry's)	1¼-oz. pkg.	136	16.3
(McCormick)	⅞-oz. pkg.	100	10.0
*(McCormick)	2-oz. serving	25	2.5
Chicken:			
*(Durkee)	1 cup (1.2-oz. dry pkg.)	104	11.2
(French's)	1¼-oz. pkg.	126	14.7
(Lawry's)	1-oz. pkg.	110	13.6
(McCormick)	⅞-oz. pkg.	95	D.N.A.
*(McCormick)	2-oz. serving	20	3.0
(Swiss)	1¼-oz. pkg.	107	22.7
(Swiss)	⅞-oz. pkg.	75	15.9
(Wyler's)	1-oz. pkg.	D.N.A.	15.0
*Herb (McCormick)	2-oz. serving	22	2.5
Mushroom:			
*(Durkee)	1 cup (1-oz. dry pkg.)	100	13.6
(French's)	¾-oz. pkg.	16	6.0
(Lawry's)	1.3-oz. pkg.	145	15.6
*(McCormick)	2-oz. serving	17	2.5
(Wyler's)	¾-oz. pkg.	D.N.A.	8.0
Onion:			
*(Durkee)	1 cup (1-oz. dry pkg.)	112	14.4
(French's)	1-oz. pkg.	72	12.0
*(Kraft)	1 oz.	11	1.9
*(McCormick)	2-oz. serving	29	3.5
(Wyler's)	¾-oz. pkg.	D.N.A.	11.0

GREEN PEA (See **PEA**)

GRENADINE SYRUP:

(Garnier) non-alcoholic	1 fl. oz.	103	26.0
(Giroux) non-alcoholic	1 fl. oz.	100	25.0
(Leroux) 25 proof	1 fl. oz.	81	15.2

GRITS (See **HOMINY GRITS**)

GROUND-CHERRY, Poha or Cape Gooseberry:

Whole (USDA)	1 lb. (weighed with husks & stems)	221	46.7
Flesh only (USDA)	4 oz.	60	12.7

(USDA): United States Department of Agriculture
DNA: Data Not Available
*Prepared as Package Directs

Food and Description	Measure or Quantity	Calories	Carbohydrates (grams)
GROUPER, raw (USDA):			
Whole	1 lb. (weighed whole)	170	0.
Meat only	4 oz.	99	0.
GUAVA, COMMON, fresh:			
Whole (USDA)	1 lb. (weighed untrimmed)	273	66.0
Whole (USDA)	1 guava (2.8 oz.)	50	12.0
Flesh only (USDA)	4 oz.	70	17.0
GUAVA, STRAWBERRY, fresh:			
Whole (USDA)	1 lb. (weighed untrimmed)	289	70.2
Flesh only (USDA)	4 oz.	74	17.9
GUINEA HEN, raw (USDA):			
Ready-to-cook	1 lb. (weighed ready-to-cook)	594	0.
Flesh & skin	4 oz.	179	0.

H

HADDOCK:			
Raw:			
Whole (USDA)	1 lb. (weighed whole)	172	0.
Meat only (USDA)	4 oz.	90	0.
Meat only (Booth)	4 oz.	90	0.
Fried (USDA)	4 oz.	187	6.6
Fried (USDA)	4″ x 3″ x ½″ fillet (3.5 oz.)	165	5.8
Frozen (Taste O'Sea)	4 oz.	80	0.
*Smoked, canned or not (USDA)	4 oz.	117	0.
HADDOCK DINNER, frozen:			
(Banquet)	9-oz. dinner	424	44.8
(Swanson)	12¼-oz. dinner	397	36.5
Low calorie (Taste O'Sea)	12-oz. dinner	245	D.N.A.
HAKE, raw (USDA):			
Whole	1 lb. (weighed whole)	144	0.
Meat only	4 oz.	84	0.

(USDA): United States Department of Agriculture
DNA: Data Not Available
*Prepared as Package Directs

Food and Description	Measure or Quantity	Calories	Carbo-hydrates (grams)
HALF & HALF (milk & cream) (See **CREAM**)			
HALF & HALF SOFT DRINK:			
Sweetened:			
(Canada Dry)	6 fl. oz.	82	21.4
(Dr. Brown's)	6 fl. oz.	75	18.8
(Hoffman)	6 fl. oz.	78	19.5
(Kirsch)	6 fl. oz.	81	20.3
(Yukon Club)	6 fl. oz.	90	22.5
Low calorie (Hoffman)	6 fl. oz.	3	.8
HALF & HALF WINE:			
(Gallo) 20% alcohol	3 fl. oz.	100	5.7
(Lejon) 18.5% alcohol	3 fl. oz.	116	6.7
HALIBUT:			
Atlantic & Pacific:			
Raw:			
Whole (USDA)	1 lb. (weighed whole)	268	0.
Meat only (USDA)	4 oz.	114	0.
Broiled (USDA)	4 oz.	194	0.
Broiled (USDA)	4″ x 3″ x ½″ steak (4.4 oz.)	214	0.
Smoked (USDA)	4 oz.	254	0.
California, raw meat only (USDA)	4 oz.	110	0.
Greenland, raw (USDA):			
Whole	1 lb. (weighed whole)	344	0.
Meat only	4 oz.	166	0.
Frozen, Northern (Van de Kamp's)	1 pkg.	477	D.N.A.
HAM (See also **PORK**):			
Cooked:			
Luncheon meat (USDA)	1 oz.	66	0.
Slice pak (Oscar Mayer)	1 slice	24	D.N.A.
Canned:			
(USDA)	1 oz.	55	3
(Armour Golden Star)	1 oz.	36	D.N.A.
(Armour Star)	1 oz.	53	D.N.A.

(USDA): United States Department of Agriculture
DNA: Data Not Available
*Prepared as Package Directs

Food and Description	Measure or Quantity	Calories	Carbohydrates (grams)
(Hormel)	1 oz. (8-lb. can)	57	.2
(Hormel)	1 oz. (6-lb. 8-oz. can)	44	.2
(Hormel)	1 oz. (4-lb. can)	48	.2
(Hormel)	1 oz. (1-lb. 8-oz. can)	48	.2
(Oscar Mayer)	1 oz.	43	D.N.A.
(Wilson)	1 oz.	45	.3
(Wilson) *Corn King*	1 oz.	49	.3
Chopped, canned:			
(USDA)	1 oz.	65	1.2
(Armour Star)	12-oz. can	996	4.4
(Hormel)	1 oz. (8-lb. can)	69	.3
(Hormel)	1 oz. (12-oz. can)	71	.4
Deviled, canned:			
(USDA)	1 oz.	99	0.
(Armour Star)	1 oz.	79	0.
(Hormel)	1 oz. (3-oz. can)	73	.2
(Underwood)	1 T.	45	Tr.
Frozen, sliced with barbecue sauce			
(Banquet) cookin' bag	4½ oz.	184	19.0
Smoked, canned (Oscar Mayer)	3 oz.	170	D.N.A.
Spiced, canned:			
(USDA)	1 oz.	83	.4
(Hormel)	1 oz. (3-lb. can)	52	.1
(Hormel)	1 oz. (5-lb. can)	78	.4
HAM CHEDDERTON (Lipton)	1 pkg. (5⅝ oz.)	654	91.5
HAM DINNER, frozen:			
(Banquet)	10-oz. dinner	352	53.2
(Morton)	10-oz. dinner	383	54.4
(Swanson)	10¼-oz. dinner	366	42.1
HAMBURGER (See **BEEF,** Ground)			
HAWAIIAN PUNCH, soft drink	6 fl. oz.	83	20.6
HAWS, SCARLET, raw (USDA):			
Whole	1 lb. (weighed with core)	316	75.5
Flesh & skin	4 oz.	99	23.6
HAZELNUT (See **FILBERT**)			

(USDA): United States Department of Agriculture
DNA: Data Not Available
*Prepared as Package Directs

Food and Description	Measure or Quantity	Calories	Carbo-hydrates (grams)
HEADCHEESE:			
(USDA)	1 oz.	76	.3
(Sugardale)	1-oz. slice	77	Tr.
HEART (USDA):			
Beef:			
Lean, raw	1 lb.	490	3.2
Lean, braised	4 oz.	213	.8
Lean with visible fat, raw	1 lb.	1148	.5
Lean with visible fat, braised	4 oz.	422	.1
Calf, raw	1 lb.	562	8.2
Calf, braised	4 oz.	236	2.0
Chicken, raw	1 lb.	608	.5
Chicken, simmered	4 oz.	196	.1
Hog, raw	1 lb.	513	1.8
Hog, braised	4 oz.	221	.3
Lamb, raw	1 lb.	735	4.5
Lamb, braised	4 oz.	295	1.1
Turkey, raw	1 lb.	776	.9
Turkey, simmered	4 oz.	245	.2
HERB SAUCE CASSEROLE			
BASE (Pennsylvania Dutch)	6¾-oz. pkg. (3 cups cooked)	854	116.1
HERRING (USDA):			
Raw:			
Atlantic, whole	1 lb. (weighed whole)	407	0.
Atlantic, meat only	4 oz.	200	0.
Pacific, meat only	4 oz.	111	0.
Canned:			
Plain, solids & liq.	4 oz.	236	0.
In tomato sauce, solids & liq.	4 oz.	200	4.2
Pickled, Bismarck type	4 oz.	253	0.
Salted or brined	4 oz.	247	0.
Smoked:			
Bloaters	4 oz.	222	0.
Hard	4 oz.	340	0.
Kippered	4 oz.	239	0.
HICKORY NUT (USDA):			
Whole	1 lb. (weighed in shell)	1068	20.3
Shelled	4 oz.	764	14.5

(USDA): United States Department of Agriculture
DNA: Data Not Available
*Prepared as Package Directs

Food and Description	Measure or Quantity	Calories	Carbo-hydrates (grams)
HI-SPOT, soft drink (Canada Dry)	6 fl. oz.	73	18.8
HO-HO (Hostess)	1 cake	120	16.1
HOMINY GRITS:			
Dry:			
(USDA)	1 oz.	103	22.1
(USDA)	½ cup (2.8 oz.)	282	60.9
(Aunt Jemima)	⅙ cup (1 oz.)	103	23.0
(Quaker)	⅙ cup (1 oz.)	103	23.0
Cooked:			
Degermed (USDA)	⅔ cup (5.6 oz.)	82	17.7
Enriched (Albers)	⅔ cup	82	17.7
Quick or regular (Aunt Jemima)	⅔ cup	103	23.0
Quick or regular (Quaker)	⅔ cup	103	23.0
HONEY, strained:			
(USDA)	½ cup (5.7 oz.)	496	134.1
(USDA)	1 T.	64	17.3
HONEY CAKE (Holland Honey Cake)	½" slice	63	D.N.A.
HONEYCOMB, cereal (Post)	1 cup	83	18.8
HONEYDEW, fresh (USDA):			
Whole	1 lb. (weighed whole)	94	22.0
Wedge	2" x 7" wedge (5.2 oz.)	50	12.8
Flesh only	4 oz.	37	8.7
Flesh only, diced	1 cup (5.9 oz.)	55	12.9
HORSERADISH:			
Raw (USDA):			
Whole	1 lb. (weighed un-pared)	288	65.2
Pared	1 oz.	25	5.6
Dehydrated (Heinz)	1 T.	26	5.2
Prepared:			
(USDA)	1 oz.	11	2.7
(Gold's)	1 tsp.	3	D.N.A.
(Kraft)	1 oz.	7	.4
Cream style (Kraft)	1 oz.	23	.7
Oil style (Kraft)	1 oz.	23	.5

(USDA): United States Department of Agriculture
DNA: Data Not Available
*Prepared as Package Directs

Food and Description	Measure or Quantity	Calories	Carbohydrates (grams)
HOT DOG BEAN SOUP, condensed (Campbell)	8 oz. (by wt.)	347	40.8
HYACINTH BEAN (USDA):			
Young pod, raw:			
Whole	1 lb. (weighed untrimmed)	140	29.1
Trimmed	4 oz.	40	8.3
Dry seeds	4 oz.	383	69.2

I

Food and Description	Measure or Quantity	Calories	Carbohydrates (grams)
ICE CREAM and **FROZEN CUSTARD** (See also listing by flavor or brand name, e.g., **CHOCOLATE ICE CREAM** or *DREAMSICLE* or *GOOD HUMOR*)			
Sweetened:			
10% fat (USDA)	8 oz. (by wt.)	438	47.2
12% fat (USDA)	1 pt. (10 oz. by wt.)	588	58.5
12% fat (USDA)	2½-oz. slice (⅛ of qt. brick)	147	14.6
12% fat (USDA)	Small container (3½ fl. oz.)	128	12.8
16% fat (USDA)	8 oz. (by wt.)	504	40.9
Deluxe (Carnation)	1 pt.	537	64.5
Dietetic (Carnation)	1 pt.	480	D.N.A.
ICE CREAM BAR, chocolate-coated:			
(Popsicle Industries)	3 fl. oz.	180	D.N.A.
(Rosedale)	3 oz.	180	D.N.A.
(Sealtest)	1 bar (3 fl. oz.)	162	14.5
ICE CREAM CONE, cone only:			
(USDA)	1 oz.	107	22.1
(Comet)	1 piece (5 grams)	19	3.9
Assorted colors (Comet)	1 piece (5 grams)	19	3.9
Pilot (Comet)	1 piece (5 grams)	19	3.9
Rolled sugar (Comet), any color	1 piece (8 grams)	37	7.7
ICE CREAM CUP, cup only (Comet), any color	1 piece (4 grams)	20	4.1

(USDA): United States Department of Agriculture
DNA: Data Not Available
*Prepared as Package Directs

Food and Description	Measure or Quantity	Calories	Carbo-hydrates (grams)
ICE CREAM SANDWICH			
(Sealtest)	1 sandwich (2.6 oz.)	208	30.8
ICE MILK:			
(USDA)	1 pt. (13.2 oz. by wt.)	568	83.8
(USDA)	1 cup (6.6 oz. by wt.)	284	41.9
Vanilla (Borden) *Lite Line*	1 pt.	431	68.6
ICE MILK BAR, chocolate-coated:			
(Popsicle Industries)	3 fl. oz.	133	D.N.A.
(Rosedale)	2½ oz.	130	D.N.A.
(Sealtest)	1 bar (3 fl. oz.)	144	16.0
ICE STICK, twin pop (Rosedale)	3 oz.	75	D.N.A.
ICING (See **CAKE ICING**)			
INCONNU or SHEEFISH, raw:			
Whole (USDA)	1 lb. (weighed whole)	417	0.
Flesh only (USDA)	4 oz.	166	0.
INDIAN PUDDING, New England (B & M)	½ cup (4.5 oz.)	150	23.6
INSTANT BREAKFAST (See individual brand name or company listings)			
IRISH WHISKEY (See **DISTILLED LIQUOR**)			
ITALIAN DINNER, frozen:			
(Banquet)	11-oz. dinner	414	44.0
(Swanson)	14-oz. dinner	448	54.1

(USDA): United States Department of Agriculture
DNA: Data Not Available
*Prepared as Package Directs

Food and Description	Measure or Quantity	Calories	Carbohydrates (grams)

J

JACKFRUIT, fresh (USDA):
Whole	1 lb. (weighed with seeds & skin)	124	32.3
Flesh only	4 oz.	111	28.8

JACK MACKEREL, raw, flesh only (USDA)
	4 oz.	162	0.

JACK ROSE MIX (Bar-Tender's)
	1 serving (⅝ oz.)	70	17.2

JALAPENO BEAN DIP (Frito-Lay)
	1 oz.	36	3.6

JAM, sweetened (See also individual listings by flavor):
(USDA)	1 oz.	77	19.8
(USDA)	1 T.	54	14.0

JAPANESE-STYLE VEGETABLES, frozen (Birds Eye)
	⅓ pkg. (3⅓ oz.)	99	6.3

JELLY, sweetened (See also individual listings by flavor):
(USDA)	1 oz.	77	20.0
(USDA)	1 T.	54	14.1
All flavors (Crosse & Blackwell)	1 T.	51	12.8
All flavors (Kraft)	1 oz.	74	18.4
All flavors (Polaner)	1 T.	54	13.0
All flavors (Smucker's)	1 oz.	84	D.N.A.

JELLY ROLL (Van de Kamp's):
Lemon	9-oz. cake	879	D.N.A.
Raspberry	9-oz. cake	589	D.N.A.

JERUSALEM ARTICHOKE (USDA):
Unpared	1 lb. (weighed with skin)	207	52.3
Pared	4 oz.	75	18.9

(USDA): United States Department of Agriculture
DNA: Data Not Available
*Prepared as Package Directs

[171]

Food and Description	Measure or Quantity	Calories	Carbohydrates (grams)
JOHANNISBERGER RIESLING WINE:			
(Deinhard) 11% alcohol	3 fl. oz.	72	4.5
(Louis M. Martini) 12.5% alcohol	3 fl. oz.	90	.2
JORDAN ALMOND (See **CANDY**)			
JUICE (See individual flavors)			
JUJUBE or CHINESE DATE (USDA):			
Fresh, whole	1 lb. (weighed with seeds)	443	116.4
Fresh, flesh only	4 oz.	119	31.3
Dried, whole	1 lb. (weighed with seeds)	1159	297.1
Dried, flesh only	4 oz.	325	83.5
JUNIOR FOOD (See **BABY FOOD**)			
JUNIORS (Tastykake):			
Chocolate	1 pkg. (2¾ oz.)	397	70.8
Chocolate devil food	1 pkg. (2¾ oz.)	284	45.2
Coconut	1 pkg. (2¾ oz.)	415	83.5
Coconut devil food	1 pkg. (2¾ oz.)	318	60.4
Jelly square	1 pkg. (3¼ oz.)	429	91.7
Koffee Kake	1 pkg. (2½ oz.)	395	59.7
Lemon	1 pkg. (2¾ oz.)	422	84.8
JUNKET (See individual flavors)			

K

Food and Description	Measure or Quantity	Calories	Carbohydrates (grams)
KABOOM, cereal	1 oz.	109	24.9
KAFE VIN (Lejon) 19.7% alcohol	3 fl. oz.	183	22.8
KALE:			
Raw, leaves (USDA)	1 lb. (weighed untrimmed)	154	26.1
Boiled, leaves including stems (USDA)	½ cup (1.9 oz.)	15	2.2
Frozen: (USDA)	4 oz.	36	6.2

Food and Description	Measure or Quantity	Calories	Carbohydrates (grams)
Boiled, drained solids (USDA)	½ cup (3.2 oz.)	28	5.0
Chopped (Birds Eye)	½ cup (3.3 oz.)	29	4.3
KARO, syrup:			
Dark corn, light corn or pancake & waffle syrup	1 pt.	1900	474.0
Dark corn, light corn, or pancake & waffle syrup	1 T.	60	14.6
KETCHUP (See **CATSUP**)			
KIDNEY (USDA):			
Beef, raw	4 oz.	148	1.0
Beef, braised	4 oz.	286	.9
Calf, raw	4 oz.	128	.1
Hog, raw	4 oz.	120	1.2
Lamb, raw	4 oz.	119	1.0
KIELBASA SAUSAGE (Usinger's)	1 oz.	88	Tr.
KINGFISH, raw (USDA):			
Whole	1 lb. (weighed whole)	210	0.
Meat only	4 oz.	119	0.
KIPPERS (See **HERRING**)			
KIRSCH LIQUEUR, (Garnier)			
96 proof	1 fl. oz.	83	8.8
KIRSCHWASSER, (Leroux)			
96 proof	1 fl. oz.	80	0.
KIX, cereal	1⅓ cup (1 oz.)	112	23.0
KNOCKWURST (USDA)	1 oz.	79	.6
KOHLRABI (USDA):			
Raw, whole	1 lb. (weighed with skin, without leaves)	96	21.9
Raw, diced	1 cup (4.8 oz.)	40	9.1
Boiled, drained solids	4 oz.	27	6.0
Boiled, drained solids	1 cup (5.4 oz.)	37	8.2

(USDA): United States Department of Agriculture
DNA: Data Not Available
*Prepared as Package Directs

Food and Description	Measure or Quantity	Calories	Carbo-hydrates (grams)
KOOL-AID (General Foods)	6 fl. oz.	74	18.9
KOOL-POPS (General Foods)	1 bar (1.3 oz.)	27	6.8
KOTTBULLAR (Hormel)	1 oz. (1-lb. can)	48	.9
KRIMPETS (Tastykake):			
Apple spice	1 cake (.9 oz.)	135	25.2
Butterscotch	1 cake (.9 oz.)	123	22.9
Chocolate	1 cake (.9 oz.)	119	21.6
Jelly	1 cake (.9 oz.)	103	21.0
Lemon	1 cake (.9 oz.)	113	21.4
Orange	1 cake (.9 oz.)	114	21.5
KUMMEL LIQUEUR:			
(Garnier) 70 proof	1 fl. oz.	75	4.3
(Hiram Walker) 70 proof	1 fl. oz.	71	3.2
(Leroux) 70 proof	1 fl. oz.	75	4.1
(Old Mr. Boston) 70 proof	1 fl. oz.	78	2.0
KUMQUAT, fresh (USDA):			
Whole	1 lb. (weighed with seeds)	274	72.1
Flesh only	4 oz.	74	19.4
Flesh only	5-6 med. kumquats	65	17.1

L

LAKE COUNTRY WINE (Taylor):			
White dinner, 12.5% alcohol	3 fl. oz.	81	2.2
Red dinner, 12.5% alcohol	3 fl. oz.	81	2.9
LAKE HERRING, raw (USDA):			
Whole	1 lb.	226	0.
Fillet	4 oz.	493	0.
LAKE TROUT, raw (USDA):			
Drawn	1 lb. (weighed with head, fins & bones)	282	0.
Meat only	4 oz.	191	0.
LAKE TROUT or SISCOWET, raw (USDA):			
Less than 6.5 lb. whole	1 lb. (weighed whole)	404	0.

(USDA): United States Department of Agriculture
DNA: Data Not Available
*Prepared as Package Directs

Food and Description	Measure or Quantity	Calories	Carbo-hydrates (grams)
Less than 6.5 lb. whole	4 oz. (meat only)	273	0.
More than 6.5 lb. whole	1 lb. (weighed whole)	856	0.
More than 6.5 lb. whole	4 oz. (meat only)	594	0.
LAMB, choice grade (USDA):			
Chops, broiled:			
Loin. One 5-oz. chop (weighed before cooking with bone) will give you:			
Lean & fat	2.8 oz.	280	0.
Lean only	2.3 oz.	122	0.
Rib. One 5-oz. chop (weighed before cooking with bone) will give you:			
Lean & fat	2.9 oz.	334	0.
Lean only	2 oz.	118	0.
Fat, separable, cooked	1 oz.	202	0.
Leg:			
Raw, lean & fat	1 lb. (weighed with bone)	845	0.
Roasted, lean & fat	4 oz.	316	0.
Roasted, lean only	4 oz.	211	0.
Shoulder:			
Raw, lean & fat	1 lb. (weighed with bone)	1082	0.
Roasted, lean & fat	4 oz.	323	0.
Roasted, lean only	4 oz.	234	0.
LAMB KABOB, frozen (Colonial)	6-oz. kabob	365	D.N.A.
LAMB'S-QUARTERS (USDA):			
Raw, trimmed	1 lb.	195	33.1
Boiled, drained	4 oz.	36	5.7
LAMB STEW, canned (B & M)	1 cup (8.9 oz.)	247	13.2
LARD:			
(USDA)	1 lb.	4091	0.
(USDA)	1 cup (7.8 oz.)	1984	0.
(USDA)	1 T.	126	0.
LASAGNE:			
Canned (Chef Boy-Ar-Dee)	8 oz. (⅕ of 40-oz. can)	241	29.7

(USDA): United States Department of Agriculture
DNA: Data Not Available
*Prepared as Package Directs

Food and Description	Measure or Quantity	Calories	Carbohydrates (grams)
Canned (Nalley's)	8 oz.	227	27.2
Frozen, with meat sauce (Buitoni)	7½ oz.	318	43.0
*Mix, dinner (Chef Boy-Ar-Dee)	8¾-oz. pkg.	290	37.7
LEEKS, raw (USDA):			
Whole	1 lb. (weighed untrimmed)	123	26.4
Trimmed	4 oz.	59	12.7
LEMON, fresh (USDA)	1 med. (2⅕″ dia.)	20	6.0
LEMONADE:			
Sweetened (Sealtest)	½ cup	52	13.4
Frozen, concentrate, sweetened:			
(USDA)	6-fl.-oz. can	430	112.0
*Diluted with 4⅓ parts water			
(USDA)	½ cup (4.2 oz.)	53	13.8
*(Minute Maid)	½ cup	49	13.1
*(Seneca)	½ cup	52	13.6
*(7L)	½ cup	55	14.0
*(Snow Crop)	½ cup	49	13.1
*(Treesweet)	½ cup	50	D.N.A.
*Pink (Birds Eye)	½ cup	51	13.5
*Pink (Treesweet)	½ cup	50	D.N.A.
Mix:			
*Twist (General Foods)	6 fl. oz.	66	15.6
*(Salada)	6 fl. oz.	79	19.2
*(Wyler's)	6 fl. oz.	63	15.8
*(Wyler's) pink	6 fl. oz.	63	15.8
LEMON CAKE MIX:			
(Betty Crocker) Sunkist	1-lb. 2.5-oz. pkg.	2202	368.2
*(Duncan Hines)	1 cake	2368	384.0
Chiffon (Betty Crocker) Sunkist	1-lb. 2.5-oz. pkg.	2202	416.2
Coconut (Betty Crocker)	1-lb. 3-oz. pkg.	2299	423.7
Coconut (Betty Crocker)	1 oz.	121	22.3
Cream moist cake (Pillsbury)	1 oz.	122	21.8
Pudding cake (Betty Crocker) Sunkist	11-oz. pkg.	1265	270.6
LEMON EXTRACT, pure (Ehlers)	1 tsp.	14	D.N.A.
LEMON FLAVORING, imitation (Ehlers)	1 tsp.	3	D.N.A.

(USDA): United States Department of Agriculture
DNA: Data Not Available
*Prepared as Package Directs

Food and Description	Measure or Quantity	Calories	Carbo-hydrates (grams)
LEMON JUICE:			
Fresh:			
(USDA)	1 cup (8.8 oz.)	62	19.7
(USDA)	1 T.	4	1.2
(Sunkist)	1 lemon	11	4.0
(Sunkist)	1 T.	4	1.0
Canned, unsweetened (USDA)	1 cup (8.6 oz.)	56	18.6
Canned, unsweetened (USDA)	1 T.	4	1.2
Plastic container (USDA)	¼ cup (2 oz.)	13	4.3
Plastic container, *ReaLemon*	1 T.	3	1.2
Frozen, unsweetened:			
Concentrate (USDA)	½ cup	145	46.8
Single strength (USDA)	½ cup	27	8.8
Full strength, already reconstituted (Minute Maid)	½ cup	27	8.8
Full strength, already reconstituted (Snow Crop)	½ cup	27	8.8
LEMON-LIMEADE, sweetened, concentrate, frozen:			
*(Minute Maid)	½ cup	51	13.1
*(Snow Crop)	½ cup	51	13.1
LEMON-LIME SOFT DRINK:			
Sweetened:			
Green (Canada Dry)	6 fl. oz.	90	23.4
Rickey (Canada Dry)	6 fl. oz.	71	18.4
(Dr. Brown's)	6 fl. oz.	75	18.8
(Dr. Pepper)	6 fl. oz.	72	18.0
(Key Food)	6 fl. oz.	75	18.8
(Kirsch)	6 fl. oz.	70	17.5
(Shasta)	6 fl. oz.	73	18.4
(Waldbaum)	6 fl. oz.	75	18.8
(White Rock)	6 fl. oz.	78	D.N.A.
Low calorie (Shasta)	6 fl. oz.	<1	<.1
LEMON PEEL, CANDIED:			
(USDA)	1 oz.	90	20.9
(Liberty)	1 oz.	93	22.6
LEMON PIE:			
(Tastykake)	4-oz. pie	366	52.0
Frozen (Mrs. Smith's)	⅙ of 8″ pie	354	46.3
Chiffon, home recipe (USDA)	⅙ of 9″ pie	438	61.3

(USDA): United States Department of Agriculture
DNA: Data Not Available
*Prepared as Package Directs

Food and Description	Measure or Quantity	Calories	Carbo-hydrates (grams)
Cream, frozen (Banquet)	2½ oz.	179	25.5
Cream, frozen (Mrs. Smith's)	⅙ of 8″ pie	194	22.7
Meringue, home recipe (USDA)	⅙ of 9″ pie	357	52.8
Meringue, frozen (Mrs. Smith's)	⅙ of 8″ pie	288	44.4
LEMON PIE FILLING (Lucky Leaf)	8 oz.	428	95.4
LEMON PIE FILLING MIX:			
*(Jell-O)	½ cup (4.3 oz.)	123	26.0
*Meringue (Jell-O)	⅛ of 8″ pie (including crust)	289	47.7
(My-T-Fine)	1 oz.	122	26.0
*(Royal)	⅛ of 9″ pie (including crust)	225	39.3
LEMON PUDDING (Betty Crocker)	1-lb. 2-oz. can	774	158.4
LEMON PUDDING MIX:			
Regular:			
*(Jell-O)	½ cup (4.3 oz.)	123	26.0
(My-T-Fine)	1 oz.	122	26.0
*(Thank-You)	½ cup	183	36.2
Instant:			
*(Jell-O)	½ cup (4.3 oz.)	177	30.5
(My-T-Fine)	1 oz.	82	20.6
*(Royal)	½ cup	180	31.2
*Dietetic with skim milk (Dia-Mel)	4 oz.	53	8.2
LEMON RENNET CUSTARD MIX:			
Powder:			
(Junket)	1 oz.	116	28.0
*Prepared with whole milk (Junket)	4 oz.	108	14.7
Tablet:			
(Junket)	1 tablet	1	.2
*Prepared with whole milk & sugar (Junket)	4 oz.	101	13.4
LEMON SOFT DRINK:			
Sweetened:			
(Canada Dry)	6 fl. oz.	71	18.4

(USDA): United States Department of Agriculture
DNA: Data Not Available
*Prepared as Package Directs

Food and Description	Measure or Quantity	Calories	Carbo-hydrates (grams)
(Dr. Brown's) *Tune-Up*	6 fl. oz.	75	18.8
(Hoffman)	6 fl. oz.	81	20.2
(Kirsch)	6 fl. oz.	64	16.1
Low calorie:			
(Dr. Brown's) *Slim-Ray*	6 fl. oz.	3	.8
(Hoffman)	6 fl. oz.	3	.8
(No-Cal)	6 fl. oz.	2	0.
(Shasta)	6 fl. oz.	<1	<.1
LEMON TURNOVER, frozen			
(Pepperidge Farm)	1 piece	285	D.N.A.
LENTIL:			
Whole:			
Dry:			
(USDA)	½ lb.	771	136.3
(USDA)	1 cup (6.7 oz.)	649	114.8
(Sinsheimer)	1 oz.	95	17.0
Cooked, drained solids (USDA)	½ cup (3.6 oz.)	107	19.5
Split, dry (USDA)	½ lb.	782	140.2
LENTIL SOUP, canned:			
(Crosse & Blackwell)	6½ oz. (½ can)	190	15.1
*(Manischewitz)	8 oz. (by wt.)	166	29.4
LETTUCE:			
Bibb (USDA)	1 lb. (weighed un-trimmed)	47	8.4
Bibb (USDA)	7.8-oz. head (4″ dia.)	30	6.0
Boston (USDA)	1 lb. (weighed un-trimmed)	47	8.4
Boston (USDA)	7.8-oz. head (4″ dia.)	30	6.0
Butterhead varieties (See Bibb & Boston)			
Cos (See Romaine)			
Dark green (See Romaine)			
Grand Rapids (USDA)	1 lb. (weighed un-trimmed)	52	10.2
Grand Rapids (USDA)	2 large leaves (1.8 oz.)	10	2.0
Great Lakes (USDA)	1 lb. (weighed un-trimmed)	56	12.5
Great Lakes (USDA)	1-lb. head (4¾″ dia.)	60	13.0

(USDA): United States Department of Agriculture
DNA: Data Not Available
*Prepared as Package Directs

Food and Description	Measure or Quantity	Calories	Carbohydrates (grams)
Iceberg:			
(USDA)	1 lb. (weighed untrimmed)	56	12.5
(USDA)	1-lb. head (4¾" dia.)	60	13.0
Leaves (USDA)	1 cup (2.3 oz.)	8	1.9
Chopped (USDA)	1 cup (2 oz.)	8	1.7
Chunks (USDA)	1 cup (2.6 oz.)	10	2.1
Looseleaf varieties (See Salad Bowl)			
New York (USDA)	1 lb. (weighed untrimmed)	56	12.5
New York (USDA)	1-lb. head (4¾" dia.)	60	13.0
Romaine:			
(USDA)	1 lb. (weighed untrimmed)	52	10.2
Shredded & broken into pieces (USDA)	½ cup (.8 oz.)	4	.8
Salad Bowl (USDA)	1 lb. (weighed untrimmed)	52	10.2
Salad Bowl (USDA)	2 large leaves (1.8 oz.)	10	2.0
Simpson (USDA)	1 lb. (weighed untrimmed)	52	10.2
Simpson (USDA)	2 large leaves (1.8 oz.)	10	2.0
White Paris (See Romaine)			
LIEBFRAUMILCH WINE:			
(Anheuser) 10% alcohol	3 fl. oz.	63	.9
(Deinhard) 11% alcohol	3 fl. oz.	60	3.6
(Deinhard) *Hans Christof*, 11% alcohol	3 fl. oz.	60	3.6
(Julius Kayser) Glockenspiel, 10% alcohol	3 fl. oz.	57	1.8
LIFE, cereal (Quaker)	1 cup (1.5 oz.)	160	29.8
LIKE, soft drink, low calorie (Seven-Up)	6 fl. oz.	1	.3
LIMA BEAN (See **BEAN, LIMA**)			

(USDA): United States Department of Agriculture
DNA: Data Not Available
*Prepared as Package Directs

Food and Description	Measure or Quantity	Calories	Carbo-hydrates (grams)
LIME, fresh, whole:			
(USDA)	1 lb. (weighed with skin & seeds)	107	36.2
(USDA)	1 med. (2″ dia.)	16	5.4
LIMEADE, concentrate, sweetened, frozen:			
(USDA)	6 fl. oz.	408	107.9
*Diluted with 4⅓ parts water			
(USDA)	½ cup (4.4 oz.)	50	13.6
*(Minute Maid)	½ cup	50	13.4
*(7L)	½ cup	52	13.5
*(Snow Crop)	½ cup	50	13.4
***LIMEADE MIX** (Wyler's)	6 fl. oz.	63	15.7
LIME ICE, home recipe (USDA)	8 oz. (by wt.)	177	74.0
LIME JUICE:			
Fresh (USDA)	1 cup (8.6 oz.)	64	22.1
Canned or bottled:			
(USDA)	1 cup (8.6 oz.)	64	22.1
(USDA)	1 fl. oz.	8	2.8
(Calavo)	1 fl. oz.	8	2.8
Plastic container *ReaLime*	1 T.	4	1.5
LIME PIE, Key lime, cream, frozen (Banquet)	2½ oz.	204	27.5
***LIME PIE FILLING MIX,** Key lime (Royal)	⅛ of 9″ pie (including crust)	225	39.0
LIME SHERBET or FRUIT ICE MIX (Junket):	6 serving pkg. (4 oz.)	388	108.8
LIME SOFT DRINK (Yukon Club)	6 fl. oz.	65	16.2
LINGCOD, raw (USDA):			
Whole	1 lb. (weighed whole)	130	0.
Meat only	4 oz.	95	0.
LIQUEUR (See individual kinds)			

(USDA): United States Department of Agriculture
DNA: Data Not Available
*Prepared as Package Directs

Food and Description	Measure or Quantity	Calories	Carbo-hydrates (grams)
LITCHI NUT (USDA):			
Fresh:			
Whole	4 oz. (weighed in shell, with seeds)	44	11.2
Flesh only	4 oz.	73	18.6
Dried:			
Whole	4 oz. (weighed in shell, with seeds)	145	36.9
Flesh only	2 oz.	157	40.1
LIVER (USDA):			
Beef, raw	1 lb.	635	24.0
Beef, fried	4 oz.	260	6.0
Calf, raw	1 lb.	635	18.6
Calf, fried	4 oz.	296	4.5
Chicken, raw	1 lb.	585	13.2
Chicken, simmered	4 oz.	187	3.5
Goose, raw	1 lb.	826	24.5
Hog, raw	1 lb.	594	13.2
Hog, fried	4 oz.	273	2.8
Lamb, raw	1 lb.	617	13.2
Lamb, broiled	4 oz.	296	3.2
Turkey, raw	1 lb.	626	18.1
Turkey, simmered	4 oz.	97	3.5
LIVER PATE (See **PATE**)			
LIVER SAUSAGE or LIVER-WURST (USDA):			
Fresh	1 oz.	87	.5
Smoked	1 oz.	90	.7
LOBSTER:			
Raw:			
Whole (USDA)	1 lb. (weighed whole)	107	.6
Meat only (USDA)	4 oz.	103	.6
Northern, meat only (Booth)	4 oz.	103	.6
Cooked, meat only (USDA)	4 oz.	108	.4
Canned, meat only (USDA)	4 oz.	108	.4
LOBSTER NEWBURG:			
Home recipe (USDA)	4 oz.	220	5.8
Frozen (Stouffer's)	11½-oz. pkg.	671	16.0

(USDA): United States Department of Agriculture
DNA: Data Not Available
*Prepared as Package Directs

Food and Description	Measure or Quantity	Calories	Carbo-hydrates (grams)
LOBSTER PASTE, canned (USDA)	1 oz.	51	.4
LOBSTER SALAD, home recipe (USDA)	4 oz.	125	2.6
LOBSTER SOUP, canned:			
Bisque (Crosse & Blackwell)	6½ oz. (½ can)	88	6.6
Cream of (Crosse & Blackwell)	6½ oz. (½ can)	92	6.5
LOCHON ORA, Scottish liqueur (Leroux) 70 proof	1 fl. oz.	89	7.4
LOGANBERRY (USDA):			
Fresh:			
Untrimmed	1 lb. (weighed with caps)	267	64.2
Trimmed	1 cup (5 oz.)	89	21.4
Canned, solids & liq. (USDA):			
Water pack	4 oz.	45	10.7
Juice pack	4 oz.	61	14.4
Light syrup	4 oz.	79	19.5
Heavy syrup	4 oz.	101	25.2
Extra heavy syrup	4 oz.	122	30.8
LOG CABIN, syrup:			
Buttered	1 T.	53	13.0
Maple flavored	1 T.	52	13.4
LONGAN (USDA):			
Raw:			
Whole	1 lb. (weighed with shell & seeds)	147	38.0
Flesh only	4 oz.	69	17.9
Dried:			
Whole	1 lb. (weighed with shell & seeds)	467	120.8
Flesh only	4 oz.	324	83.9
LOOK FIT, any flavor (A&P)	1 can	225	19.0
LOQUAT, fresh (USDA):			
Whole	1 lb. (weighed with seeds)	168	43.3
Flesh only	4 oz.	54	14.1

(USDA): United States Department of Agriculture
DNA: Data Not Available
*Prepared as Package Directs

Food and Description	Measure or Quantity	Calories	Carbo-hydrates (grams)
LUCKY CHARMS, cereal	1¼ cup (1 oz.)	110	23.0
LUMBERJACK, syrup (Nalley's)	1 oz.	78	19.6
LUNCHEON MEAT (See also individual listings, e.g. **BOLOGNA**):			
Meat loaf (USDA)	1 oz.	57	.9
(Eckrich):			
Beef, chopped, *Slender Sliced*	1 oz.	38	D.N.A.
Chicken chipped, *Slender Sliced*	1 oz.	77	D.N.A.
Ham, chipped, smoked *Slender Sliced*	1 oz.	45	D.N.A.
Loaves:			
Chicken breast	1 oz.	32	D.N.A.
Gourmet	1 oz.	28	D.N.A.
Honey style	1 oz.	42	D.N.A.
Peppered	1 oz.	38	D.N.A.
Pressed luncheon	1 oz.	40	D.N.A.
Pork loin, chipped, smoked, *Slender Sliced*	1 oz.	40	D.N.A.
Turkey, chipped, smoked, *Slender Sliced*	1 oz.	38	D.N.A.
(Sugardale)	1-oz. slice	77	Tr.
Old fashioned loaf (Sugardale)	1-oz. slice	76	Tr.
Pickle & pimento:			
(Hormel)	1 oz. (6-lb. can)	81	.3
(Sugardale)	1-oz. slice	78	Tr.
Spiced (Hormel)	1 oz. (6-lb. can)	101	.3
LUNG, raw (USDA):			
Beef	1 lb.	435	0.
Calf	1 lb.	481	0.
Lamb	1 lb.	467	0.

M

MACADAMIA NUT (USDA):			
Whole	1 lb. (weighed in shell)	972	22.4
Shelled	1 oz.	196	4.5

(USDA): United States Department of Agriculture
DNA: Data Not Available
*Prepared as Package Directs

Food and Description	Measure or Quantity	Calories	Carbo-hydrates (grams)
MACARONI. Plain macaroni products are essentially the same in caloric value and carbohydrate content on the same weight basis. The longer they are cooked, the more water is absorbed and this affects the nutritive values.			
Dry:			
Elbow-type (USDA)	1 cup (4.8 oz.)	502	102.3
1-inch pieces (USDA)	1 cup (3.8 oz.)	406	82.7
2-inch pieces (USDA)	1 cup (3 oz.)	317	64.6
(USDA)	1 oz.	105	21.3
Cooked (USDA):			
8-10 minutes, firm	1 cup (4.6 oz.)	192	39.1
8-10 minutes, firm	4 oz.	168	34.1
14-20 minutes, tender	1 cup (4.9 oz.)	155	32.2
14-20 minutes, tender	4 oz.	126	26.1
MACARONI & BEEF:			
(Morton House)	12¾-oz. can	745	D.N.A.
In tomato sauce (Franco-American)	4 oz.	112	12.5
With tomatoes, frozen (Stouffer's)	11½-oz. pkg.	410	39.0
MACARONI & CHEESE:			
Home recipe, baked (USDA)	1 cup (7.8 oz.)	473	44.2
Canned:			
(USDA)	8 oz.	216	24.2
(Franco-American)	8 oz.	220	25.0
(Heinz)	8 oz.	211	24.1
MacaroniO's (Franco-American)	8 oz.	170	22.2
Frozen:			
(Banquet)	20-oz. pkg.	742	82.0
(Banquet) cookin' bag	8 oz.	280	36.0
(Kraft)	8 oz.	386	35.2
(Morton) casserole	8 oz.	287	28.2
(Stouffer's)	12-oz. pkg.	477	52.1
(Swanson)	8-oz. pkg.	328	29.2
(Van de Kamp's)	1 pkg.	495	D.N.A.
MACARONI & CHEESE MIX:			
Dry (USDA)	1 oz.	113	17.8
Cheddar sauce (Betty Crocker)	8-oz. pkg.	856	144.0

(USDA): United States Department of Agriculture
DNA: Data Not Available
*Prepared as Package Directs

Food and Description	Measure or Quantity	Calories	Carbo-hydrates (grams)
Cheddar sauce (Betty Crocker)	1 oz.	107	18.0
*Mac-A-Roni & Cheddar (Golden Grain)	½ cup	157	18.4
*Stir 'n Serv, instant (Golden Grain)	½ cup (3.5 oz.)	174	22.4
MACARONI & CHILI SAUCE MIX:			
*Mac-A-Roni Fiesta (Golden Grain)	½ cup (3.5 oz.)	156	25.0
Mexi Casserole (Betty Crocker)	6-oz. pkg.	564	120.6
MACARONI CREOLE (Heinz)	7¾-oz. can	143	24.4
MACARONI DINNER:			
& beef, frozen:			
(Morton)	11-oz. dinner	414	58.3
(Swanson)	11¼-oz. dinner	302	35.0
& cheese:			
*(Chef Boy-Ar-Dee)	4½-oz. pkg.	221	33.8
*(Kraft)	4 oz.	203	26.1
*(Kraft) deluxe	4 oz.	202	27.9
Frozen (Banquet)	12-oz. dinner	342	47.0
Frozen (Morton)	12¾-oz. dinner	445	66.6
Frozen (Swanson)	12¾-oz. dinner	367	48.4
*Italian-style (Kraft)	4 oz.	119	20.5
*Mexican-style (Kraft)	4 oz.	126	22.6
Monte Bello with sauce mix (Betty Crocker)	7.5-oz. pkg.	705	150.8
MACARONI SALAD, canned (Nalley's)	4 oz.	181	13.9
MACKEREL (USDA):			
Atlantic:			
Raw:			
Whole	1 lb. (weighed whole)	468	0.
Meat only	4 oz.	217	0.
Broiled with butter	4 oz.	268	0.
Canned, solids & liq.	4 oz.	208	0.
Pacific:			
Raw:			
Dressed	1 lb. (weighed with bones & skin)	519	0.

(USDA): United States Department of Agriculture
DNA: Data Not Available
*Prepared as Package Directs

Food and Description	Measure or Quantity	Calories	Carbo-hydrates (grams)
Meat only	4 oz.	180	0.
Canned, solids & liq.	4 oz.	204	0.
Salted	4 oz.	346	0.
Smoked	4 oz.	248	0.
MACKEREL, JACK (See **JACK MACKEREL**)			
MADEIRA WINE:			
(Leacock) 19% alcohol	3 fl. oz.	120	6.3
(Leacock) *St. John*, 19% alcohol	3 fl. oz.	120	6.3
MAGGI, seasoning	1 T.	17	.1
MAI TAI COCKTAIL, 48 proof			
(Lemon Hart)	3 fl. oz.	180	15.6
MAI TAI MIX (Bar-Tender's)	1 serving (⅝ oz.)	69	17.0
MALT, dry (USDA)	1 oz.	104	21.9
MALTED MILK MIX:			
Dry powder (USDA)	1 oz.	116	20.1
*Prepared (USDA)	1 cup (9½ oz.)	280	31.6
Instant (Borden)	2 heaping tsp.	80	13.4
(Horlicks)	1 oz.	118	19.8
Instant, chocolate (Borden)	2 heaping tsp.	77	16.0
MALTED TABLETS (Horlicks)	1 tablet	6	.9
MALTEX, cereal	1 oz.	109	22.7
MALT EXTRACT, dried (USDA)	1 oz.	104	25.3
MALT LIQUOR:			
Big Cat	12 fl. oz.	155	D.N.A.
Country Club	12 fl. oz.	183	2.8
***MALT-O-MEAL*,** cereal	¾ cup	102	22.1
MAMEY or MAMMEE APPLE, raw (USDA)	1 lb. (weighed with skin & seeds)	143	35.2

(USDA): United States Department of Agriculture
DNA: Data Not Available
*Prepared as Package Directs

Food and Description	Measure or Quantity	Calories	Carbohydrates (grams)
MANDARIN ORANGE, CANNED, low calorie, solids & liq. (Diet Delight)	½ cup (4.3 oz.)	32	6.1
MANDARIN ORANGE, FRESH (See **TANGERINE**)			
MANGO, fresh (USDA):			
Whole	1 lb. (weighed with seeds & skin)	201	51.1
Whole	1 med. (7 oz.)	132	33.6
Flesh only, diced or sliced	½ cup (2.8 oz.)	54	13.8
MANHATTAN COCKTAIL:			
(Calvert) 60 proof	3 fl. oz.	161	2.0
(Hiram Walker) 55 proof	3 fl. oz.	147	3.0
MANHATTAN MIX			
(Bar-Tender's)	1 serving (⅕ oz.)	24	5.6
MANICOTTI, without sauce, frozen (Buitoni)	1 piece	82	10.0
MAPLE FLAVORING, imitation maple (Ehlers)	1 tsp.	8	D.N.A.
MAPLE RENNET CUSTARD MIX:			
Powder:			
(Junket)	1 oz.	116	27.8
*Prepared with whole milk (Junket)	4 oz.	108	14.6
Tablet:			
(Junket)	1 tablet	1	.2
*Prepared with whole milk & sugar (Junket)	4 oz.	101	13.4
MAPLE SYRUP:			
(USDA)	1 T.	50	13.0
Imitation (Karo)	1 pt.	1900	474.0
Imitation (Karo)	1 T.	60	14.4
Dietetic (Dia-Mel)	1 T.	22	5.5
MARASCHINO LIQUEUR:			
(Garnier) 60 proof	1 fl. oz.	94	11.1
(Leroux) 60 proof	1 fl. oz.	88	9.7

(USDA): United States Department of Agriculture
DNA: Data Not Available
*Prepared as Package Directs

Food and Description	Measure or Quantity	Calories	Carbo-hydrates (grams)
MARBLE CAKE MIX:			
Dry (USDA)	1 oz.	120	21.4
*With boiled white icing (USDA)	4 oz.	375	70.3
(Betty Crocker)	1/12 of cake	206	37.2
MARGARINE, salted or unsalted:			
(USDA)	1 lb.	3266	1.8
(USDA)	1 cup (8 oz.)	1633	.9
(USDA)	4 oz. (1 stick)	816	.5
(USDA)	1 T.	101	Tr.
(Blue Bonnet) regular or soft	1 T.	100	Tr.
(Borden) Danish flavor	1 T.	103	Tr.
(Fleischmann's) regular or soft	1 T.	100	Tr.
(Golden Glow)	1 T. (.4 oz.)	89	.1
(Good Luck)	1 T. (.5 oz.)	102	.1
(Good Luck) soft	1 T. (.4 oz.)	89	.1
(Imperial)	1 T. (.5 oz.)	102	.1
(Imperial)	1/4 lb.	811	1.0
(Imperial) *Soft-Spread*	1 T. (.4 oz.)	89	.1
(Mazola) polyunsaturated	1/4 cup (2 oz.)	413	.6
(Mazola) polyunsaturated	1 T. (.5 oz.)	102	.1
(Miracle) corn oil	1 T. (9 grams)	67	<.1
(Nucoa) polyunsaturated	1 T. (.5 oz.)	102	.1
(Nucoa) *Dream Soft*	1 T. (.4 oz.)	91	.1
(Nu-Maid)	1 oz.	204	.1
(Parkay) regular	1 T. (.5 oz.)	101	.1
(Parkay) soft cup	1 T. (.5 oz.)	95	.1
(Parkay) corn oil, deluxe	1 T. (.5 oz.)	101	.1
(Parkay) corn oil, soft	1 T. (.5 oz.)	95	.1
(Parkay) safflower oil, soft	1 T. (.5 oz.)	95	.1
(Saffola) regular or soft	1 T.	108	.1
(Sealtest)	1 T.	109	Tr.
MARGARINE, IMITATION, diet:			
(Fleischmann's)	1 T.	50	.1
(Imperial)	1 T. (.5 oz.)	48	0.
(Mazola)	1 T. (.5 oz.)	50	Tr.
(Nucoa)	1 T. (.5 oz.)	50	Tr.
(Parkay) soft	1 T. (.5 oz.)	55	0.
MARGARINE, WHIPPED:			
(Blue Bonnet)	1 T.	70	.1
(Imperial)	1 T. (10 grams)	68	<.1
(Miracle) cottonseed — soybean	1 T. (9 grams)	67	<.1

(USDA): United States Department of Agriculture
DNA: Data Not Available
*Prepared as Package Directs

Food and Description	Measure or Quantity	Calories	Carbohydrates (grams)
(Miracle) sticks	1 T.	67	.1
(Nucoa)	1 T.	70	.1
(Parkay) cup	1 T. (9 grams)	67	<.1
MARGARITA COCKTAIL, (Calvert) 45 proof	3 fl. oz.	176	9.5
MARGARITA MIX (Bar-Tender's)	1 serving (⅝ oz.)	70	17.3
MARGAUX, French red Bordeaux (Barton & Guestier) 12% alcohol	3 fl. oz.	62	.4
MARINADE MIX:			
(Adolph's) instant	⅘-oz. pkg.	26	6.6
(Lawry's) lemon pepper	2.7-oz. pkg.	159	29.7
MARMALADE:			
Sweetened:			
(USDA)	1 oz.	73	19.9
(USDA)	1 T.	51	14.0
(Crosse & Blackwell)	1 T.	60	14.9
(King Kelly)	1 T.	48	D.N.A.
(Kraft)	1 oz.	78	19.3
Dietetic or low calorie:			
(Dia-Mel)	1 T.	22	5.4
(Louis Sherry)	1 T.	4	1.1
(Polaner)	1 T.	6	1.2
(Slenderella)	1 T. (.6 oz.)	22	5.6
MARMALADE PLUM (USDA):			
Fresh, whole	1 lb. (with skin & seeds)	431	108.9
Fresh, flesh only	4 oz.	142	35.8
MARSALA WINE (Italian Swiss Colony-Private Stock) 19.7% alcohol	3 fl. oz.	124	7.1
MARTINI COCKTAIL:			
Gin:			
(Calvert) 60 proof	3 fl. oz.	176	Tr.
(Hiram Walker) 67.5 proof	3 fl. oz.	168	Tr.
Vodka (Hiram Walker) 60 proof	3 fl. oz.	147	Tr.

(USDA): United States Department of Agriculture
DNA: Data Not Available
*Prepared as Package Directs

Food and Description	Measure or Quantity	Calories	Carbo- hydrates (grams)
MASA HARINA (Quaker):			
Dry	⅓ cup (1.3 oz. dry)	136	26.0
*Tortillas	2 tortillas (6″)	136	26.0
MATZO:			
Regular, daily & Passover (Manischewitz)	1 matzo	121	26.0
Diet-10's (Goodman's)	1 sq.	110	23.0
Diet-10's (Goodman's)	1 cracker	12	2.6
Diet thins (Manischewitz)	1 matzo	109	23.3
Egg 'n Onion (Manischewitz)	1 matzo	112	22.8
Egg, Passover (Manischewitz)	1 matzo	136	26.6
Midgetea (Goodman's)	1 matzo	40	8.4
Round tea (Goodman's)	1 matzo	70	14.6
Tasteas (Manischewitz)	1 matzo	139	19.9
Thin tea (Manischewitz)	1 matzo	113	24.7
Unsalted (Goodman's)	1 matzo	110	23.0
Unsalted (Horowitz-Margareten)	1 matzo	135	28.2
Whole wheat, Passover (Manischewitz)	1 matzo	126	24.2
MATZO MEAL (Manischewitz)	1 cup	438	94.0
MAYONNAISE:			
(USDA)	1 oz.	204	.6
(USDA)	1 T.	101	.3
(Best Foods) *Real*	1 pt.	3100	7.0
(Best Foods) *Real*	1 T.	100	.2
(Hellmann's) *Real*	1 T.	100	.2
(Kraft)	1 oz.	204	.3
(Kraft) *Salad Bowl*	1 oz.	203	.7
(Nalley's)	1 oz.	204	.9
(Saffola)	1 T.	90	2.2
(Wesson)	1 T.	110	Tr.
Sugar-free (Chelten House)	1 T.	108	D.N.A.
MAYPO, cereal, dry, any flavor:			
Instant	1 oz.	105	19.8
1-minute	1 oz.	107	19.8
MAY WINE (Deinhard) 11% alcohol	3 fluid oz.	60	1.0

(USDA): United States Department of Agriculture
DNA: Data Not Available
*Prepared as Package Directs

Food and Description	Measure or Quantity	Calories	Carbo-hydrates (grams)
MEAL (See **CORNMEAL** or **CRACKER MEAL** or **MATZO MEAL**)			
MEATBALL:			
Cocktail (Cresca)	1 meatball	10	D.N.A.
Dinner, with Kluski noodles, frozen (Tom Thumb)	3-lb. 8-oz. tray	2362	140.5
In sauce, canned (Prince)	4 oz.	181	9.1
Stew, canned (Chef Boy-Ar-Dee)	7½ oz. (¼ of 30-oz. can)	180	11.7
Stew (Morton House)	24-oz. can	1240	D.N.A.
With gravy, canned (Chef Boy-Ar-Dee)	3⅘ oz. (¼ of 15¼-oz. can)	126	9.2
MEAT LOAF DINNER frozen:			
With tomato sauce, mashed potato & peas (USDA)	12 oz.	447	33.3
(Banquet)	11-oz. dinner	420	28.8
(Morton)	11-oz. dinner	437	23.6
(Swanson)	10-oz. dinner	419	42.2
(Swanson) 3-course	16-oz. dinner	495	51.1
MEAT LOAF SEASONING MIX (Lawry's)	1 pkg. (3½ oz.)	334	65.2
MEAT, POTTED:			
(Armour Star)	5½-oz. can	330	0.
(Armour Star)	3-oz. can	180	0.
(Hormel)	3-oz. can	169	1.0
MEAT TENDERIZER (Adolph's)			
Unseasoned	1 T.	<1	.1
Seasoned	1 T.	<1	Tr.
MEDOC WINE, (Cruse) 12% alcohol	3 fl. oz.	72	D.N.A.
MELBA TOAST:			
Garlic (Keebler)	1 piece (2 grams)	9	1.5
Garlic, rounds (Old London)	1 piece (2 grams)	9	1.6
Onion, rounds (Old London)	1 piece (2 grams)	10	1.5
Plain (Keebler)	1 piece (2 grams)	9	1.5

(USDA): United States Department of Agriculture
DNA: Data Not Available
*Prepared as Package Directs

Food and Description	Measure or Quantity	Calories	Carbo-hydrates (grams)
Pumpernickel (Old London)	1 piece (4 grams)	17	3.2
Rye:			
(Keebler)	1 piece (2 grams)	8	1.7
(Old London)	1 piece (4 grams)	17	3.3
Unsalted (Old London)	1 piece (4 grams)	18	3.3
Sesame (Keebler)	1 piece (2 grams)	11	1.4
Sesame, rounds (Old London)	1 piece (2 grams)	10	1.3
Wheat (Old London)	1 piece (4 grams)	17	3.3
Wheat, unsalted (Old London)	1 piece (4 grams)	18	3.3
White:			
(Keebler)	1 piece (4 grams)	16	3.3
(Old London)	1 piece (4 grams)	17	3.3
Rounds (Old London)	1 piece (2 grams)	9	1.6
Unsalted (Old London)	1 piece (4 grams)	17	3.3
MELON (See individual listings, e.g. **CANTALOUPE, WATER-MELON,** etc.)			
MELON BALL, in syrup, frozen:			
Cantaloupe & honeydew (USDA)	½ cup (4 oz.)	72	18.2
Mixed (Birds Eye)	¼ pkg. (4 oz.)	36	12.2
MELON BALL CRISPS, dehydrated snack (Epicure)	1 oz.	87	22.0
MENHADEN, Atlantic, canned, solids & liq. (USDA)	4 oz.	195	0.
METRECAL DINNER, any kind	9-oz. can	225	23.5
MEXICAN DINNER:			
Combination, frozen:			
(Patio)	1 dinner	586	D.N.A.
(Rosarita)	12-oz. dinner	518	D.N.A.
Mexican style, frozen:			
(Banquet)	12-oz. dinner	569	74.0
(Patio)	1 dinner	666	D.N.A.
(Rosarita)	15-oz. dinner	530	D.N.A.
(Swanson)	16¼-oz. dinner	658	67.3
MEXICAN-STYLE VEGETA-BLES, frozen (Birds Eye)	⅓ pkg. (3⅓ oz.)	214	27.7
MILK AMPLIFIER, syrup (Hershey's)	1 oz.	78	18.6

(USDA): United States Department of Agriculture
DNA: Data Not Available
*Prepared as Package Directs

Food and Description	Measure or Quantity	Calories	Carbo-hydrates (grams)
MILK, CONDENSED, sweetened, canned:			
(USDA)	1 cup	980	166.0
(Dime)	1 oz.	126	21.2
(Eagle)	1 oz.	125	20.6
(Magnolia)	1 oz.	126	21.2
(Nestlé's) *Lion's Brand*	1 oz.	96	12.8
(Sealtest)	1 cup	982	166.8
(Sealtest)	1 T.	64	10.9
MILK, DRY:			
Whole:			
(USDA)	4 T.	129	9.8
(Sealtest)	4 T.	141	10.8
Nonfat, instant:			
(USDA)	4 T.	122	17.5
*(Carnation)	1 cup	81	11.6
*(Pet)	1 cup	81	11.8
*(Sanalac)	1 cup	82	11.6
(Sealtest)	4 T.	102	14.5
MILK, EVAPORATED, canned:			
Regular:			
Unsweetened (USDA)	1 cup	345	24.0
(Carnation)	1 cup	348	24.4
(Pet)	1 cup	352	24.0
(Sealtest)	1 cup	346	24.0
Skimmed:			
(Pet)	1 cup	176	26.4
(Sunshine)	1 cup	176	24.8
MILK, FRESH:			
Whole:			
3.5% fat (USDA)	1 cup	159	12.0
3.7% fat (USDA)	1 cup	160	11.9
Homogenized, vitamin D, 3.5% fat (Borden)	1 cup	160	12.0
3.5% fat (Sealtest)	1 cup	151	11.0
3.7% fat (Sealtest)	1 cup	159	11.2
Multivitamin (Sealtest)	1 cup	151	11.0
Skim:			
(USDA)	1 cup	89	12.5
Partially skimmed with 2% nonfat milk solids added (USDA)	1 cup	145	14.7

(USDA): United States Department of Agriculture
DNA: Data Not Available
*Prepared as Package Directs

Food and Description	Measure or Quantity	Calories	Carbo-hydrates (grams)
(Sealtest)	1 cup	81	11.2
Dari Lean (Dairylea)	1 cup	135	D.N.A.
Diet (Sealtest)	1 cup	105	13.7
Light n' Lively (Sealtest)	1 cup	116	13.4
Lite Line (Borden)	1 cup	117	14.4
n-r-g (Sealtest)	1 cup	127	13.7
Vita Lure (Sealtest)	1 cup	137	13.7
Buttermilk, cultured, fresh:			
(USDA)	1 cup	90	13.0
0.1% fat (Borden)	1 cup	88	12.5
1.0% fat (Borden)	1 cup	107	12.4
3.5% fat (Borden)	1 cup	158	11.9
(Sealtest)	1 cup	100	9.5
Buttermilk, cultured, dried (USDA)	4 oz.	439	56.7
Chocolate milk drinks, fresh:			
With whole milk:			
(USDA)	1 cup	210	27.3
Dutch chocolate (Borden)	1 cup	210	26.1
(Sealtest)	1 cup	205	24.9
With skim milk:			
(USDA)	1 cup	190	27.2
(Sealtest)	1 cup	154	25.1
MILK, GOAT, whole (USDA)	1 cup	165	11.0
MILK, HUMAN (USDA)	1 oz. (by wt.)	22	2.7
MILK, REINDEER (USDA)	1 oz. (by wt.)	66	1.2
MILK SHAKE MIX, any flavor, *Great Shakes:*			
*With whole milk	1 cup (9.6 oz.)	259	37.0
*With nonfat milk	1 cup (9.7 oz.)	189	38.0
MILLET, whole-grain (USDA)	1 lb.	1483	330.7
MINCEMEAT:			
(Crosse & Blackwell)	1 T.	60	14.3
Condensed (None Such)	9-oz. block	997	211.3
Ready-to-use (None Such)	18-oz. jar	1148	265.7
MINCE PIE:			
Home recipe (USDA)	⅙ of 9″ pie (5.6 oz.)	428	65.1

(USDA): United States Department of Agriculture
DNA: Data Not Available
*Prepared as Package Directs

Food and Description	Measure or Quantity	Calories	Carbo- hydrates (grams)
Frozen:			
(Banquet)	5 oz.	401	62.8
(Marvin)	⅙ of 9″ pie	252	45.6
(Mrs. Smith's)	⅙ of 8″ pie	335	48.2
MINESTRONE SOUP:			
Condensed (USDA)	8 oz. (by wt.)	197	26.3
*Prepared with equal volume water (USDA)	1 cup (8.6 oz.)	105	14.2
Condensed (Campbell)	8 oz. (by wt.)	163	20.9
(Crosse & Blackwell)	6½ oz. (½ can)	92	14.2
*Mix (Golden Grain)	1 cup	69	11.2
MISO, cereal & soybeans (USDA)	4 oz.	194	26.6
MOCHA EXTRACT (Ehlers)	1 tsp.	2	D.N.A.
***MOCHA NUT PUDDING MIX,** instant (Royal)	½ cup (4.9 oz.)	190	30.0
MOLASSES:			
Barbados (USDA)	½ cup (5.4 oz.)	418	108.2
Barbados (USDA)	1 T.	54	14.0
Blackstrap (USDA)	½ cup (5.4 oz.)	329	85.0
Blackstrap (USDA)	1 T.	43	11.0
Light (USDA)	½ cup (5.4 oz.)	389	100.4
Light (USDA)	1 T.	50	13.0
Medium (USDA)	½ cup (5.4 oz.)	358	92.7
Medium (USDA)	1 T.	46	12.0
(Brer Rabbit) Gold Label	1 T.	50	13.0
(Brer Rabbit) Green Label	1 T.	46	12.0
Unsulphured (Grandma's)	1 T.	57	15.0
MOR (Wilson) canned luncheon meat	3 oz.	267	1.6
MORTADELLA, sausage (USDA)	1 oz.	89	.2
MOSELMAID, German Moselle wine (Deinhard) 11% alcohol	3 fl. oz.	60	1.0
MOUNTAIN WINE (Louis M. Martini) 12.5% alcohol, red, Riesling, vin rosé or white	3 fl. oz.	90	.2

(USDA): United States Department of Agriculture
DNA: Data Not Available
*Prepared as Package Directs

Food and Description	Measure or Quantity	Calories	Carbo-hydrates (grams)
MOXIE, soft drink	6 fl. oz.	90	22.2
MR. ENERGY, soft drink	6 fl. oz.	114	D.N.A.
MRS. BUTTERWORTH'S SYRUP	1 T.	55	12.8
MUFFIN:			
Blueberry, home recipe (USDA)	1.6-oz. muffin (2¾″ dia.)	135	20.1
Bran:			
Home recipe (USDA)	1.6-oz. muffin (2¾″ dia.)	125	20.7
(Van de Kamp's)	1 muffin (1.9 oz.)	168	D.N.A.
Corn:			
Home recipe, prepared with whole-ground cornmeal (USDA)	1.6-oz. muffin (2¾″ dia.)	138	20.4
Home recipe, prepared with degermed cornmeal (USDA)	1.6-oz. muffin (2¾″ dia.)	151	23.1
(Thomas')	1 muffin	180	25.8
English:			
(Cain's)	1 muffin	145	28.0
(Di Carlo)	1 muffin	145	28.0
(Hostess)	1 muffin	145	28.0
King size (Newly Weds)	1 muffin	189	35.7
Queen size (Newly Weds)	1 muffin	106	20.0
(Thomas')	1 muffin	140	28.7
(Wonder)	1 muffin	145	28.0
Golden Egg (Arnold)	1 muffin	156	24.0
Plain, home recipe (USDA)	1.6-oz. muffin (2¾″ dia.)	141	20.3
MUFFIN MIX:			
Apple cinnamon (Betty Crocker)	14-oz. pkg.	1708	306.6
Banana nut (Betty Crocker) *Chiquita*	14-oz. pkg.	1778	285.6
Blueberry:			
Wild (Betty Crocker)	13.5-oz. pkg.	1242	228.2
(Duncan Hines)	1 pkg.	1210	204.0
*(Duncan Hines)	1 muffin	101	17.0
Without berries (Duncan Hines)	1 pkg.	1160	D.N.A.

(USDA): United States Department of Agriculture
DNA: Data Not Available
*Prepared as Package Directs

Food and Description	Measure or Quantity	Calories	Carbo- hydrates (grams)
Coffee nut (Betty Crocker)	14-oz. pkg.	1820	274.4
Corn:			
With enriched flour (USDA)	1 oz.	118	20.4
*Prepared with enriched flour, egg & milk (USDA)	1.6-oz. muffin (2¾" dia.)	156	24.0
With cake flour & nonfat dry milk (USDA)	1 oz.	196	34.4
*Prepared with egg & water (USDA)	1.6-oz. muffin (2¾" dia.)	143	24.9
(Betty Crocker)	14-oz. pkg.	1610	288.4
*(Dromedary)	1.9-oz. muffin	192	27.4
(Flako)	1.3-oz. muffin (1/12 of pkg.)	134	21.0
(Pillsbury) golden	1 oz.	112	18.8
Date (Betty Crocker)	14-oz. pkg.	1666	306.6
Honey bran (Betty Crocker)	14-oz. pkg.	1638	303.8
Oatmeal (Betty Crocker)	14-oz. pkg.	1778	277.2
Orange (Betty Crocker) Sunkist	14-oz. pkg.	1652	312.2
MULLET, raw (USDA):			
Whole	1 lb. (weighed whole)	351	0.
Meat only	4 oz.	166	0.
MUNG BEAN SPROUT (See **BEAN SPROUT**)			
MUSCATEL WINE:			
(Gallo) 14% alcohol	3 fl. oz.	86	7.8
(Gallo) 16% alcohol	3 fl. oz.	101	7.2
(Gallo) 20% alcohol	3 fl. oz.	111	8.4
(Gold Seal) 19% alcohol	3 fl. oz.	158	9.4
(Italian Swiss Colony-Gold Medal) 19.7% alcohol	3 fl. oz.	130	9.0
(Italian Swiss Colony-Private Stock) golden, 19.7% alcohol	3 fl. oz.	138	10.8
(Taylor) 19.5% alcohol	3 fl. oz.	147	11.1
MUSHROOM:			
Raw (USDA):			
Whole	½ lb. (weighed untrimmed)	62	9.7
Trimmed	½ cup (1.2 oz.)	10	1.4

(USDA): United States Department of Agriculture
DNA: Data Not Available
*Prepared as Package Directs

Food and Description	Measure or Quantity	Calories	Carbo-hydrates (grams)
Slices	½ cup (1.2 oz.)	10	1.4
Canned:			
Solids & liq. (USDA)	1 cup (8.6 oz.)	41	5.8
Solids & liq. (USDA)	4 oz.	19	2.7
Sliced, chopped or whole, broiled in butter (B in B)	4 oz.	28	4.1
Sliced or stems & pieces or whole (Green Giant)	4 oz.	12	D.N.A.
(Oxford Royal)	4 oz.	17	2.4
Frozen:			
Whole (Birds Eye)	⅓ pkg. (1.5 oz.)	11	1.9
Whole, in butter sauce (Green Giant)	4 oz.	78	8.8
MUSHROOM SOUP:			
(Green Giant)	8 oz. (by wt.)	152	D.N.A.
*Barley (Manischewitz)	8 oz. (by wt.)	72	12.3
Bisque (Crosse & Blackwell)	6½ oz. (½ can)	103	8.3
Cream of:			
Condensed (USDA)	8 oz. (by wt.)	252	19.1
*Prepared with equal volume water (USDA)	1 cup (8.4 oz.)	134	10.1
*Prepared with equal volume milk (USDA)	1 cup (8.4 oz.)	211	15.8
Condensed (Campbell)	8 oz. (by wt.)	261	17.0
(Heinz) *Great American*	1 cup	120	11.4
*(Heinz)	1 cup	141	9.9
*Dietetic (Claybourne)	8 oz. (by wt.)	80	10.7
Low sodium (Campbell)	8¼-oz. can	138	9.0
Golden, condensed (Campbell)	8 oz. (by wt.)	159	15.9
MUSHROOM SOUP MIX:			
*(Golden Grain)	1 cup	121	16.0
(Lipton)	1 pkg. (1¼ oz.)	127	24.1
*(Wyler's)	6 fl. oz.	113	7.0
MUSKELLUNGE, raw (USDA):			
Whole	1 lb. (weighed whole)	242	0.
Meat only	4 oz.	124	0.

MUSKMELON (See **CANTALOUPE, CASABA** or **HONEYDEW**)

(USDA): United States Department of Agriculture
DNA: Data Not Available
*Prepared as Package Directs

Food and Description	Measure or Quantity	Calories	Carbohydrates (grams)
MUSKRAT, roasted (USDA)	4 oz.	174	0.
MUSSEL (USDA):			
Atlantic & Pacific raw, in shell	1 lb. (weighed in shell)	153	7.2
Atlantic & Pacific, raw, meat only	4 oz.	108	3.8
Pacific, canned, drained solids	4 oz.	129	1.7
MUSTARD, prepared:			
Brown:			
(USDA)	1 tsp.	8	.5
(Gulden's)	¼-oz. packet (1 scant tsp.)	7	.4
(Heinz)	1 tsp.	11	.6
Dusseldorf (Kraft)	1 oz.	.30	1.7
Horseradish (Kraft)	1 oz.	29	1.6
Salad (Kraft)	1 oz.	23	1.7
Yellow:			
(USDA)	1 tsp.	8	.6
(Gulden's)	¼-oz. packet (1 scant tsp.)	5	.5
(Heinz)	1 tsp.	10	.1
(Kraft)	1 oz.	23	1.7
MUSTARD GREENS:			
Raw, whole (USDA)	1 lb. (weighed untrimmed)	98	17.8
Boiled, drained solids (USDA)	1 cup (7.8 oz.)	51	8.8
Frozen:			
Not thawed (USDA)	4 oz.	23	3.6
Boiled, drained solids (USDA)	½ cup (3.8 oz.)	21	3.3
Chopped (Birds Eye)	½ cup (3.3 oz.)	19	2.2
MUSTARD SPINACH (USDA):			
Raw	1 lb.	100	17.7
Boiled, drained solids	4 oz.	18	3.2

N

NASSAU DRY WINE (Gallo) 20% alcohol	3 fl. oz.	106	7.5
NATTO, fermented soybean (USDA)	4 oz.	189	13.0

(USDA): United States Department of Agriculture
DNA: Data Not Available
*Prepared as Package Directs

Food and Description	Measure or Quantity	Calories	Carbo-hydrates (grams)
NEAR BEER (See **BEER, NEAR**)			
NEAPOLITAN CREAM PIE, frozen:			
(Banquet)	2½ oz.	188	27.2
(Mrs. Smith's)	⅙ of 8″ pie	209	25.5
NECTARINE, fresh (USDA):			
Whole	1 lb. (weighed with pits)	267	71.4
Flesh only	4 oz.	73	19.4
NEW ZEALAND SPINACH (USDA):			
Raw	1 lb.	86	14.1
Boiled, drained solids	4 oz.	15	2.4
NIERSTEINER, German Rhine wine (Julius Kayser) 10% alcohol	3 fl. oz.	54	.9
NOODLE. Plain noodle products are essentially the same in caloric value and carbohydrate content on the same weight basis. The longer they are cooked, the more water is absorbed and this affects the nutritive values. (USDA):			
Dry, 1½″ strips	1 cup (2.6 oz.)	283	52.6
Dry	1 oz.	110	20.4
Cooked	1 cup (5.6 oz.)	200	37.2
Cooked	1 oz.	35	6.6
NOODLE & BEEF, canned:			
(Heinz)	8-oz. can	133	18.1
(Nalley's)	4 oz.	159	5.9
With gravy (College Inn)	4 oz.	318	59.1
With tomato sauce (College Inn)	4 oz.	319	47.4
NOODLE with CHICKEN:			
Canned (College Inn)	4 oz.	302	52.9
*Mix (Kraft)	4 oz.	122	18.9

(USDA): United States Department of Agriculture
DNA: Data Not Available
*Prepared as Package Directs

Food and Description	Measure or Quantity	Calories	Carbo-hydrates (grams)
NOODLE, CHOW MEIN, canned:			
(USDA)	1 oz.	139	16.4
(Chun King)	1 oz.	145	16.0
(Hung's)	1 oz.	148	16.1
NOODLE DINNER:			
Cantong dinner mix (Betty Crocker)	5-oz. pkg.	590	88.5
With chicken, canned (Lynden)	14 oz.	421	33.0
With chicken & vegetables, canned (Lynden)	15 oz.	550	50.0
With chicken, frozen (Swanson)	10¾-oz. dinner	370	46.0
*Romanoff dinner mix (Kraft)	4 oz.	214	19.6
Stroganoff dinner mix (Betty Crocker)	5.5-oz. pkg.	654	100.1
With turkey, canned (Lynden)	15 oz.	369	28.0
NOODLE MIX:			
Almondine (Betty Crocker)	6-oz. pkg.	726	101.4
*Almondine *Noodle-Roni*	½ cup (3.5 oz.)	126	19.1
*Casserole *Noodle-Roni*	½ cup	85	14.6
Italiano (Betty Crocker)	6-oz. pkg.	606	106.8
*Parmesano *Noodle-Roni*	½ cup	87	15.0
Romanoff (Betty Crocker)	5.5-oz. pkg.	666	95.2
*Romanoff *Noodle-Roni*	½ cup (3.5 oz.)	158	19.8
Scallop-A-Roni	½ cup	88	13.4
Twist-A-Roni	½ cup (3.5 oz.)	120	18.0
NOODLE SOUP:			
Beef (See **BEEF SOUP**)			
Chicken (See **CHICKEN SOUP**)			
With ground beef, condensed, canned (Campbell)	8 oz. (by wt.)	181	18.4
N-RICH, cream substitute	⅑ oz.	10	1.7
NUITS ST. GEORGE, French red Burgundy (Barton & Guestier) 13.5% alcohol	3 fl. oz.	70	.5
NUT, mixed (See also individual kinds):			
Dry roasted:			
(Planters)	1 oz.	175	6.2

Food and Description	Measure or Quantity	Calories	Carbo-hydrates (grams)
(Skippy)	1 oz.	172	6.9
Oil roasted:			
With peanuts (Planters)	1 oz.	185	6.2
Without peanuts (Planters)	1 oz.	180	6.0
(Skippy)	1 oz.	181	4.2
NUT LOAF (See **BREAD, CANNED**)			
NUTMEG (Ehlers)	1 tsp.	12	D.N.A.
NUTRAMENT (Drackett):			
Liquid:			
Cherry	1 can (12½ fl. oz.)	423	56.0
Chocolate or chocolate marshmallow	1 can (12½ fl. oz.)	399	50.0
Dutch chocolate	1 can (12½ fl. oz.)	422	56.0
Strawberry	1 can (12½ fl. oz.)	375	44.0
Vanilla	1 can (12½ fl. oz.)	387	47.0
Powder:			
Chocolate or chocolate malt	1 packet (2 oz.)	214	37.3
Strawberry or vanilla	1 packet (2 oz.)	214	38.3

O

Food and Description	Measure or Quantity	Calories	Carbo-hydrates (grams)
OAT FLAKES, cereal:			
(USDA)	1 cup (1.4 oz.)	162	29.0
(Post) fortified	1 cup (1.5 oz.)	164	28.4
OATMEAL:			
Instant:			
Dry:			
(H-O)	1 cup	250	42.4
(H-O)	1 T.	15	2.6
(Quaker)	1-oz. packet (¾ cup cooked)	107	19.0
(3 Minute)	1 oz.	109	19.0
With apple & cinnamon (Quaker)	1.1-oz. packet (¾ cup cooked)	119	24.0
With maple & brown sugar (Quaker)	1⅝-oz. packet (¾ cup cooked)	177	36.0

(USDA): United States Department of Agriculture
DNA: Data Not Available
*Prepared as Package Directs

Food and Description	Measure or Quantity	Calories	Carbo-hydrates (grams)
With raisins & spice (Quaker)	1.5-oz. packet (¾ cup cooked)	154	32.0
Cooked (3 Minute)	1 cup	175	31.0
Quick:			
Dry:			
(H-O)	1 cup	250	42.4
(H-O)	1 T.	15	2.6
(Ralston Oats)	5 T. (1 oz.)	107	18.3
Cooked:			
*(USDA)	1 cup (8.3 oz.)	130	22.9
*(Albers)	1 cup	148	26.0
*(Quaker)	1 cup	160	28.4
*(Ralston Oats)	1 cup	160	27.5
Regular:			
Dry:			
(USDA)	1 cup (2.5 oz.)	280	49.1
(USDA)	1 T.	18	3.1
Old fashioned (H-O)	1 cup	250	42.4
Old fashioned (H-O)	1 T.	15	2.6
(Ralston Oats)	5 T.	107	18.3
(Ralston Oats)	1 T.	21	3.7
Cooked:			
*(USDA)	1 cup (8.3 oz.)	130	22.9
*Old fashioned (Albers)	1 cup	148	26.0
*Old fashioned (Quaker)	1 cup (1.5-oz. dry)	160	28.4
*(Ralston Oats)	1 cup	160	27.5
OCEAN PERCH (USDA):			
Atlantic:			
Raw, whole	1 lb. (weighed whole)	124	0.
Fried	4 oz.	257	7.7
Frozen, breaded, fried, reheated	4 oz.	362	18.7
Pacific, raw:			
Whole	1 lb. (weighed whole)	116	0.
Meat only	4 oz.	108	0.
OCEAN PERCH DINNER, frozen (Banquet)	9-oz. dinner	472	49.2
OCTOPUS, raw, meat only (USDA)	4 oz.	83	0.

(USDA): United States Department of Agriculture
DNA: Data Not Available
*Prepared as Package Directs

Food and Description	Measure or Quantity	Calories	Carbohydrates (grams)
OESTRICHLER LENCHEN RIESLING, German Rhine wine (Deinhard) 11% alcohol	3 fl. oz.	72	4.5
OIL, salad or cooking:			
(USDA) including olive	½ cup (3.7 oz.)	928	0.
(USDA) including olive	1 T.	115	0.
Buttery flavor (Wesson)	1 T.	125	0.
Corn (Mazola)	1 pt.	3915	0.
Corn (Mazola)	1 T.	125	0.
Cottonseed, winterized (Kraft)	1 oz.	257	0.
Peanut (Planters)	1 T.	125	0.
Safflower (Kraft)	1 oz.	257	0.
Safflower (*Saff-O-Life*)	1 oz.	255	0.
(Saffola)	1 T.	120	0.
(Wesson)	1 T.	125	0.
OKRA:			
Raw, whole (USDA)	1 lb. (weighed untrimmed)	140	29.6
Boiled, drained solids (USDA):			
Whole	½ cup (3.1 oz.)	26	5.3
Pods	8 pods (3″ x ⅝″)	24	5.1
Slices	½ cup (2.8 oz.)	23	4.8
Canned, with tomatoes (King Pharr)	½ cup	26	5.0
Frozen:			
Cut & pods, uncooked (USDA)	4 oz.	44	10.2
Cut, drained solids, boiled (USDA)	½ cup (3.2 oz.)	35	8.1
Whole, drained, solids, boiled (USDA)	½ cup (2.4 oz.)	26	6.1
Cut & whole, uncooked, (Birds Eye)	½ cup (3.3 oz.)	36	7.6
OKS, cereal (Kellogg's)	1 cup (¾ oz.)	73	14.9
OLD FASHIONED COCKTAIL (Hiram Walker) 62 proof	3 fl. oz.	165	3.0
OLD FASHIONED MIX (Bar-Tender's)	1 serving (⅙ oz.)	20	4.7
OLD MANSE SYRUP	1 T.	50	13.2

(USDA): United States Department of Agriculture
DNA: Data Not Available
*Prepared as Package Directs

Food and Description	Measure or Quantity	Calories	Carbo-hydrates (grams)
OLEOMARGARINE (See **MARGARINE**)			
OLIVE:			
Green:			
(USDA)	1 oz.	32	.4
(USDA)	4 med. or 3 extra large or 2 giant	15	Tr.
(USDA)	1 olive (13⁄16″ x 11⁄16″)	8	.1
(La Manna, Azema & Farnan)	1 med.-size manzanilla	4	.1
(La Manna, Azema & Farnan)	1 queen size	5	.1
Ripe, by variety:			
Ascolano, any size (USDA)	4 oz.	146	2.9
Greek style, with pits, drained (USDA)	4 oz.	307	8.0
Manzanilla, any size (USDA)	4 oz.	146	2.9
Mission, any size (USDA)	4 oz.	209	3.6
Mission (USDA)	3 small or 2 large	15	Tr.
Mission, slices (USDA)	1⁄2 cup (2.2 oz.)	115	2.0
Sevillano, any size (USDA)	4 oz.	105	3.1
Ripe, by size:			
Select (Lindsay)	1 olive	3	.1
Medium (Lindsay)	1 olive	4	.1
Large (Lindsay)	1 olive	5	.1
Extra large (Lindsay)	1 olive	5	.1
Mammoth (Lindsay)	1 olive	6	.1
Giant (Lindsay)	1 olive	8	.2
Jumbo (Lindsay)	1 olive	10	.2
Colossal (Lindsay)	1 olive	13	.3
Supercolossal (Lindsay)	1 olive	16	.3
Super supreme (Lindsay)	1 olive	18	.3
ONION:			
Raw (USDA):			
Whole	1 lb. (weighed untrimmed)	157	35.9
Whole	3.9-oz. onion (21⁄2″ dia.)	41	9.6
Chopped	1⁄2 cup (3 oz.)	32	7.5
Chopped	1 T.	4	1.0
Grated or ground	1 T.	5	1.2
Slices	1⁄2 cup (2 oz.)	21	4.9

(USDA): United States Department of Agriculture
DNA: Data Not Available
*Prepared as Package Directs

Food and Description	Measure or Quantity	Calories	Carbohydrates (grams)
Boiled, drained solids (USDA):			
Whole	½ cup (3.7 oz.)	30	6.8
Halves or pieces	½ cup (3.2 oz.)	26	5.8
Cream sauce:			
Canned (Durkee) *O & C*	15½-oz. can	352	36.6
Frozen (Birds Eye)	½ cup (3 oz.)	127	12.2
Dehydrated flakes (USDA)	1 oz.	99	23.0
Frozen:			
Chopped (Birds Eye)	¼ pkg. (4 oz.)	43	9.8
Whole, small (Birds Eye)	⅓ pkg. (3.3 oz.)	42	9.9
French-fried rings:			
(Durkee) *O & C*	2 cups (3½-oz. can)	618	44.5
Frozen (Birds Eye)	¼ pkg. (2 oz.)	168	17.3
Frozen (Commodore)	1 oz.	55	2.9
Frozen (Mrs. Paul's)	1 oz.	41	D.N.A.
Pickled, cocktail (Crosse & Blackwell)	1 T.	1	.3
Pickled, sweet Dutch (Smucker's)	1 onion	4	1.0
ONION BOUILLON:			
Cube (Herb-Ox)	1 cube	12	1.3
Cube (Wyler's)	1 cube	5	1.2
Instant (Herb-Ox)	1 packet	15	1.2
ONION, GREEN, raw (USDA):			
Whole	1 lb. (weighed untrimmed)	157	35.7
Bulb & entire top	2 oz.	20	4.6
Bulb without green top	3 small onions (.8 oz.)	10	2.6
Slices, bulb & white portion of top	½ cup (1.7 oz.)	22	5.2
Tops only	1 oz.	8	1.6
ONION JUICE (McCormick)	1 tsp.	<1	D.N.A.
ONION SOUP:			
Condensed (USDA)	8 oz. (by wt.)	123	9.8
*Prepared with equal volume water (USDA)	1 cup (8.4 oz.)	65	5.3
Condensed (Campbell)	8 oz. (by wt.)	84	6.1
(Crosse & Blackwell)	6½ oz. (½ can)	46	4.8
(Hormel)	15-oz. can	145	5.5

(USDA): United States Department of Agriculture
DNA: Data Not Available
*Prepared as Package Directs

Food and Description	Measure or Quantity	Calories	Carbo-hydrates (grams)
ONION SOUP MIX:			
Dry (USDA)	1 oz.	99	15.3
*Prepared (USDA)	1 cup (8.1 oz.)	34	5.2
French (Croyden House)	1 tsp.	11	2.3
*(Golden Grain)	1 cup	41	7.0
(Lipton)	1 pkg. (1.4 oz.)	145	22.1
*(Wyler's)	6 fl. oz.	28	5.0
ONION, WELCH, raw (USDA):			
Whole	1 lb. (weighed untrimmed)	100	19.2
Trimmed	4 oz.	39	7.4
OPOSSUM, roasted, meat only			
(USDA)	4 oz.	251	0.
ORANGE, fresh:			
All varieties:			
Peeled (USDA)	4 oz.	56	13.8
Sections (USDA)	1 cup (8.6 oz.)	120	29.8
Sections, chilled, bottled (Kraft)	4 oz.	58	12.6
California Navel:			
Whole (USDA)	1 lb. (weighed with rind & seeds)	157	39.2
(USDA)	6.3-oz. orange (2⅘" dia.)	63	15.4
Flesh only (USDA)	4 oz.	58	14.4
Sections (USDA)	1 cup (8.6 oz.)	124	31.0
Wedge, unpeeled (Sunkist)	⅙ orange	10	4.0
Cut, bite-size (Sunkist)	½ cup	62	16.0
California Valencia (USDA):			
Whole	1 lb. (weighed with rind & seeds)	174	42.2
Flesh only	4 oz.	58	14.1
Sections	1 cup (8.6 oz.)	124	30.2
Florida, all varieties (USDA):			
Whole	1 lb. (weighed with rind & seeds)	158	40.3
Whole	7.4-oz. orange (3" dia.)	75	19.0
Sections	1 cup (8.6 oz.)	114	29.2
ORANGEADE:			
(Sealtest) container	½ cup	62	15.6

(USDA): United States Department of Agriculture
DNA: Data Not Available
*Prepared as Package Directs

Food and Description	Measure or Quantity	Calories	Carbo-hydrates (grams)
Frozen, sweetened:			
*(Minute Maid)	½ cup	63	15.1
*(Snow Crop)	½ cup	63	15.1
*Mix (General Foods) *Twist*	1 cup	87	20.9
*Mix (Salada)	6 fl. oz.	80	19.4
ORANGE-APRICOT JUICE DRINK, canned:			
(USDA)	1 cup (8.8 oz.)	124	31.6
(BC)	1 cup	120	D.N.A.
ORANGE-BANANA JUICE DRINK, canned (BC)	1 cup	120	D.N.A.
ORANGE CAKE MIX:			
(Betty Crocker) *Sunkist*	1-lb. 2.75-oz. pkg.	2194	429.4
(Betty Crocker) *Sunkist*	1 oz.	117	22.9
Chiffon (Betty Crocker) *Sunkist*	1-lb. 2.5-oz. pkg.	2109	414.4
*(Duncan Hines)	1 cake	2369	384.0
(Pillsbury)	1 oz.	120	21.9
ORANGE DRINK:			
Canned (Hi-C)	6 fl. oz.	89	22.2
Canned (Sealtest)	6 fl. oz.	83	20.2
*Mix (Wyler's)	6 fl. oz.	63	15.8
ORANGE EXTRACT (Ehlers)	1 tsp.	14	D.N.A.
ORANGE-GRAPEFRUIT JUICE:			
Canned (Treesweet)	½ cup	62	D.N.A.
Frozen, concentrate:			
(USDA)	6-oz. can	327	77.2
*Diluted with 3 parts water (USDA)	½ cup (4.4 oz.)	55	13.1
*(Birds Eye)	½ cup (4.2 oz.)	48	12.5
*(7L)	½ cup	55	13.0
*(Treesweet)	½ cup	62	D.N.A.
*Unsweetened (Minute Maid)	½ cup	50	12.7
*Unsweetened (Snow Crop)	½ cup	50	12.7
ORANGE-GRAPEFRUIT JUICE DRINK, canned (BC)	6 fl. oz.	90	D.N.A.
ORANGE ICE (Sealtest)	⅙ qt.	177	43.5

(USDA): United States Department of Agriculture
DNA: Data Not Available
*Prepared as Package Directs

Food and Description	Measure or Quantity	Calories	Carbohydrates (grams)
ORANGE JUICE:			
Fresh:			
All varieties (USDA)	½ cup (4.3 oz.)	55	12.8
California Navel (USDA)	½ cup (4.3 oz.)	59	13.8
California Valencia (USDA)	½ cup (4.3 oz.)	58	12.9
Florida, early or midseason (USDA)	½ cup (4.3 oz.)	49	11.4
Florida Temple (USDA)	½ cup (4.3 oz.)	66	15.8
Florida Valencia (USDA)	½ cup (4.3 oz.)	55	12.9
(Sunkist)	½ cup	52	13.0
Canned, sweetened:			
(USDA)	½ cup	65	15.8
(Heinz)	5½-oz. can	69	15.1
(Stokely-Van Camp)	½ cup	65	15.8
(Treesweet)	½ cup	65	15.8
Canned or bottled, unsweetened:			
(USDA)	½ cup (4.4 oz.)	60	14.0
Chilled (Kraft)	½ cup	52	11.2
(Sealtest)	½ cup	64	14.4
(Stokely-Van Camp)	½ cup	60	14.0
Dehydrated, crystals:			
(USDA)	4-oz. can	429	100.5
*Reconstituted (USDA)	1 cup (8.7 oz.)	114	26.8
Frozen, concentrate:			
(USDA)	6-oz. can	330	80.0
*Diluted with 3 parts water (USDA)	½ cup (4.3 oz.)	55	13.5
*(Birds Eye)	½ cup (4.2 oz.)	48	12.6
*Imitation (Birds Eye)	½ cup (4 oz.)	67	16.6
*(Lake Hamilton)	½ cup	58	13.2
*(Minute Maid)	½ cup	60	14.3
*(Seald-Sweet)	½ cup	56	13.3
*(7L)	½ cup	55	13.5
*(Snow Crop)	½ cup	60	14.3
*(Treesweet)	½ cup	62	D.N.A.

ORANGE, MANDARIN (See **MANDARIN ORANGE** & **TANGERINE**)

Food and Description	Measure or Quantity	Calories	Carbohydrates (grams)
ORANGE PEEL, CANDIED:			
(USDA)	1 oz.	90	22.8
(Liberty)	1 oz.	93	22.6

(USDA): United States Department of Agriculture
DNA: Data Not Available
*Prepared as Package Directs

Food and Description	Measure or Quantity	Calories	Carbo-hydrates (grams)
ORANGE-PINEAPPLE DRINK, canned:			
(BC)	6 fl. oz.	96	D.N.A.
(Hi-C)	6 fl. oz.	88	21.8
ORANGE-PINEAPPLE PIE			
(Tastykake)	4-oz. pie	374	56.2
ORANGE RENNET CUSTARD MIX:			
Powder:			
(Junket)	1 oz.	116	27.7
*Prepared with whole milk (Junket)	4 oz.	108	14.6
Tablet:			
(Junket)	1 tablet	1	.2
*Prepared with whole milk & sugar (Junket)	4 oz.	101	13.4
ORANGE SHERBET (See SHERBET)			
ORANGE SOFT DRINK:			
Sweetened:			
(Canada Dry)	6 fl. oz.	96	24.7
(Clicquot Club)	6 fl. oz.	105	25.1
(Cott)	6 fl. oz.	105	25.1
(Dr. Brown's)	6 fl. oz.	87	21.9
(Dr. Pepper)	6 fl. oz.	102	25.2
Fanta	6 fl. oz.	96	24.0
(Hires)	6 fl. oz.	87	21.9
(Hoffman)	6 fl. oz.	96	24.0
(Key Food)	6 fl. oz.	87	21.9
(Kirsch)	6 fl. oz.	88	21.9
(Mission)	6 fl. oz.	105	25.1
(Nedick's)	6 fl. oz.	87	21.9
Orangette	6 fl. oz.	94	24.3
(Shasta)	6 fl. oz.	95	24.0
(Waldbaum)	6 fl. oz.	87	21.9
(White Rock)	6 fl. oz.	90	D.N.A.
(Yoo-Hoo)	6 fl. oz.	90	18.0
High-protein (Yoo-Hoo)	6 fl. oz.	114	24.6
(Yukon Club)	6 fl. oz.	90	22.5

(USDA): United States Department of Agriculture
DNA: Data Not Available
*Prepared as Package Directs

Food and Description	Measure or Quantity	Calories	Carbo-hydrates (grams)
Low calorie:			
(Dr. Brown's) *Slim-Ray*	6 fl. oz.	3	.8
(Hoffman)	6 fl. oz.	3	.8*
(No-Cal)	6 fl. oz.	4	0.
(Shasta)	6 fl. oz.	<1	<.1
ORGEAT SYRUP (Julius Wile)	1 fl. oz.	103	26.0
ORVIETO WINE, Italian white:			
(Antinori) 12% alcohol	3 fl. oz.	84	6.3
(Antinori) *Castello La Scala,* 12½% alcohol	3 fl. oz.	87	6.3
OVALTINE, dry:			
Natural	4 heaping tsp.	77	16.6
Swiss chocolate	4 heaping tsp.	77	17.7
OXTAIL CONSOMME MIX, instant (Knorr Swiss)	1 tsp.	11	D.N.A.
OXTAIL SOUP (Crosse & Blackwell)	6½ oz. (½ can)	134	7.4
OYSTER:			
Raw:			
Eastern:			
Meat only (USDA)	13-19 med. oysters (8.5 oz.)	160	8.0
Meat only (USDA)	1 cup (8.5 oz.)	160	8.0
Meat only (USDA)	4 oz.	75	3.9
(Epicure)	1 cup	220	13.0
Pacific, meat only (USDA)	4 oz.	103	7.3
Canned, solids & liq. (USDA)	4 oz.	86	5.5
Fried (USDA)	4 oz.	271	21.1
Smoked, Japanese baby (Cresca)	3⅔-oz. can	222	D.N.A.
OYSTER CRACKER (See **CRACKER**)			
OYSTER STEW:			
Home recipe (USDA):			
1 part oysters to 1 part milk by volume	1 cup (6-8 oysters)	244	14.2
1 part oysters to 2 parts milk by volume	4 oz.	110	5.1

(USDA): United States Department of Agriculture
DNA: Data Not Available
*Prepared as Package Directs

Food and Description	Measure or Quantity	Calories	Carbo-hydrates (grams)
1 part oysters to 3 parts milk by volume	4 oz.	98	5.3
1 part oysters to 3 parts milk by volume	1 cup (3-4 oysters)	198	10.8
Canned, condensed (Campbell)	8 oz. (by wt.)	129	12.0
Frozen:			
Condensed (USDA)	8 oz. (by wt.)	232	15.6
*Prepared with equal volume water (USDA)	4 oz. (by wt.)	58	3.9
*Prepared with equal volume milk (USDA)	4 oz. (by wt.)	95	6.7
Condensed (Campbell)	8 oz. (by wt.)	232	15.6

P

PAGAN PINK WINE (Gallo) 11% alcohol	3 fl. oz.	81	6.6
PAISANO WINE (Gallo) 13% alcohol	3 fl. oz.	53	1.2
PANCAKE, home recipe (USDA)	4″ pancake (1 oz.)	62	9.2
PANCAKE BATTER (Perx)	1⅓ oz. (4″ pancake)	57	8.9
PANCAKE & WAFFLE MIX (See also **PANCAKE & WAFFLE MIX, DIETETIC**):			
Blueberry (Pillsbury)	1 oz.	98	20.6
Buckwheat:			
(USDA)	1 cup (4.8 oz.)	442	94.9
(USDA)	1 oz.	93	19.9
*Prepared with egg & milk (USDA)	4″ pancake (1 oz.)	57	6.7
*(Aunt Jemima)	4″ pancake (1.2 oz.)	64	8.1
Hungry Jack (Pillsbury)	1 oz.	95	20.2
Buttermilk:			
(USDA)	1 cup (4.8 oz.)	480	102.2
(USDA)	1 oz.	101	21.5
*Prepared with milk (USDA)	1 pancake (1 oz.)	57	9.0
*Prepared with milk & egg (USDA)	1 pancake (1 oz.)	64	9.2
*(Aunt Jemima)	4″ pancake (1 oz.)	71	9.3
(Betty Crocker)	1 oz.	99	21.7

(USDA): United States Department of Agriculture
DNA: Data Not Available
*Prepared as Package Directs

Food and Description	Measure or Quantity	Calories	Carbo-hydrates (grams)
Complete (Betty Crocker)	1 oz.	106	21.2
*(Duncan Hines)	4" pancake	105	14.0
Hungry Jack (Pillsbury)	1 oz.	98	20.5
Plain:			
(USDA)	1 cup (4.8 oz.)	480	102.2
(USDA)	1 oz.	101	21.5
*Prepared with milk (USDA)	1 pancake (1 oz.)	57	9.0
*Prepared with milk & egg (USDA)	1 pancake (1 oz.)	64	9.2
*(Aunt Jemima)	4" pancake (1 oz.)	61	8.0
*(Aunt Jemima) Deluxe Easy Pour	4" pancake (1.2 oz.)	79	11.0
(Albers)	1 cup	459	99.2
(Golden Mix)	1 cup	459	80.8
(Golden Mix)	1 oz.	107	18.8
Hungry Jack (Pillsbury)	1 oz.	97	19.9
Hungry Jack, extra light (Pillsbury)	1 oz.	97	20.2
Sweet cream (Pillsbury)	1 oz.	101	20.2

PANCAKE & WAFFLE MIX, DIETETIC:

Buttermilk (Tillie Lewis)	1 oz.	93	18.1
*Buttermilk (Tillie Lewis)	4" pancake (1.2 oz.)	42	8.0
Plain (Tillie Lewis)	1 oz.	93	18.1
*Plain (Tillie Lewis)	4" pancake (1.2 oz.)	42	8.0

PANCAKE & WAFFLE SYRUP:

Sweetened (Polaner)	1 T.	54	13.5
Sweetened (Smucker's)	1 T.	44	D.N.A.
Dietetic or low calorie:			
(Dia-Mel)	1 T.	22	5.5
(Diet Delight)	1 T.	6	1.2
(Tillie Lewis)	1 T.	13	3.0

PANCREAS, raw (USDA):

Beef, lean only	4 oz.	160	0.
Beef, medium-fat	4 oz.	321	0.
Calf	4 oz.	183	0.
Hog or hog sweetbread	4 oz.	274	0.

PAPAW, raw (USDA):

Whole	1 lb. (weighed with rind & seeds)	289	57.2
Flesh only	4 oz.	96	18.9

Food and Description	Measure or Quantity	Calories	Carbo-hydrates (grams)
PAPAYA:			
Fresh (USDA):			
Whole	1 lb. (weighed with skin & seeds)	119	30.4
Flesh only	4 oz.	44	11.3
Cubed	1 cup (½" cubes)	71	18.2
Concentrate (Karika):			
*3 to 1 blend	6 fl. oz.	14	D.N.A.
*4 to 1 blend	6 fl. oz.	11	D.N.A.
*5 to 1 blend	6 fl. oz.	9	D.N.A.
PARSLEY, fresh (USDA):			
Whole	½ lb.	100	19.3
Chopped	1 T.	1	Tr.
PARSNIP (USDA):			
Raw, whole	1 lb. (weighed unpared)	293	67.5
Boiled, drained solids, cut in pieces	½ cup (3.7 oz.)	70	15.8
PASHA TURKISH COFFEE, Turkish liqueur (Leroux) 53 proof	1 fl. oz.	97	13.3
PARTY FRUIT, soft drink (Kirsch)	6 fl. oz.	88	22.1
PARTY PUNCH, undiluted (Mogen David) 12% alcohol	3 fl. oz.	156	21.3
PASSION FRUIT, fresh (USDA):			
Whole	1 lb. (weighed with shell)	212	50.0
Pulp & seeds	4 oz.	102	24.0
PASTINAS, dry (USDA):			
Carrot	1 oz.	105	21.5
Egg	1 oz.	109	20.4
Spinach	1 oz.	104	21.2
PASTRAMI (Vienna)	1 oz.	57	.4
PASTRY SHELL (See also **PIE CRUST**):			
Frozen (Pepperidge Farm)	1 shell	226	15.5
(Stella D'oro)	1 shell	143	16.2

(USDA): United States Department of Agriculture
DNA: Data Not Available
*Prepared as Package Directs

Food and Description	Measure or Quantity	Calories	Carbo-hydrates (grams)
Pot pie (Keebler)	4″ shell	236	29.6
Tart, sweet (Keebler)	3″ shell	158	16.6
PATE, canned:			
De foie gras (USDA)	1 oz.	131	1.4
De foie gras (USDA)	1 T.	69	.7
Liver (Hormel)	1 oz.	78	1.1
(Sell's)	1 T.	43	9.9
Swiss Parfait with herbs or truffles (Cresca)	1 oz.	73	D.N.A.
PEA, GREEN:			
Raw (USDA):			
In pod	1 lb. (weighed in pod)	145	24.8
Shelled	1 lb.	381	65.3
Shelled	½ cup (2.4 oz.)	58	9.9
Boiled, drained solids (USDA)	½ cup (2.8 oz.)	58	9.8
Canned, regular pack:			
Alaska, Early or June, solids & liq. (USDA)	½ cup (4.4 oz.)	82	15.5
Alaska, Early or June, drained solids (USDA)	½ cup (3 oz.)	76	14.4
Alaska, Early or June, drained liq. (USDA)	4 oz.	29	5.9
Alaska, drained solids (Butter Kernel)	½ cup	69	12.8
Alaska or Early, solids & liq. (Stokely-Van Camp)	½ cup	82	15.5
Early June, drained solids (Cannon)	4 oz.	100	19.1
Early June, drained solids (Fall River)	½ cup	69	12.8
Sweet, drained solids (Butter Kernel)	½ cup	60	10.4
Sweet, drained solids (Cannon)	4 oz.	91	17.0
Sweet, drained solids (Fall River)	½ cup	60	10.4
(Green Giant)	½ cup	69	12.8
(King Pharr)	½ cup	98	17.0
Canned, dietetic pack:			
Solids & liq. (USDA)	4 oz.	62	11.1
Drained solids (USDA)	4 oz.	88	16.2
Drained liq. (USDA)	4 oz.	25	4.6

Food and Description	Measure or Quantity	Calories	Carbo- hydrates (grams)
Solids & liq. (Blue Boy)	4 oz.	46	7.6
Solids & liq. (Diet Delight)	½ cup (4.4 oz.)	45	7.6
(S and W) *Nutradiet*	4 oz.	40	6.8
(Tillie Lewis)	½ cup (4.4 oz.)	59	8.6
Frozen:			
Uncooked (USDA)	4 oz.	82	14.5
Uncooked (USDA)	1 cup (5.1 oz.)	106	18.6
Boiled, drained solids (USDA)	½ cup (2.9 oz.)	57	9.8
(Blue Goose)	4 oz.	76	12.4
(Stokely-Van Camp)	4 oz.	82	14.5
Sweet or tender tiny (Birds Eye)	½ cup (3.3 oz.)	70	12.2
In butter sauce (Birds Eye)	½ cup (3.3 oz.)	90	10.6
In butter sauce, baby peas (Green Giant)	4 oz.	109	12.5
In butter sauce, sweet (Green Giant)	4 oz.	116	13.4
With cream sauce (Birds Eye)	½ cup (2.7 oz.)	129	13.1
With cream sauce (Green Giant) boil-in-the-bag	4 oz.	88	10.1

PEA, MATURE SEED:
Dry:			
Whole (USDA)	1 lb.	1542	273.5
Whole (USDA)	1 cup (7 oz.)	680	120.6
Split:			
(USDA)	1 lb.	1579	284.4
(USDA)	1 cup (7.2 oz.)	706	127.3
(Sinsheimer)	1 oz.	99	17.5
Cooked, split, drained solids (USDA)	½ cup (3.4 oz.)	112	11.4

PEA POD, edible-podded or Chinese:
Raw (USDA)	1 lb. (weighed untrimmed)	228	51.7
Boiled, drained solids (USDA)	4 oz.	49	10.7

PEA & CARROT:
Canned, dietetic pack; solid & liq.:			
(Blue Boy)	4 oz.	33	5.5
(Diet Delight)	½ cup (4.1 oz.)	40	6.7
(S and W) *Nutradiet*	4 oz.	37	6.4
Frozen:			
Not thawed (USDA)	4 oz.	62	11.8

(USDA): United States Department of Agriculture
DNA: Data Not Available
*Prepared as Package Directs

Food and Description	Measure or Quantity	Calories	Carbohydrates (grams)
Boiled, drained solids (USDA)	4 oz.	60	11.5
Boiled, drained solids (USDA)	½ cup (3 oz.)	46	8.8
(Birds Eye)	½ cup (3.3 oz.)	55	10.7
(Blue Goose)	4 oz.	57	10.0
PEA & CELERY, frozen (Birds Eye)	½ cup (3.3 oz.)	58	10.6
PEA & ONION:			
Canned (Green Giant)	4 oz.	75	D.N.A.
Frozen (Birds Eye)	½ cup (3.3 oz.)	67	12.4
PEA & POTATO, with cream sauce, frozen (Birds Eye)	½ cup (2.7 oz.)	136	14.3
PEA with SAUTEED MUSHROOM, frozen (Birds Eye)	½ cup (3.3 oz.)	67	11.8
PEA SOUP, GREEN:			
Canned, low sodium (Campbell)	8½-oz. can (by wt.)	152	25.0
Canned, condensed:			
(USDA)	8 oz. (by wt.)	241	41.8
*Prepared with equal volume water (USDA)	1 cup (8.6 oz.)	130	22.5
*Prepared with equal volume milk (USDA)	1 cup (8.6 oz.)	208	28.6
(Campbell)	8 oz. (by wt.)	263	42.0
Dry mix:			
(USDA)	1 oz.	103	17.5
*(USDA)	1 cup (8.5 oz.)	121	20.3
*(Golden Grain)	1 cup	115	14.4
(Lipton)	1 pkg. (4 oz.)	418	67.4
Frozen, condensed:			
With ham (USDA)	8 oz. (by wt.)	257	36.3
*With ham, prepared with equal volume water (USDA)	8 oz. (by wt.)	129	18.2
With ham (Campbell)	8 oz. (by wt.)	247	32.9
PEA SOUP, SPLIT:			
Canned, regular pack:			
Condensed (USDA)	8 oz. (by wt.)	268	38.6
*Prepared with equal volume water (USDA)	1 cup	145	20.6

(USDA): United States Department of Agriculture
DNA: Data Not Available
*Prepared as Package Directs

Food and Description	Measure or Quantity	Calories	Carbo-hydrates (grams)
With ham, condensed			
(Campbell)	8 oz. (by wt.)	320	43.3
*(Manischewitz)	8 oz. (by wt.)	133	22.6
*With ham (Heinz)	1 cup	150	21.2
With smoked ham (Heinz)			
Great American	1 cup	166	21.4
Canned, dietetic:			
*Condensed (Claybourne)	1 cup	98	19.1
(Tillie Lewis)	1 cup	150	26.6

PEACH:
Fresh:

Food and Description	Measure or Quantity	Calories	Carbo-hydrates (grams)
Whole (USDA)	1 lb. (weighed unpeeled)	150	38.3
Whole (USDA)	4-oz. peach (2″ dia.)	35	10.0
Diced (USDA)	½ cup (4.6 oz.)	51	12.9
Sliced (USDA)	½ cup (3 oz.)	33	8.5
Chilled, bottled (Kraft)	4 oz.	66	17.2
Canned, regular pack, solids & liq.:			
Juice pack (USDA)	4 oz.	51	13.2
Light syrup (USDA)	4 oz.	66	17.1
Heavy syrup (USDA)	2 med. halves & 2 T. syrup	91	23.5
Heavy syrup, halves (USDA)	½ cup (4.4 oz.)	99	25.6
Heavy syrup, sliced (USDA)	½ cup (4.4 oz.)	98	25.4
Extra heavy syrup (USDA)	4 oz.	110	28.4
Halves (Hunt's)	4 oz.	51	13.2
Spiced (Hunt's)	4 oz.	110	28.5
(Stokely-Van Camp)	2 med. halves & 2 T. syrup	91	23.5
(White House)	½ cup (4.5 oz.)	100	25.6
Canned, dietetic or unsweetened pack:			
Water pack, solids & liq. (USDA)	½ cup (4.3 oz.)	38	9.9
(Blue Boy) sliced, solids & liq.	4 oz.	32	7.4
(Del Monte) cling	4 oz.	35	D.N.A.
(Diet Delight) cling, halves	½ cup (4.4 oz.)	31	5.9
(Diet Delight) cling, slices	½ cup (4.3 oz.)	33	6.4
(Diet Delight) freestone, halves	½ cup (4.3 oz.)	32	5.8
(Diet Delight) freestone, slices	½ cup (4.2 oz.)	30	5.5
(Libby's) halves or slices	4 oz.	34	9.2
(Naturmade)	4 oz.	32	7.8

(USDA): United States Department of Agriculture
DNA: Data Not Available
*Prepared as Package Directs

Food and Description	Measure or Quantity	Calories	Carbohydrates (grams)
(S and W) *Nutradiet*, cling, halves, unsweetened	2 halves	25	5.7
(S and W) *Nutradiet*, cling, slices, unsweetened	4 oz.	27	5.8
(Yes Madame) Elberta, halves & slices	4 oz.	34	8.1
Dehydrated:			
(USDA)	1 oz.	96	24.9
Cooked, solids & liq. with added sugar (USDA)	½ cup (4.4 oz.)	151	39.1
Peach Crisps, dehydrated snack (Epicure)	1 oz.	88	22.4
Slices (Vacu-Dry)	1 oz.	96	24.9
Dried:			
(USDA)	1 lb.	1188	309.8
(USDA)	½ cup (3.6 oz.)	230	60.1
Cooked, unsweetened (USDA)	½ cup (5-6 halves & 3 T. liq.)	110	29.0
Cooked, with added sugar (USDA)	½ cup (5-6 halves & 3 T. liq.)	181	47.0
Frozen:			
Not thawed (USDA)	12-oz. pkg.	300	77.0
Not thawed (USDA)	16-oz. can	400	103.0
Quick thaw (Birds Eye)	½ cup (5 oz.)	87	22.3
(Spiegl)	½ cup	88	22.5
With whole strawberries, quick thaw (Birds Eye)	½ cup (5 oz.)	81	20.4
PEACH LIQUEUR:			
(Bols) 60 proof	1 fl. oz.	96	8.9
(Hiram Walker) 60 proof	1 fl. oz.	81	8.0
(Leroux) 60 proof	1 fl. oz.	85	8.9
PEACH NECTAR, canned (USDA)	1 cup (8.4 oz.)	115	29.6
PEACH PIE:			
Home recipe (USDA)	⅙ of 9″ pie (5.6 oz.)	403	60.4
(Tastykake)	4-oz. pie	360	52.8
Frozen (Banquet)	5 oz.	320	45.5
Frozen (Mrs. Smith's)	⅙ of 8″ pie	299	42.1
PEACH PIE FILLING:			
(Lucky Leaf)	8 oz.	300	74.0
(Musselman's)	1 cup	292	D.N.A.

(USDA): United States Department of Agriculture
DNA: Data Not Available
*Prepared as Package Directs

Food and Description	Measure or Quantity	Calories	Carbo-hydrates (grams)
PEACH PRESERVE, dietetic or low calorie:			
(Dia-Mel)	1 T.	22	5.4
(Kraft)	1 oz.	9	2.0
(Tillie Lewis)	1 T.	9	2.1
PEACH TURNOVER, frozen			
(Pepperidge Farm)	1 turnover	285	D.N.A.
PEANUT:			
Raw (USDA):			
Whole	1 lb. (weighed in shell)	1868	61.6
With skins	1 oz.	160	5.2
Without skins	1 oz.	161	5.0
Roasted:			
Whole (USDA)	1 lb. (weighed in shell)	1769	62.6
Shelled, with skins (USDA)	1 oz.	164	5.8
Salted (USDA)	1 oz.	166	5.3
Halves, salted (USDA)	½ cup (2.5 oz.)	421	13.5
Chopped (USDA)	½ cup (2.4 oz.)	404	13.0
Chopped, salted (USDA)	1 T.	52	1.6
Dry (Franklin)	1 oz.	163	5.4
Dry (Frito-Lay)	1 oz.	179	2.5
Dry (Planters)	1 oz. (jar)	170	5.4
Dry (Planters) *Peanut Crisps*	1-oz. bag	150	6.2
Dry (Skippy)	1 oz.	169	5.8
Oil (Planters) cocktail	¾-oz. bag	130	3.7
Oil (Planters) cocktail	1 oz. (can)	185	5.0
Oil (Skippy)	1 oz.	181	3.6
(Nab)	1 packet (1.5 oz.)	267	8.0
Spanish, dry roasted (Planters)	1 oz. (jar)	175	3.4
Spanish, oil roasted (Planters)	1 oz. (can)	180	3.4
PEANUT BUTTER:			
(USDA)	½ cup (4.4 oz.)	739	23.6
(USDA)	1 T.	93	2.8
(The Peanut Kids)	1 oz.	165	5.5
(Peter Pan)	1 T.	100	3.9
(Planters)	1 T.	100	3.8
(Skippy)	1 oz.	179	4.2
(Skippy)	1 T.	100	2.0
Diet spread (Peter Pan)	1 T.	100	2.0

(USDA): United States Department of Agriculture
DNA: Data Not Available
*Prepared as Package Directs

Food and Description	Measure or Quantity	Calories	Carbohydrates (grams)
PEAR:			
Fresh, whole:			
(USDA)	1 lb. (weighed with stems & core)	252	63.2
(USDA)	6.4-oz. pear (3" x 2½" dia.)	100	25.0
Slices (USDA)	½ cup (2.8 oz.)	50	12.5
Canned, regular pack:			
Light syrup, solids & liq. (USDA)	4 oz.	69	17.7
Heavy syrup, halves or slices (USDA)	½ cup (with syrup)	87	22.5
Heavy syrup (USDA)	2 med. halves & 2 T. syrup	90	23.0
Extra heavy syrup, solids & liq. (USDA)	4 oz.	104	26.8
(Hunt's) Bartlett	4 oz.	52	13.4
(Stokely-Van Camp)	2 med. halves & 2 T. syrup	90	23.0
Canned, unsweetened or low calorie:			
Solids & liq. (USDA)	½ cup (4.2 oz.)	39	10.1
Solids & liq. (Blue Boy) Bartlett	4 oz.	33	9.6
(Del Monte)	4 oz.	36	D.N.A.
(Diet Delight) solids and liq.	½ cup	39	7.6
(Dole)	½ cup & 2 T. liq.	38	D.N.A.
(Libby's) halves	4 oz.	31	9.4
(S and W) *Nutradiet*, quartered	4 oz.	30	7.3
(Yes Madame) Bartlett, halves	½ cup	32	8.6
Dried:			
(USDA)	1 lb.	1216	305.3
Cooked, without added sugar, solids & liq. (USDA)	4 oz.	143	36.0
Cooked, with added sugar solids & liq. (USDA)	4 oz.	171	43.0
PEAR, CANDIED (USDA)	1 oz.	86	22.0
PEAR NECTAR, sweetened (USDA)	½ cup (8.2 oz.)	62	15.8
PECAN:			
In shell (USDA)	1 lb. (weighed in shell)	1652	35.1

(USDA): United States Department of Agriculture
DNA: Data Not Available
*Prepared as Package Directs

Food and Description	Measure or Quantity	Calories	Carbohydrates (grams)
Shelled (USDA):			
Whole	1 lb.	3116	66.2
Halves	½ cup (1.9 oz.)	371	7.9
Chopped	½ cup (1.8 oz.)	360	7.6
Chopped	1 T.	52	1.0
Dry roasted (Planters)	1 oz.	206	3.4
PECAN PIE:			
Home recipe (USDA)	⅙ of 9″ pie (4.9 oz.)	585	71.8
Frozen (Mrs. Smith's)	⅙ of 8″ pie	422	52.0
PEPPER, BLACK:			
(USDA)	¼ tsp.	1	.3
(Lawry's) seasoned	1 tsp.	8	1.6
PEPPER, HOT CHILI:			
Green, (USDA):			
Raw, whole	4 oz.	31	7.5
Raw, without seeds	4 oz.	42	10.3
Canned, chili sauce	1 oz.	5	1.4
Canned pods, without seeds, solids & liq.	4 oz.	28	6.9
Red, (USDA):			
Raw, whole	4 oz. (weighed with seeds)	101	19.7
Raw, trimmed, pods only	4 oz.	54	13.1
Canned, chili sauce	1 oz.	6	1.1
Canned, pods, without seeds, solids & liq.	⅛ cup	7	1.8
Dried:			
Pods (USDA)	1 oz.	91	17.0
Pods (Chili Products)	1 oz.	88	16.9
Powder with added seasoning (USDA)	1 oz.	96	16.0
Powder with added seasoning (USDA)	1 T.	50	8.0
PEPPER POT SOUP, condensed (Campbell's)	8 oz. (by wt.)	188	17.2
PEPPER, SWEET:			
Green:			
Raw:			
Whole (USDA)	1 lb. (weighed untrimmed)	82	17.9

(USDA): United States Department of Agriculture
DNA: Data Not Available
*Prepared as Package Directs

Food and Description	Measure or Quantity	Calories	Carbo-hydrates (grams)
Without stem & seeds (USDA)	1 med. pepper (2.2 oz.)	15	3.0
Chopped (USDA)	½ cup (2.6 oz.)	16	3.6
Slices (USDA)	½ cup (1.4 oz.)	9	2.0
Strips (USDA)	½ cup (1.7 oz.)	11	2.4
Boiled, strips, drained solids (USDA)	½ cup (2.4 oz.)	12	2.6
Parboiled then baked (USDA)	1 med. pepper (2.2 oz.)	17	3.9
Canned, halves (Cannon)	4 oz.	20	D.N.A.
Red:			
Raw, whole (USDA)	1 lb. (weighed with stems & seeds)	112	25.8
Raw, without stem & seeds (USDA)	1 med. pepper (2.1 oz.)	20	4.0
Canned, diced (Cannon)	4 oz.	31	D.N.A.
PEPPER, STUFFED:			
Home recipe, with beef & crumbs (USDA)	4 oz.	193	19.1
Frozen, with beef, in creole sauce (Holloway House)	1 pepper (7 oz.)	279	58.0
PEPPERMINT EXTRACT (Ehlers)	1 tsp.	12	D.N.A.
PEPPERMINT SCHNAPPS (See **SCHNAPPS**)			
PEP WHEAT FLAKES, cereal (Kellogg's)	1 cup (1 oz.)	106	23.0
PERCH, raw (USDA):			
White, whole	1 lb. (weighed whole)	193	0.
White, meat only	4 oz.	134	0.
Yellow, whole	1 lb. (weighed whole)	161	0.
Yellow, meat only	4 oz.	103	0.
PERNOD (Julius Wile)	1 fl. oz.	79	1.1

(USDA): United States Department of Agriculture
DNA: Data Not Available
*Prepared as Package Directs

Food and Description	Measure or Quantity	Calories	Carbo- hydrates (grams)
PERSIMMON (USDA):			
Japanese or Kaki, fresh:			
With seeds	1 lb. (weighed with skin, calyx & seeds)	286	73.3
Seedless	1 lb. (weighed with skin & calyx)	293	75.1
Seedless	4.4-oz. persimmon (2½″ dia.)	75	20.0
Native, fresh, whole	1 lb. (weighed with seeds & calyx)	472	124.6
Native, fresh, flesh only	4 oz.	144	37.9
PERX, cream substitute	1 tsp.	5	.6
PETITE MARMITE SOUP,			
canned (Crosse & Blackwell)	6½ oz. (½ can)	33	3.7
PETTIJOHNS (Quaker):			
Rolled whole wheat, dry	⅓ cup (1 oz.)	96	21.0
*Rolled whole wheat, cooked	⅔ cup	96	21.0
PHEASANT, raw (USDA):			
Ready-to-cook	1 lb. (weighed ready-to-cook)	596	0.
Flesh & skin	4 oz.	172	0.
Flesh only	4 oz.	184	0.
PICKEREL, raw (USDA):			
Whole	1 lb. (weighed whole)	194	0.
Meat only	4 oz.	95	0.
PICKLE:			
Chowchow (See **CHOWCHOW**)			
Cucumber, fresh or bread & butter:			
(USDA)	½ cup (3 oz.)	62	15.2
(USDA)	1 oz.	21	5.1
(USDA)	3 slices (¼″ x 1½″)	15	3.8
(Durkee)	½ cup	59	D.N.A.
(Durkee)	3 slices (¼″ x 1½″)	15	D.N.A.
(Heinz)	3 slices	15	3.6
Dill:			
(USDA)	4.8-oz. pickle (4″ x 1¾″)	14	3.0

(USDA): United States Department of Agriculture
DNA: Data Not Available
*Prepared as Package Directs

Food and Description	Measure or Quantity	Calories	Carbo-hydrates (grams)
(USDA)	1 oz.	3	.6
(Albro)	1 oz.	3	.5
(Durkee)	1 pickle (4″ x 1¾″)	15	D.N.A.
(Heinz)	1 pickle (4″)	12	2.0
Processed (Heinz)	1 pickle (3″)	2	.2
(Smucker's)	1 oz.	3	.8
Dill, candied sticks (Smucker's)	.7-oz. pickle	38	9.5
Dill, hamburger (Heinz)	3 slices	1	.1
Dill, hamburger (Smucker's)	1 oz.	3	.8
Kosher dill (Smucker's)	1 oz.	3	.8
Sour:			
Cucumber (USDA)	4.8-oz. pickle (1¾″ x 4″)	14	2.7
Cucumber (USDA)	1 oz.	3	.6
(Albro)	1 oz.	3	.5
(Durkee)	1 pickle (¾″ x 4″)	15	D.N.A.
(Heinz)	1 pickle (2″)	9	1.6
Sweet:			
Cucumber (USDA):			
Whole	1 oz.	41	10.3
Whole	.7-oz. pickle (2¾″ x ¾″)	29	7.3
Chopped	½ cup (2.6 oz.)	108	27.0
Chopped	1 T.	13	3.3
(Albro)	1 oz.	24	5.9
(Durkee)	1 pickle (2¾″ x ¾″)	20	D.N.A.
(Smucker's)	1 pickle (.5 oz.)	25	6.2
Candied, midgets (Smucker's)	1 pickle	10	2.5
Chips, fresh pack (Smucker's)	1 slice	7	1.8
Chopped (Durkee)	½ cup	112	D.N.A.
Chopped (Durkee)	1 T.	14	D.N.A.
Gherkin (Heinz)	1 pickle (2″)	29	7.0
Mixed (Durkee)	1 pickle (1¾″ x 4″)	15	D.N.A.
Mixed (Heinz)	3 slices	23	5.4
Mixed (Smucker's)	1 pickle (.5 oz.)	23	5.8
Mixed, chopped (Durkee)	½ cup	112	D.N.A.
Mixed, chopped (Durkee)	1 T.	14	D.N.A.
Mustard (Heinz)	1 T.	30	6.8
Relish (See RELISH)			
Sticks, fresh pack (Smucker's)	1 pickle (.5 oz.)	16	4.0

PIE (See individual kinds)

(USDA): United States Department of Agriculture
DNA: Data Not Available
*Prepared as Package Directs

Food and Description	Measure or Quantity	Calories	Carbohydrates (grams)
PIECRUST (See also **PASTRY SHELL**)			
Home recipe, baked, 9″ pie (USDA)	1 crust	675	59.1
Home recipe, baked, 9″ pie (USDA)	2 crusts	1350	118.2
Frozen:			
(Mrs. Smith's)	1 pkg. (2 crusts)	1180	93.6
8″ shell (Mrs. Smith's)	⅙ of 8″ shell	132	10.4
Graham cracker (Mrs. Smith's)	1 shell	665	79.4
PIECRUST MIX:			
Dry (USDA)	1 oz.	148	14.0
*Prepared with water (USDA)	4 oz.	526	49.9
(Betty Crocker)	11-oz. pkg.	1738	138.6
Graham cracker (Betty Crocker)	6.5-oz. pkg.	884	124.2
*(Flako)	⅙ of 9″ shell (.8 oz. dry)	124	12.0
PIE FILLING (See individual kinds)			
PIESPORTER RIESLING,			
German Moselle wine (Julius Kayser) 10% alcohol	3 fl. oz.	57	1.7
PIGEON (See **SQUAB**)			
PIGEONPEA (USDA):			
Raw, immature seeds in pods	1 lb.	207	37.7
Dry seeds	1 lb.	1551	288.9
PIGNOLIA (See **PINE NUT**)			
PIGS FEET, pickled:			
(USDA)	4 oz.	226	0.
(Hormel)	1-pt. can	440	.2
PIKE, raw (USDA):			
Blue, whole	1 lb. (weighed whole)	180	0.
Blue, meat only	4 oz.	102	0.
Northern, whole	1 lb. (weighed whole)	104	0.

(USDA): United States Department of Agriculture
DNA: Data Not Available
*Prepared as Package Directs

Food and Description	Measure or Quantity	Calories	Carbohydrates (grams)
Northern, meat only	4 oz.	100	0.
Walleye, whole	1 lb. (weighed whole)	240	0.
Walleye, meat only	4 oz.	106	0.
PILI NUT (USDA):			
In shell	1 lb. (weighed in shell)	546	6.9
Shelled	4 oz.	759	9.5
PILLSBURY INSTANT BREAKFAST:			
Chocolate	1 oz.	101	19.0
Chocolate malt	1 oz.	101	18.8
Strawberry	1 oz.	104	19.2
Vanilla	1 oz.	101	17.9
PIMIENTO, canned:			
Drained solids (USDA)	1 med. pod (1.3 oz.)	10	2.0
Solids & liq. (USDA)	4 oz.	31	6.6
Diced, solids & liq. (Cannon)	4 oz.	31	6.6
Pieces, pods, slices (Dromedary)	4 oz.	31	4.6
PIMM'S CUP (Julius Wile):			
#1	1 fl. oz.	69	3.3
#2 & #3	1 fl. oz.	68	3.0
#4	1 fl. oz.	59	.9
#5	1 fl. oz.	60	1.0
#6	1 fl. oz.	63	1.8
PINEAPPLE:			
Fresh:			
Whole (USDA)	1 lb. (weighed untrimmed)	123	32.3
Diced (USDA)	½ cup (2.8 oz.)	41	10.7
Slices (USDA)	3-oz. slice (¾" x 3 ½")	44	11.5
Diced (Calavo)	½ cup	38	9.5
Canned, regular pack:			
Juice pack:			
Solids & liq. (USDA)	4 oz.	66	17.1
Chunks or crushed (Dole)	½ cup (includes 2 T. juice)	64	D.N.A.

(USDA): United States Department of Agriculture
DNA: Data Not Available
*Prepared as Package Directs

Food and Description	Measure or Quantity	Calories	Carbo-hydrates (grams)
Sliced (Dole)	2 slices & 2 T. juice	64	D.N.A.
Light syrup, solids & liq. (USDA)	4 oz.	67	17.5
Heavy syrup:			
Chunks (Dole)	½ cup (includes 2 T. syrup)	84	D.N.A.
Crushed solids & liq. (USDA)	½ cup (4.6 oz.)	96	25.4
Crushed (Dole)	½ cup (includes 2 T. syrup)	94	D.N.A.
Crushed (Stokely-Van Camp)	½ cup (includes 2 T. syrup)	96	25.4
Slices, solids & liq. (USDA)	4 oz.	84	22.0
Slices (USDA)	2 small or 1 large slice & 2 T. syrup	90	23.7
Slices (Dole)	1 large slice & 2 T. syrup	76	D.N.A.
Slices (Dole)	2 med. slices & 2 T. syrup	84	D.N.A.
Slices (Stokely-Van Camp)	2 small slices & 2 T. syrup	90	23.7
Spears (Dole)	2 spears & 2 T. syrup	52	D.N.A.
Tidbits, solids & liq. (USDA)	½ cup (4.6 oz.)	95	25.0
Tidbits (Dole)	½ cup (includes 2 T. syrup)	94	D.N.A.
Extra heavy syrup, solids & liq. (USDA)	4 oz.	102	26.5
Canned, unsweetened, low calorie or dietetic:			
Water pack (USDA)	4 oz.	44	11.6
Chunks, low calorie (Diet Delight)	½ cup (4.4 oz.)	60	11.4
Chunks, low calorie (Dole)	½ cup (includes 2 T. liq.)	54	D.N.A.
Crushed, solids & liq. (Diet Delight)	½ cup (4.3 oz.)	60	13.1
Slices:			
(Del Monte)	4 oz.	44	D.N.A.
Solids & liq. (Diet Delight)	½ cup (4.3 oz.)	44	8.6
(Dole)	2 slices & 2 T. liq.	54	D.N.A.
In pineapple juice (Dole)	2 slices & 2 T. juice	56	D.N.A.
(Libby's)	4 oz.	48	11.6

(USDA): United States Department of Agriculture
DNA: Data Not Available
*Prepared as Package Directs

Food and Description	Measure or Quantity	Calories	Carbo-hydrates (grams)
(S and W) *Nutradiet*	2½ slices (3.5 oz.)	69	16.6
(White Rose)	4 oz.	67	16.2
Tidbits:			
(Diet Delight)	½ cup (4.4 oz.)	50	10.8
In pineapple juice (Dole)	½ cup (includes 2 T. juice)	77	D.N.A.
(S and W) *Nutradiet*	4 oz.	78	18.8
Frozen:			
Chunks, sweetened, solids & liq. (USDA)	½ cup (4.3 oz.)	105	27.3
Chunks in heavy syrup (Dole)	½ cup (includes 2 T. syrup)	92	D.N.A.
PINEAPPLE CAKE MIX:			
(Betty Crocker) *Dole*	1-lb. 2.5-oz. pkg.	2164	421.8
(Betty Crocker) *Dole*	1 oz.	117	22.8
Chiffon (Betty Crocker) *Dole*	1-lb. 2.5-oz. pkg.	2183	416.2
Upside down (Betty Crocker) *Dole*	1-lb. 5.5-oz. pkg.	2064	397.8
*(Duncan Hines)	1 cake	2369	384.0
(Pillsbury)	1 oz.	122	21.8
PINEAPPLE, CANDIED:			
(USDA)	1 oz.	90	22.6
(Liberty)	1 oz.	93	22.6
PINEAPPLE CRISPS, deyhdrated snack (Epicure)	1 oz.	86	22.5
PINEAPPLE FLAVORING, imitation (Ehlers)	1 tsp.	12	D.N.A.
PINEAPPLE & GRAPEFRUIT DRINK, canned:			
(USDA)	½ cup	68	17.0
(Dole)	½ cup	62	D.N.A.
(Hi-C)	½ cup	59	15.8
Ping (Stokely-Van Camp)	½ cup	61	D.N.A.
Pink grapefruit (Dole)	½ cup	62	D.N.A.
*PINEAPPLE & GRAPEFRUIT JUICE, unsweetened, frozen (Dole)	½ cup	51	D.N.A.

(USDA): United States Department of Agriculture
DNA: Data Not Available
*Prepared as Package Directs

Food and Description	Measure or Quantity	Calories	Carbohydrates (grams)
PINEAPPLE JUICE:			
Canned, unsweetened:			
(USDA)	½ cup (4.4 oz.)	68	17.0
(Dole)	½ cup	74	D.N.A.
(Heinz)	5½-oz. can	86	19.8
(S and W) *Nutradiet*	4 oz.	66	16.0
(Stokely-Van Camp)	½ cup	68	17.0
Frozen, concentrate:			
Unsweetened, undiluted			
(USDA)	6-fl.-oz. can	387	95.7
*Unsweetened, diluted with 3 parts water (USDA)	½ cup	65	16.0
*Unsweetened, diluted (Dole)	½ cup	67	D.N.A.
PINEAPPLE & ORANGE DRINK, canned:			
(USDA)	½ cup	68	16.9
Pong (Stokely-Van Camp)	½ cup	61	D.N.A.
PINEAPPLE & ORANGE JUICE:			
(Kraft)	½ cup	56	12.6
*Unsweetened, frozen (Dole)	½ cup	51	D.N.A.
PINEAPPLE-PAPAYA FRUIT SPREAD (Vita)	1 T.	9	D.N.A.
PINEAPPLE PIE:			
Home recipe:			
(USDA)	⅙ of 9″ pie (5.6 oz.)	400	60.2
Chiffon (USDA)	⅙ of 9″ pie (4.9 oz.)	403	54.7
Custard (USDA)	⅙ of 9″ pie (5.4 oz.)	334	48.8
(Tastykake)	4-oz. pie	389	57.8
With cheese (Tastykake)	4-oz. pie	436	59.4
Frozen:			
(Banquet)	5 oz.	371	55.0
(Mrs. Smith's)	⅙ of 8″ pie	305	44.0
PINEAPPLE PIE FILLING			
(Lucky Leaf)	8 oz.	240	59.0

(USDA): United States Department of Agriculture
DNA: Data Not Available
*Prepared as Package Directs

Food and Description	Measure or Quantity	Calories	Carbohydrates (grams)
PINEAPPLE PRESERVE, low calorie:			
(Dia-Mel)	1 T.	22	5.4
(Tillie Lewis)	1 T.	9	2.1
PINEAPPLE SOFT DRINK:			
(Hires)	6 fl. oz.	90	22.5
(Kirsch)	6 fl. oz.	89	22.3
(Nedick's)	6 fl. oz.	90	22.5
(Yoo-Hoo)	6 fl. oz.	90	18.0
High-protein (Yoo-Hoo)	6 fl. oz.	114	24.6
PINE NUT (USDA):			
Pignolias, shelled	4 oz.	626	13.2
Piñon, whole	4 oz. (weighed in shell)	418	14.0
Piñon, shelled	4 oz.	720	23.3
PINOT CHARDONNAY WINE			
(Louis M. Martini) 12.5% alcohol	3 fl. oz.	90	.2
PINOT NOIR WINE			
(Louis M. Martini) 12.5% alcohol	3 fl. oz.	90	.2
PISTACHIO NUT:			
Whole (USDA)	4 oz. (weighed in shell)	337	10.8
Shelled (USDA)	½ cup (2.2 oz.)	371	11.8
Shelled (USDA)	1 T.	46	1.5
*PISTACHIO NUT PUDDING, instant (Royal)	½ cup (5 oz.)	185	30.5
PITANGA, fresh (USDA):			
Whole	1 lb. (weighed whole)	187	45.9
Flesh only	4 oz.	58	14.2
PIZZA PIE:			
Home recipe, with cheese topping (USDA)	4 oz.	267	32.1
Home recipe, with sausage topping (USDA)	4 oz.	265	33.6
Chilled, partially baked (USDA)	4 oz.	236	35.0

(USDA): United States Department of Agriculture
DNA: Data Not Available
*Prepared as Package Directs

Food and Description	Measure or Quantity	Calories	Carbo-hydrates (grams)
Chilled, baked (USDA)	4 oz.	278	41.2
Frozen:			
Partially baked (USDA)	4 oz.	260	37.5
Baked (USDA)	4 oz.	278	40.1
Baked (USDA)	⅛ of 14″ pie (2.6 oz.)	184	26.6
Instant (Buitoni)	1 piece	140	21.0
Little, with cheese (Chef Boy-Ar-Dee)	1 pie (2½ oz.)	164	22.7
With cheese (Chef Boy-Ar-Dee)	⅙ of 12½-oz. pie	133	18.3
With pepperoni (Chef Boy-Ar-Dee)	⅙ of 14-oz. pie	151	18.1
Little, with sausage (Chef Boy-Ar-Dee)	1 pie (2½ oz.)	170	22.3
With sausage (Chef Boy-Ar-Dee)	⅙ of 13¼-oz. pie	146	18.1
PIZZA PIE MIX:			
*With cheese (Chef Boy-Ar-Dee)	⅕ of 15½-oz. pie	182	26.5
*With cheese (Kraft)	4 oz.	265	26.1
*With sausage (Chef Boy-Ar-Dee)	⅕ of 17-oz. pie	203	25.7
PIZZA SAUCE, canned:			
(Buitoni)	1 cup	158	21.2
(Chef Boy-Ar-Dee)	5¼ oz. (½ of 10½-oz. can)	110	7.0
(Contadina)	1 cup	143	21.4
PLANTAIN, raw (USDA):			
Whole	1 lb. (weighed with skin)	389	101.9
Flesh only	4 oz.	135	35.4
PLUM:			
Damson, fresh (USDA):			
Whole	1 lb. (weighed with pits)	272	75.3
Flesh only	4 oz.	75	20.2
Japanese hybrid, fresh (USDA):			
Whole	1 lb. (weighed with pits)	205	52.4

Food and Description	Measure or Quantity	Calories	Carbo-hydrates (grams)
Whole	2.1-oz. plum (2″ dia.)	27	6.9
Diced	½ cup (2.9 oz.)	39	10.1
Halves	½ cup (3.1 oz.)	42	10.8
Slices	½ cup (3 oz.)	40	10.3
Prune-type, fresh (USDA):			
Whole	1 lb. (weighed with pits)	160	42.0
Halves	½ cup (2.8 oz.)	60	15.8
Canned, regular pack, solids & liq.:			
Purple, light syrup (USDA)	4 oz.	71	18.8
Purple, heavy syrup:			
(USDA)	4 oz.	94	24.4
(USDA)	½ cup (4.1 oz.)	97	25.3
(USDA)	3 plums & 2 T. syrup	101	26.3
Purple, extra heavy syrup, solids & liq. (USDA)	4 oz.	116	30.3
Canned, unsweetened or low calorie:			
Greengage, water pack (USDA)	4 oz.	37	9.8
Purple:			
Solids & liq. (USDA)	4 oz.	52	13.5
Solids & Liq. (Diet Delight)	½ cup (4.4 oz.)	64	12.6
Whole (Yes Madame)	½ cup	52	12.4
PLUM PIE (Tastykake)	4-oz. pie	364	53.8
PLUM PRESERVE, DAMSON, low calorie (Polaner)	1 T.	6	.3
PLUM PUDDING (Crosse & Blackwell)	4 oz.	340	62.4
POHA (See **GROUND-CHERRY**)			
POKE SHOOTS (USDA):			
Raw	1 lb.	104	16.8
Boiled, drained solids	4 oz.	23	3.5
POLISH-STYLE SAUSAGE:			
(USDA)	3 oz.	258	1.0
(Wilson)	3 oz.	245	1.0

(USDA): United States Department of Agriculture
DNA: Data Not Available
*Prepared as Package Directs

Food and Description	Measure or Quantity	Calories	Carbo-hydrates (grams)
POLLOCK (USDA):			
Raw, drawn	1 lb. (weighed with head, tail, fins & bones)	194	0.
Cooked, creamed	4 oz.	145	4.5
POMEGRANATE, raw (USDA):			
Whole	1 lb. (weighed whole)	160	41.7
Pulp only	4 oz.	71	18.6
POMMARD WINE, French red Burgundy:			
(Barton & Guestier) 13% alcohol	3 fl. oz.	67	.4
(Chanson) *St. Vincent*, 11½% alcohol	3 fl. oz.	81	6.3
(Cruse) 12% alcohol	3 fl. oz.	72	D.N.A.
POMPANO, raw (USDA):			
Whole	1 lb. (weighed whole)	422	0.
Meat only	4 oz.	188	0.
POPCORN:			
Unpopped (USDA)	1 oz.	102	20.4
Popped (USDA):			
Plain	1 oz.	109	21.8
Plain	1 cup (.4 oz.)	54	10.7
Oil & salt added	1 oz.	129	16.8
Oil & salt added	1 cup (.5 oz.)	64	8.2
Sugar-coated	1 oz.	109	24.2
(Jiffy Pop)	2½ oz. (½ pkg.)	332	29.8
Balls (Pophitt)	1 oz.	91	D.N.A.
Buttered (Wise)	½ cup	21	2.9
Butter flavor (Jiffy Pop)	2½ oz. (½ pkg.)	337	29.4
Cracker Jack, regular-size pack	1⅜-oz. pkg. (approx. 1 cup)	193	32.4
Cracker Jack, pass around pack	6-oz. pkg. (approx. 4 cups)	750	131.0
Fiddle Faddle (Ovaltine)	1 oz.	125	23.0
Caramel-coated:			
Peanut (Wise)	½ cup	64	13.5
Pixies with peanuts (Wise)	1 oz.	103	23.0
(Old London)	1 oz.	117	22.2

(USDA): United States Department of Agriculture
DNA: Data Not Available
*Prepared as Package Directs

Food and Description	Measure or Quantity	Calories	Carbo-hydrates (grams)
(Wise)	½ cup	53	14.8
Cheese-flavored (Old London)	1 oz.	114	21.9
Cheese-flavored (Wise)	½ cup	25	2.8
POPOVER, home recipe (USDA)	1 average popover (1.8 oz.)	112	12.9
***POPOVER MIX** (Flako)	2.3-oz. popover (⅙ of pkg.)	166	22.0
POPSICLE (Popsicle Industries):			
All flavors, except chocolate	3 fl. oz.	70	17.5
Chocolate	3 fl. oz.	106	D.N.A.
POP-UP (See **TOASTER CAKE**)			
PORGY, raw (USDA):			
Whole	1 lb. (weighed whole)	208	0.
Meat only	4 oz.	127	0.
PORK, medium-fat:			
Fresh (USDA):			
Boston butt:			
Raw	1 lb. (weighed with bone & skin)	1220	0.
Roasted, lean & fat	4 oz.	400	0.
Roasted, lean only	4 oz.	277	0.
Chop:			
Cooked	1 chop (4 oz., weighed with bone)	295	0.
Cooked, lean & fat	1 chop (3 oz., weighed without bone)	335	0.
Cooked, lean only	1 chop (3 oz., weighed without bone)	230	0.
Fat, separable, cooked	1 oz.	221	0.
Ham:			
Raw	1 lb. (weighed with bone & skin)	1188	0.
Roasted, lean & fat	4 oz.	424	0.
Roasted, lean only	4 oz.	246	0.

(USDA): United States Department of Agriculture
DNA: Data Not Available
*Prepared as Package Directs

Food and Description	Measure or Quantity	Calories	Carbo-hydrates (grams)
Loin:			
Raw	1 lb. (weighed with bone)	1065	0.
Roasted, lean & fat	4 oz.	411	0.
Roasted, lean only	4 oz.	291	0.
Picnic:			
Raw	1 lb. (weighed with bone & skin)	1083	0.
Simmered, lean & fat	4 oz.	424	0.
Simmered, lean only	4 oz.	240	0.
Spareribs:			
Raw	1 lb. (weighed with bone)	976	0.
Braised, lean & fat	4 oz.	499	0.
Cured, light commercial cure:			
Bacon (See **BACON**)			
Boston Butt (USDA):			
Raw	1 lb. (weighed with bone & skin)	1227	0.
Roasted, lean & fat	4 oz.	374	0.
Roasted, lean only	4 oz.	276	0.
Ham:			
Raw (USDA)	1 lb. (weighed with bone & skin)	1100	0.
Roasted, lean & fat (USDA)	4 oz.	327	0.
Roasted, lean only (USDA)	4 oz.	212	0.
Fully cooked, boneless:			
Parti-Style (Armour Star)	3 oz.	125	.1
(Wilson)	3 oz.	140	0.
Picnic:			
Raw (USDA)	1 lb. (weighed with bone & skin)	1060	0.
Raw (Wilson)	3 oz.	188	0.
Roasted, lean & fat (USDA)	4 oz.	366	0.
Roasted, lean only (USDA)	4 oz.	239	0.
PORK & BEANS (See **BEANS & PORK**)			
PORK & BEEF, luncheon meat (USDA)	1 oz.	95	0.
PORK, CANNED, chopped luncheon meat: (USDA)	1 oz.	83	.4

(USDA): United States Department of Agriculture
DNA: Data Not Available
*Prepared as Package Directs

Food and Description	Measure or Quantity	Calories	Carbohydrates (grams)
Chopped (USDA)	1 cup (4.8 oz.)	400	1.8
Diced (USDA)	1 cup (5 oz.)	415	1.8
(Hormel)	1 oz.	70	.3
PORK DINNER, loin of pork, frozen (Swanson)	10-oz. dinner	460	40.5
PORK & GRAVY, canned (USDA)	4 oz.	290	7.1
PORK KABOB, frozen (Colonial Beef)	6-oz. kabob	500	D.N.A.
PORK RINDS, fried, *Baken•ets* (See also other brand names)	1 oz.	151	D.N.A.
PORK SAUSAGE:			
Uncooked, links or bulk (USDA)	1 oz.	142	Tr.
(Armour Star)	1-oz. sausage	131	D.N.A.
Little Friers (Oscar Mayer)	1 link	55	D.N.A.
(Wilson)	1 oz.	134	0.
Cooked, links or bulk (USDA)	2 oz.	270	Tr.
Canned, solids & liq. (USDA)	1 oz.	118	.7
Canned, drained solids (USDA)	1 oz.	108	.5
PORK, SWEET & SOUR, frozen (Chun King)	1 oz.	38	D.N.A.
PORT WINE:			
(Gallo) 16% alcohol	3 fl. oz.	94	7.8
(Gallo) ruby, 20% alcohol	3 fl. oz.	112	8.7
(Gallo) tawny, Old Decanter, 20% alcohol	3 fl. oz.	112	8.4
(Gallo) white, 20% alcohol	3 fl. oz.	111	8.4
(Gold Seal) 19% alcohol	3 fl. oz.	158	9.4
(Great Western) Solera, 19% alcohol	3 fl. oz.	154	11.6
(Great Western) Solera, tawny, 19% alcohol	3 fl. oz.	152	11.0
(Great Western) white, 19% alcohol	3 fl. oz.	156	12.3
(Italian Swiss Colony-Gold Medal) 19.7% alcohol	3 fl. oz.	130	8.7

(USDA): United States Department of Agriculture
DNA: Data Not Available
*Prepared as Package Directs

Food and Description	Measure or Quantity	Calories	Carbo- hydrates (grams)
(Italian Swiss Colony-Gold Medal) white, 19.7% alcohol	3 fl. oz.	132	9.3
(Italian Swiss Colony-Private Stock) 19.7% alcohol	3 fl. oz.	138	10.8
(Italian Swiss Colony-Private Stock) tawny, 19.7% alcohol	3 fl. oz.	137	10.5
(Louis M. Martini) 19½% alcohol	3 fl. oz.	165	2.0
(Louis M. Martini) tawny, 19½% alcohol	3 fl. oz.	165	2.0
(Robertson's) ruby, 20% alcohol	3 fl. oz.	138	9.9
(Robertson's) tawny, *Dry Humour*, 21% alcohol	3 fl. oz.	145	9.9
(Robertson's) tawny, *Game Bird*, 21% alcohol	3 fl. oz.	145	9.9
(Robertson's) *Rebello Valente*, 20½% alcohol	3 fl. oz.	141	9.9
(Taylor) 19.5% alcohol	3 fl. oz.	150	10.9
(Taylor) tawny, 19.5% alcohol	3 fl. oz.	144	10.0
POST TOASTIES, cereal	1 cup (1 oz.)	110	24.0
POSTUM, instant	1 cup (5.5 oz.)	9	2.9
POTATO:			
Raw, whole (USDA)	1 lb. (weighed unpared)	279	62.8
Au gratin (USDA)	4 oz.	164	15.4
Baked, peeled after baking (USDA)	1 med. (3 raw to 1 lb.)	92	20.8
Boiled, peeled after boiling (USDA)	1 med. (3 raw to 1 lb.)	103	23.2
Boiled, peeled before boiling (USDA)	1 med. (3 raw to 1 lb.)	79	17.6
French-fried in deep fat (USDA)	10 pieces (2″ x ½″ x ½″)	156	20.5
Hash-browned, after holding overnight (USDA)	4 oz.	260	33.0
Mashed, milk added (USDA)	½ cup (3.6 oz.)	68	13.5
Mashed, milk & butter added	½ cup (3.6 oz.)	98	12.8
Pan-fried from raw (USDA)	1 cup (6 oz.)	456	55.4

(USDA): United States Department of Agriculture
DNA: Data Not Available
*Prepared as Package Directs

Food and Description	Measure or Quantity	Calories	Carbohydrates (grams)
Pan-fried from raw (USDA)	4 oz.	304	37.0
Scalloped (USDA)	4 oz.	118	16.7
Canned:			
Solids & liq. (USDA)	1 cup (8.8 oz.)	110	24.5
Solids & liq. (USDA)	4 oz.	50	11.1
White (Butter Kernel)	3-4 small potatoes	96	22.0
Whole, new (Hunt's)	4 oz.	50	11.1
& ham (Morton House)	12¾-oz. can	660	D.N.A.
Dehydrated, mashed:			
Flakes, without milk (USDA):			
Dry	½ cup (.8 oz.)	84	19.3
*Prepared with water, milk & fat	½ cup (3.8 oz.)	100	15.5
Granules, without milk (USDA):			
Dry	½ cup (3.5 oz.)	352	80.4
*Prepared with water, milk & fat	½ cup (3.7 oz.)	101	15.1
Granules with milk (USDA):			
Dry	½ cup (3.5 oz.)	358	77.7
*Prepared with water & fat	½ cup (3.7 oz.)	83	13.8
Frozen:			
Au gratin (Stouffer's)	11½-oz. pkg.	304	35.6
Au gratin (Swanson)	8-oz. pkg.	241	16.8
Diced for hash-browning, not thawed (USDA)	4 oz.	83	19.7
Diced, hash-browned (USDA)	4 oz.	254	32.9
French-fried:			
Not thawed (USDA)	9-oz. pkg.	434	66.6
Not thawed (USDA)	4 oz.	193	29.6
Heated (USDA)	10 pieces (2″ x ½″ x ½″)	125	19.2
(Birds Eye)	17 pieces (3 oz.)	144	22.0
Crinkle-cut (Birds Eye)	17 pieces (3 oz.)	144	22.0
Fanci-fries (Birds Eye)	¼ pkg. (3 oz.)	173	21.0
(Mrs. Paul's)	4 oz.	250	38.8
Mashed, not thawed (USDA)	4 oz.	85	19.4
Mashed, heated (USDA)	4 oz.	105	17.8
Potato puffs, French-fried (Birds Eye)	⅓ pkg. (2.7 oz.)	149	14.6
Scalloped (Swanson)	8-oz. pkg.	257	12.9
Shredded for hash-browns (Birds Eye)	⅓ pkg. (3 oz.)	63	14.7
Stuffed, baked, with cheese topping (Holloway House)	1 potato (6 oz.)	251	28.0

(USDA): United States Department of Agriculture
DNA: Data Not Available
*Prepared as Package Directs

Food and Description	Measure or Quantity	Calories	Carbo-hydrates (grams)
Stuffed, baked, with sour cream			
& chives (Holloway House)	1 potato (6 oz.)	256	27.4
Tiny Taters (Birds Eye)	⅙ pkg. (2.7 oz.)	109	11.6
POTATO CHIP:			
(USDA)	1 oz.	161	14.2
(USDA)	10 chips (2″ dia.)	113	10.0
(Lay's)	1 oz.	157	13.9
(Nalley's)	1 oz.	154	13.9
(Ruffles)	1 oz.	157	13.9
(Wise)	1 oz.	160	14.2
Barbecue flavored (Wise)	1 oz.	160	14.2
Onion-garlic chips (Wise)	1 oz.	160	14.2
Ridgies (Wise)	1 oz.	160	14.2
POTATO MIX:			
Au gratin (French's)	5.5-oz. pkg.	672	95.0
*Au gratin (French's)	½ cup	112	16.0
Au gratin, with sauce (Betty Crocker)	5.5-oz. pkg.	588	105.1
Buds, instant (Betty Crocker)	5-oz. pkg.	500	114.0
Escalloped, with sauce (Betty Crocker)	5.5-oz. pkg.	534	113.3
Mashed, country style (French's)	1⅓ cups (2⅔-oz. pkg.)	267	60.0
*Mashed, country style (French's)	½ cup	137	16.5
Mashed, instant (French's)	3.5-oz. pkg.	352	73.0
*Mashed, instant (French's)	½ cup	114	16.0
Scalloped (French's)	5⅝-oz. pkg.	552	117.0
*Scalloped (French's)	½ cup	109	20.0
Scalloped (Pillsbury)	1 oz.	97	20.2
POTATO PANCAKE MIX:			
(French's)	3-oz. pkg.	284	62.0
*(French's)	¼ pkg. (3 small pancakes)	90	15.5
POTATO SALAD:			
Home recipe, with cooked salad dressing (USDA)	4 oz.	112	18.5
Home recipe, with mayonnaise & French dressing, hard-cooked eggs (USDA)	4 oz.	164	15.2
Canned (Nalley's)	4 oz.	159	20.3

(USDA): United States Department of Agriculture
DNA: Data Not Available
*Prepared as Package Directs

Food and Description	Measure or Quantity	Calories	Carbohydrates (grams)
POTATO SOUP, Cream of:			
Canned, condensed (Campbell)	8 oz. (by wt.)	132	20.7
Frozen:			
Condensed (USDA)	8 oz. (by wt.)	197	22.7
*Prepared with equal volume water (USDA)	8 oz. (by wt.)	100	11.1
*Prepared with equal volume milk (USDA)	8 oz. (by wt.)	173	17.0
Condensed (Campbell)	8 oz. (by wt.)	204	22.9
POTATO SOUP MIX:			
(Lipton)	1 pkg.	305	57.4
*With leek (Wyler's)	6 fl. oz.	116	9.0
POTATO STICK:			
(USDA)	1 oz.	154	14.4
O & C (Durkee)	1½ cups (1¾-oz. can)	282	24.8
O & C (Durkee)	1 oz.	161	14.2
Julienne (Wise)	1 oz.	136	15.0
POUILLY-FUISSE WINE, French white Burgundy:			
(Barton & Guestier) 12% alcohol	3 fl. oz.	64	.3
(Chanson) *St. Vincent*, 12% alcohol	3 fl. oz.	84	6.3
(Cruse) 12% alcohol	3 fl. oz.	72	D.N.A.
POUILLY-FUME, French white Loire Valley (Barton & Guestier) 12% alcohol	3 fl. oz.	60	.1
POUND CAKE:			
Home recipe, old fashioned (USDA)	1.1-oz. slice (2¾" x 3" x ⅝")	142	14.1
Marble (Drake's)	1 slice	186	31.2
Plain (Drake's)	1 slice	181	40.0
Raisin (Drake's)	1 slice	232	40.2
POUND CAKE MIX:			
(Betty Crocker)	1-lb. 1-oz. pkg.	2346	333.2
*(Dromedary)	1" slice	278	36.2
PREAM, cream substitute	1 tsp.	11	1.1

(USDA): United States Department of Agriculture
DNA: Data Not Available
*Prepared as Package Directs

Food and Description	Measure or Quantity	Calories	Carbo-hydrates (grams)
PRESERVE (See also individual listings by flavor):			
Sweetened:			
(USDA)	1 oz.	77	19.8
(USDA)	1 T.	54	14.0
(Crosse & Blackwell)	1 T.	59	14.8
(Kraft)	1 oz.	78	19.3
(Polaner)	1 T.	54	13.5
(Smucker's)	1 oz.	84	D.N.A.
Low calorie (Kraft)	1 oz.	9	2.0
PRETZEL:			
(USDA)	1 oz.	111	21.5
(USDA)	1 small stick (1 gram)	4	.8
(Keebler) Log	1 piece (4 grams)	16	3.4
(Keebler) Stix	1 piece (<1 gram)	2	.4
(Keebler) Twist	1 piece (6 grams)	23	4.3
(Nab) Pretzelette	1 packet (1 oz.)	108	21.7
(Nab) *Very-Thin* Sticks	1 packet (¾ oz.)	79	16.7
(Nabisco) Pretzelette	1 piece (2 grams)	6	1.3
(Nabisco) *Mister Salty* Dutch	1 piece (.4 oz.)	51	11.2
(Nabisco) *Mister Salty* 3-ring	1 piece (3 grams)	12	2.3
(Nabisco) *Mister Salty Veri-Thin*	1 piece (5 grams)	20	4.1
(Nabisco) *Mister Salty Veri-Thin* Stick	1 piece (<1 gram)	1	.2
(Old London) *Chick-a-Dees*	1 oz.	106	21.9
(Quinlan)	5 pieces (1 oz.)	100	D.N.A.
(Quinlan) Rods	2 pieces (1 oz.)	100	D.N.A.
(Quinlan) Sticks	35 pieces (1 oz.)	100	D.N.A.
(Quinlan) Thick, beer-type	3 pieces (1 oz.)	100	D.N.A.
(Quinlan) Thin	6 pieces (1 oz.)	100	D.N.A.
(Rold Gold) Stix	1 pkg. (1⅛ oz.)	110	24.4
(Sunshine) Extra thin	1 piece (5 grams)	20	4.0
PRICKLY PEAR, fresh (USDA)	1 lb. (weighed with rind & seeds)	84	21.8
PRINCE BLANC WINE, French white Bordeaux (Barton & Guestier) 12% alcohol	3 fl. oz.	62	.6
PRINCE NOIR WINE, French red Bordeaux (Barton & Guestier) 12% alcohol	3 fl. oz.	61	.4

(USDA): United States Department of Agriculture
DNA: Data Not Available
*Prepared as Package Directs

Food and Description	Measure or Quantity	Calories	Carbo-hydrates (grams)
PRODUCT 19, cereal (Kellogg's)	1 cup (1 oz.)	106	23.0
PRUNE:			
Dried, "softenized":			
Small (USDA)	4 oz. (about 21 prunes)	237	62.7
Medium (USDA)	4 oz. (about 17 prunes)	246	64.5
Medium (USDA)	4 prunes (1.1 oz.)	70	18.0
Large (USDA)	4 oz. (about 13 prunes)	255	67.3
Dried, cooked, unsweetened (USDA)	1 cup (17-18 med. with ⅓ cup liq.)	295	78.0
Canned, diet (Dia-Mel)	4 prunes	54	13.1
Dehydrated:			
Nugget-type & pieces (USDA)	4 oz.	390	103.5
Nugget-type & pieces, cooked with sugar, solids & liq. (USDA)	½ cup (4.4 oz.)	227	59.3
Pitted (Vacu-Dry)	1 oz.	98	25.9
PRUNE JUICE, canned:			
(USDA)	½ cup (4.5 oz.)	99	24.3
(Heinz)	5½-oz. can	119	28.5
RealPrune	½ cup	98	24.1
(Santa Clara)	4 oz.	100	24.0
PRUNE WHIP, home recipe (USDA)	1 cup (4.8 oz.)	210	49.8
PUDDING or PUDDING MIX (See individual kinds)			
PUFF (See **CRACKER** or individual kinds of hors d'oeuvres, such as **CHICKEN PUFF**)			
PUFFA PUFFA RICE, cereal (Kellogg's)	1 cup (1 oz.)	120	23.9
PUFFED OAT CEREAL (USDA):			
Plain	1 oz.	112	21.3
Sugar-coated	1 oz.	112	24.1

(USDA): United States Department of Agriculture
DNA: Data Not Available
*Prepared as Package Directs

Food and Description	Measure or Quantity	Calories	Carbo-hydrates (grams)
PUFFED RICE CEREAL (See **RICE, PUFFED**)			
PULIGNY MONTRACHET WINE, French white Burgundy: (Barton & Guestier) 12%			
alcohol	3 fl. oz.	61	.3
(Chanson) 12% alcohol	3 fl. oz.	84	6.3
PUMPKIN:			
Fresh, whole (USDA)	1 lb. (weighed with rind & seeds)	83	20.6
Fresh, flesh only (USDA)	4 oz.	37	9.0
Canned (USDA)	½ cup (4.3 oz.)	40	9.6
Canned (Stokely-Van Camp)	½ cup	40	9.6
PUMPKIN PIE:			
Home recipe (USDA)	⅙ of 9″ pie (5.4 oz.)	321	37.2
(Tastykake)	4-oz. pie	368	50.5
Frozen (Banquet)	5 oz.	306	46.5
Frozen (Mrs. Smith's)	⅙ of 8″ pie	229	33.6
PUMPKIN SEED, dry (USDA):			
Whole	4 oz. (weighed in hull)	464	12.6
Hulled	4 oz.	627	17.0
*PUNCH DRINK MIX (Salada)	6 fl. oz.	80	19.4
PURPLE PASSION, soft drink (Canada Dry)	6 fl. oz.	85	22.2
PURSLANE (USDA):			
Raw	1 lb.	95	17.2
Boiled, drained solids	4 oz.	17	3.2
PUSSYCAT MIX (Bar-Tender's)	1 serving (⅔ oz.)	75	18.5

Q

QUAIL, raw (USDA):			
Ready-to-cook	1 lb. (weighed with bones)	686	0.
Flesh & skin only	4 oz.	195	0.

(USDA): United States Department of Agriculture
DNA: Data Not Available
*Prepared as Package Directs

Food and Description	Measure or Quantity	Calories	Carbo-hydrates (grams)
QUAKE, cereal (Quaker)	1 cup (1 oz.)	118	23.0
QUIK (See individual kinds)			
QUINCE, fresh (USDA):			
Untrimmed	1 lb. (weighed with skin & seeds)	158	42.3
Flesh only	4 oz.	65	17.4
QUININE SOFT DRINK or TONIC WATER:			
Sweetened:			
(Canada Dry)	6 fl. oz.	71	18.4
(Dr. Brown's)	6 fl. oz.	66	16.5
Fanta	6 fl. oz.	63	15.0
(Hoffman)	6 fl. oz.	66	16.5
(Schweppes)	6 fl. oz.	66	16.5
(Shasta)	6 fl. oz.	59	14.6
(Yukon Club)	6 fl. oz.	66	16.5
Low calorie:			
(Hoffman)	6 fl. oz.	3	.8
(No-Cal)	6 fl. oz.	2	0.
QUISP, cereal (Quaker)	1 cup (⅞ oz.)	103	19.7

R

RABBIT (USDA):			
Domesticated, ready-to-cook	1 lb. (weighed with bones)	581	0.
Domesticated, stewed, flesh only	4 oz.	245	0.
Wild, raw, flesh only	4 oz.	153	0.
RACCOON, roasted, meat only (USDA)	4 oz.	289	0.
RADISH (USDA):			
Common, raw:			
Without tops	½ lb. (weighed untrimmed)	35	7.4
Trimmed, whole	4 small radishes (1.4 oz.)	6	1.4
Trimmed, sliced	½ cup (2 oz.)	10	2.1

(USDA): United States Department of Agriculture
DNA: Data Not Available
*Prepared as Package Directs

Food and Description	Measure or Quantity	Calories	Carbo-hydrates (grams)
Oriental, raw, without tops	½ lb. (weighed unpared)	34	7.5
Oriental, raw, trimmed & pared	4 oz.	22	4.8

RAISIN:
Dried:

Whole (USDA)	4 oz.	328	88.0
Whole (USDA)	½ cup (2.5 oz.)	208	55.7
Whole (USDA)	1 T.	28	7.7
Chopped (USDA)	½ cup (2.8 oz.)	234	62.6
Ground (USDA)	½ cup (4.7 oz.)	388	104.1
Seedless, California Thompson (Sun Maid)	½ cup	236	62.6
Seedless, California Thompson (Sun Maid)	1 T.	29	7.8
Cooked, added sugar, solids & liq. (USDA)	½ cup (4.3 oz.)	260	68.8

RAISIN PIE:

Home recipe (USDA)	⅙ of 9″ pie (5.6 oz.)	427	67.9
(Tastykake)	4-oz. pie	391	60.8
Frozen (Mrs. Smith's)	⅙ of 8″ pie	315	42.1

RAISIN PIE FILLING (Lucky Leaf)

	8 oz.	292	67.8

RAJA FISH (See **SKATE**)

RALSTON, cereal, dry:

Instant	4 T. (1 oz.)	97	20.2
Regular	3⅓ T. (1 oz.)	97	20.2

RASPBERRY:
Black:
Fresh:

(USDA)	½ lb. (weighed with caps & stems)	161	34.6
(USDA)	4 oz. (weighed with caps & stems removed)	83	17.8
(USDA)	½ cup (2.4 oz.)	49	10.5
Canned, water pack, unsweetened, solids & liq. (USDA)	4 oz.	58	12.1

(USDA): United States Department of Agriculture
DNA: Data Not Available
*Prepared as Package Directs

Food and Description	Measure or Quantity	Calories	Carbohydrates (grams)
Red:			
Fresh:			
(USDA)	½ lb. (weighed with caps & stems)	126	29.9
(USDA)	½ cup (2.6 oz.)	41	9.8
Canned, water pack, un- sweetened or low calorie:			
Solids & liq. (USDA)	4 oz.	40	10.0
Solids & liq. (Blue Boy)	4 oz.	48	11.2
Frozen:			
Not thawed (USDA)	10-oz. pkg.	277	69.7
Sweetened, not thawed (USDA)	½ cup (4.4 oz.)	122	30.8
Quick thaw (Birds Eye)	½ cup (5 oz.)	129	32.2
*RASPBERRY DRINK MIX (Wyler's)	6 fl. oz.	63	15.8
RASPBERRY JAM, dietetic, black (Slenderella)	1 T.	24	6.0
RASPBERRY LIQUEUR, (Leroux) 50 proof	1 fl. oz.	74	8.3
RASPBERRY PRESERVE, dietetic:			
Red (Polaner)	1 T.	6	1.5
Black seedless (Dia-Mel)	1 T.	22	5.4
Black (Kraft)	1 oz.	9	1.9
RASPBERRY, RED, PIE FILLING (Lucky Leaf)	8 oz.	324	79.0
RASPBERRY RENNET CUSTARD MIX:			
Powder:			
(Junket)	1 oz.	115	28.0
*Prepared with whole milk (Junket)	4 oz.	108	14.7
Tablet:			
(Junket)	1 tablet	1	.2
*Prepared with whole milk & sugar (Junket)	4 oz.	101	13.4

(USDA): United States Department of Agriculture
DNA: Data Not Available
*Prepared as Package Directs

Food and Description	Measure or Quantity	Calories	Carbo- hydrates (grams)
RASPBERRY SHERBET & FRUIT ICE MIX (Junket)	6 serving pkg. (4 oz.)	388	108.8
RASPBERRY SOFT DRINK:			
Sweetened:			
(Canada Dry)	6 fl. oz.	100	26.2
(Hoffman)	6 fl. oz.	90	22.5
(Yukon Club)	6 fl. oz.	90	22.5
Black:			
(Dr. Brown's)	6 fl. oz.	87	21.9
(Key Food)	6 fl. oz.	87	21.9
(Kirsch)	6 fl. oz.	88	22.1
(Waldbaum)	6 fl. oz.	87	21.9
Low calorie (Hoffman)	6 fl. oz.	3	.8
Low calorie (No-Cal)	6 fl. oz.	3	<.1
RASPBERRY SYRUP, dietetic:			
(Dia-Mel)	1 T.	22	5.4
(No-Cal)	1 tsp.	<1	Tr.
RASPBERRY TURNOVER, frozen (Pepperidge Farm)	1 turnover	285	D.N.A.
RAVIOLI:			
Canned:			
Beef or meat:			
(Buitoni)	1 cup	269	28.3
(Chef Boy-Ar-Dee)	8 oz. (1/5 of 40-oz. can)	210	30.2
(Nalley's)	8 oz.	284	62.4
(Prince)	8 oz.	302	38.6
Cheese:			
(Buitoni)	1 cup	215	31.2
(Chef Boy-Ar-Dee)	7½ oz. (½ of 15-oz. can)	255	31.5
(Prince)	8 oz.	202	29.4
Chicken (Nalley's)	8 oz.	261	82.4
Frozen:			
Beef (Kraft)	8 oz.	272	31.2
Cheese, without sauce (Buitoni)	1 cup	117	16.0
Cheese (Kraft)	8 oz.	270	30.4
Meat, without sauce (Buitoni) *Raviolettes*	1 cup	140	16.0

(USDA): United States Department of Agriculture
DNA: Data Not Available
*Prepared as Package Directs

Food and Description	Measure or Quantity	Calories	Carbo-hydrates (grams)
READY GRAVY	1 fl. oz.	22	3.7
REDFISH (See **DRUM, RED** & **OCEAN PERCH,** Atlantic)			
RED & GRAY SNAPPER, raw:			
Whole (USDA)	1 lb. (weighed whole)	219	0.
Meat only (USDA)	4 oz.	105	0.
Meat only (Booth)	4 oz.	105	0.
REDHORSE, SILVER, raw (USDA):			
Drawn	1 lb. (weighed eviscerated)	204	0.
Flesh only	4 oz.	111	0.
REINDEER, raw, lean only (USDA)	4 oz.	144	0.
RELISH:			
Barbecue (Crosse & Blackwell)	1 T.	22	5.4
Barbecue (Heinz)	1 T.	32	3.0
Corn (Crosse & Blackwell)	1 T.	15	3.6
Hamburger (Crosse & Blackwell)	1 T.	20	4.7
Hamburger (Heinz)	1 T.	17	4.2
Hot dog (Crosse & Blackwell)	1 T.	22	5.4
Hot dog (Heinz)	1 T.	22	5.1
Hot pepper (Crosse & Blackwell)	1 T.	22	5.4
India (Crosse & Blackwell)	1 T.	26	6.3
India (Heinz)	1 T.	28	6.5
Onion, spicy (Crosse & Blackwell)	1 T.	21	5.0
Piccalilli (Crosse & Blackwell)	1 T.	26	6.3
Piccalilli (Heinz)	1 T.	19	4.4
Picnic, tangy (Crosse & Blackwell)	1 T.	24	6.0
Sour (USDA)	1 oz.	5	.8
Sweet:			
(USDA)	1 T.	21	5.1
(Crosse & Blackwell)	1 T.	26	6.3
(Heinz)	1 T.	25	5.7
(Smucker's)	½ oz.	20	5.0

RENNIN CUSTARD PRODUCTS
(See individual flavors)

(USDA): United States Department of Agriculture
DNA: Data Not Available
*Prepared as Package Directs

Food and Description	Measure or Quantity	Calories	Carbohydrates (grams)
RHINESKELLER WINE, (Italian Swiss Colony-Gold Medal) 12.4% alcohol	3 fl. oz.	73	3.0
RHINE WINE:			
(Deinhard) Rheinritter, 11% alcohol	3 fl. oz.	60	3.6
(Gallo) 12% alcohol	3 fl. oz.	50	.9
(Gallo) Rhine Garten, 12% alcohol	3 fl. oz.	60	3.0
(Great Western) Dutchess, 12% alcohol	3 fl. oz.	80	2.6
(Gold Seal) 12% alcohol	3 fl. oz.	82	.4
(Italian Swiss Colony-Gold Medal) 11.6% alcohol	3 fl. oz.	59	.6
(Italian Swiss Colony-Private Stock) 12% alcohol	3 fl. oz.	61	.5
(Louis M. Martini) 12.5% alcohol	3 fl. oz.	90	.2
(Taylor) 12.5% alcohol	3 fl. oz.	69	Tr.
RHUBARB:			
Fresh:			
Partly trimmed (USDA)	1 lb. (weighed with part leaves, ends & trimmings)	54	12.6
Trimmed (USDA)	4 oz.	18	4.2
Diced (USDA)	½ cup (2.2 oz.)	10	2.2
Cooked, sweetened (USDA)	½ cup (4.2 oz.)	169	43.2
Frozen, sweetened:			
Not thawed (USDA)	½ cup (3.9 oz.)	82	20.4
Cooked, added sugar (USDA)	½ cup (4.4 oz.)	177	44.9
(Birds Eye)	¼ pkg. (4 oz.)	138	34.9
RHUBARB PIE, home recipe (USDA)	⅙ of 9″ pie (5.6 oz.)	400	60.4
RICE:			
Brown:			
Raw (USDA)	½ cup (3.6 oz.)	374	80.4
Raw (USDA)	1 oz.	102	21.9
Cooked:			
(USDA)	4 oz.	135	28.9
(Carolina)	4 oz.	135	28.9
(River Brand)	4 oz.	135	28.9

(USDA): United States Department of Agriculture
DNA: Data Not Available
*Prepared as Package Directs

Food and Description	Measure or Quantity	Calories	Carbo-hydrates (grams)
(Water Maid)	4 oz.	135	28.9
White:			
Instant or Precooked:			
Dry long-grain (USDA)	1 oz.	106	23.4
Cooked:			
Long-grain (USDA)	½ cup (2.9 oz.)	89	19.8
(Carolina)	4 oz.	124	27.4
(Minute Rice)	½ cup (3 oz.)	92	20.1
Long-grain (Uncle Ben's Quick)	½ cup	96	22.0
Parboiled:			
Dry, long-grain (USDA)	1 oz.	105	23.0
Cooked:			
Long-grain (USDA)	4 oz.	120	26.4
(Aunt Caroline)	4 oz.	120	26.4
Long-grain (Uncle Ben's Converted)	½ cup	84	19.0
Regular:			
Raw (USDA)	½ cup (3.5 oz.)	359	79.6
Cooked:			
(USDA)	½ cup (3 oz.)	92	20.3
Extra long-grain (Carolina)	4 oz.	124	27.4
(Mahatma)	4 oz.	124	27.4
(River Brand)	4 oz.	124	27.4
(Water Maid)	4 oz.	124	27.4
Wild (See **WILD RICE**)			
RICE BRAN (USDA)	1 oz.	78	14.4
RICE CHEX, cereal (Ralston Purina)	1⅛ cups (1 oz.)	111	24.8
RICE FLAKES, dietetic cereal (Van Brode)	1 oz.	109	25.4
RICE, FRIED, frozen:			
(Chun King)	4 oz.	145	28.8
Shrimp (Temple)	9-oz. pkg.	394	D.N.A.
RICE HONEYS, cereal (Nabisco)	1 cup (1⅓ oz.)	151	32.7
RICE KRISPIES, cereal (Kellogg's)	1 cup (1 oz.)	106	24.6

(USDA): United States Department of Agriculture
DNA: Data Not Available
*Prepared as Package Directs

Food and Description	Measure or Quantity	Calories	Carbo-hydrates (grams)
RICE MIX:			
Beef:			
Rice-A-Roni	½ cup (3.5 oz.)	159	26.7
*(Uncle Ben's)	½ cup	102	21.3
*(Village Inn)	½ cup	116	24.4
*Cheese *Rice-A-Roni*	½ cup (3.5 oz.)	151	20.5
Chicken:			
Rice-A-Roni	½ cup (3.5 oz.)	156	25.7
*Drumstick (Minute Rice)	½ cup	150	D.N.A.
*(Uncle Ben's)	½ cup	104	21.2
*(Village Inn)	½ cup	116	24.4
*Chinese, fried, *Rice-A-Roni*	½ cup (3.5 oz.)	199	24.5
*Curry (Uncle Ben's)	½ cup	106	22.9
*Curry (Village Inn)	½ cup	116	24.4
*Drumstick (Minute Rice)	½ cup	153	24.0
*Ham *Rice-A-Roni*	½ cup (3.5 oz.)	102	14.5
*Herb (Village Inn)	½ cup	116	24.4
Keriyaki dinner (Betty Crocker)	5.5-oz. pkg.	644	106.7
*Long & wild grain (Uncle Ben's)	½ cup	100	21.4
*Long & wild grain (Village Inn)	½ cup	116	24.4
Milanese (Betty Crocker)	5-oz. pkg.	545	90.5
Provence (Betty Crocker)	5.5-oz. pkg.	600	108.9
Rib Roast (Minute Rice)	½ cup	149	24.1
Spanish:			
Rice-A-Roni	½ cup (3.5 oz.)	116	18.1
*(Minute Rice)	½ cup	150	25.0
*(Uncle Ben's)	½ cup	115	24.0
*(Village Inn)	½ cup	116	24.4
*Turkey *Rice-A-Roni*	½ cup (3.5 oz.)	178	25.3
*Wild *Rice-A-Roni*	½ cup (3.5 oz.)	138	21.0
*Yellow (Village Inn)	½ cup	116	24.4
RICE & PEAS with MUSH-ROOMS, frozen (Birds Eye)	½ cup (1.8 oz.)	37	7.4
RICE POLISH (USDA)	1 oz.	75	16.4
RICE, PUFFED, cereal:			
(USDA)	1 cup (.4 oz.)	52	11.6
(Checker)	½ oz.	56	14.4
(Kellogg's)	1 cup (.5 oz.)	55	12.8
(Quaker)	1 cup (.4 oz.)	45	10.4
(Van Brode) dietetic	1 oz.	109	25.2

(USDA): United States Department of Agriculture
DNA: Data Not Available
*Prepared as Package Directs

Food and Description	Measure or Quantity	Calories	Carbo-hydrates (grams)
RICE PUDDING, cinnamon, canned (Bounty)	4 oz.	195	29.0
RICE, SPANISH:			
Home recipe, cooked (USDA)	4 oz.	99	18.8
Canned:			
(College Inn)	4 oz.	231	48.3
(Heinz)	4 oz.	61	10.0
(Nalley's)	4 oz.	85	32.4
RICE, SPANISH, SEASONING MIX (Lawry's)	1½-oz. pkg.	125	20.7
RIESLING WINE, Alsatian:			
(Willm) 11-14% alcohol	3 fl. oz.	66	3.6
(Willm) Grand Reserve			
Exceptionelle, 11-14% alcohol	3 fl. oz.	66	3.6
RIPPLE WINE (Gallo):			
Red, 11% alcohol	3 fl. oz.	56	3.3
White, 11% alcohol	3 fl. oz.	55	3.3
ROCKFISH (USDA):			
Raw, flesh only	1 lb.	440	0.
Oven-steamed, flesh only	4 oz.	121	2.2
ROCK & RYE LIQUEUR:			
(Garnier) 60 proof	1 fl. oz.	70	6.2
(Hiram Walker) 60 proof	1 fl. oz.	87	9.5
(Leroux) 60 proof	1 fl. oz.	74	8.3
(Leroux)Irish Moss, 70 proof	1 fl. oz.	110	13.0
(Old Mr. Boston) 48 proof	1 fl. oz.	72	6.0
(Old Mr. Boston) 60 proof	1 fl. oz.	94	5.8
ROE (USDA):			
Raw, carp, cod, haddock, herring, pike or shad	4 oz.	148	1.7
Raw, salmon, sturgeon, turbot	4 oz.	235	1.6
Baked or broiled, cod & shad	4 oz.	143	2.2
Canned, cod, haddock or herring, solids & liq.	4 oz.	134	.4
ROLAIDS (Warner-Lambert)	1 piece	4	1.4

(USDA): United States Department of Agriculture
DNA: Data Not Available
*Prepared as Package Directs

Food and Description	Measure or Quantity	Calories	Carbohydrates (grams)
ROLL & BUN:			
Barbeque (Arnold)	1 piece (1.3 oz.)	111	18.8
Brown & serve:			
Unbrowned (USDA)	1 oz.	85	14.4
Browned (USDA)	1 oz.	93	15.6
(Wonder)	1 roll	80	12.5
Cinnamon, iced (Van de Kamp's)	1 roll (1.3 oz.)	127	D.N.A.
Club, brown & serve (Pepperidge Farm)	1 roll (1.4 oz.)	96	20.0
Deli Twists (Arnold)	1 roll (1.2 oz.)	109	17.2
Dinner (Arnold)	1 roll (.6 oz.)	61	9.6
Dinner, fully baked (Pepperidge Farm)	1 roll (.7 oz.)	58	9.6
Dutch Egg sandwich buns (Arnold)	1 bun (1¼ oz.)	119	16.1
Finger (Arnold)	1 roll (.6 oz.)	60	9.5
Finger, butter (Van de Kamp's)	1 roll (1.1 oz.)	105	D.N.A.
Frankfurter:			
(USDA)	1 roll (1.4 oz.)	116	20.7
(Arnold)	1 bun (1.3 oz.)	104	17.8
New England (Arnold)	1 roll (1.3 oz.)	108	18.5
French, brown & serve:			
(Pepperidge Farm)	1 roll (5 oz.)	361	75.0
(Pepperidge Farm)	1 roll (3 oz.)	241	50.0
Giraffe sandwich buns (Arnold)	1 bun (1.6 oz.)	135	22.7
Golden Twist, brown & serve (Pepperidge Farm)	1 roll (1 oz.)	112	13.2
Hamburger (USDA)	1 roll (1.4 oz.)	116	20.7
Hard (USDA)	1 roll (1.8 oz.)	162	30.9
Hard (Levy's)	1 roll (2.5 oz.)	130	37.4
Hearth, brown & serve (Pepperidge Farm)	1 roll (.7 oz.)	54	9.9
Hot Cross bun (Van de Kamp's)	1 bun (1.1 oz.)	63	D.N.A.
Parker (Arnold)	1 roll (.6 oz.)	62	9.7
Plain (USDA)	1 roll (1.3 oz.)	113	20.1
Poppy finger (Arnold)	1 roll (.6 oz.)	61	9.4
Raisin (USDA)	1 bun (1.5 oz.)	118	24.3
Sesame crisp, brown & serve (Pepperidge Farm)	1 roll (.8 oz.)	63	11.3
Sourdough, French (Van de Kamp's)	1 roll (1.5 oz.)	130	D.N.A.
Sweet (USDA)	1 bun (1.5 oz.)	136	21.2
Tea (Arnold)	1 roll (.4 oz.)	36	5.7
Whole-wheat (USDA)	1 roll (1.3 oz.)	98	19.9

(USDA): United States Department of Agriculture
DNA: Data Not Available
*Prepared as Package Directs

Food and Description	Measure or Quantity	Calories	Carbohydrates (grams)
ROLL DOUGH:			
Frozen, unraised (USDA)	1 oz.	76	13.4
Frozen, baked (USDA)	1 oz.	88	15.9
Refrigerated:			
Cinnamon with icing (Pillsbury)	1 oz.	100	14.0
Dinner (Pillsbury):			
Butterflake	1 oz.	80	11.9
Crescent	1 oz.	94	10.8
Parkerhouse	1 oz.	76	12.6
Snowflake	1 oz.	84	11.9
ROLL MIX:			
Dry (USDA)	1 oz.	111	20.5
*Prepared (USDA)	1 oz.	85	15.4
(Pillsbury)	1 oz.	113	19.2
***ROMAN MEAL CEREAL**	¾ cup (1.2 oz. dry)	126	22.8
***ROOT BEER DRINK MIX**			
(Wyler's)	6 fl. oz.	92	23.0
ROOT BEER SOFT DRINK:			
Sweetened:			
(Canada Dry)	6 fl. oz.	78	20.4
(Clicquot Club)	6 fl. oz.	78	19.5
(Cott)	6 fl. oz.	78	19.5
(Dad's)	6 fl. oz.	79	19.6
(Dr. Brown's)	6 fl. oz.	81	20.2
(Dr. Pepper)	6 fl. oz.	90	22.8
Fanta	6 fl. oz.	90	24.0
(Hires)	6 fl. oz.	78	19.5
(Hoffman)	6 fl. oz.	81	20.2
(Key Food)	6 fl. oz.	81	20.2
(Kirsch)	6 fl. oz.	71	17.7
(Mason's)	6 fl. oz.	60	15.0
(Mission)	6 fl. oz.	78	19.5
(Shasta)	6 fl. oz.	84	21.3
(Waldbaum)	6 fl. oz.	81	20.2
(Yukon Club)	6 fl. oz.	81	20.2
Low calorie:			
(Dad's)	6 fl. oz.	1	.1
(Hoffman)	6 fl. oz.	3	.8
(No-Cal)	6 fl. oz.	<1	<.1
Draft (Shasta)	6 fl. oz.	<1	<.1

(USDA): United States Department of Agriculture
DNA: Data Not Available
*Prepared as Package Directs

Food and Description	Measure or Quantity	Calories	Carbohydrates (grams)
ROSE APPLE, raw (USDA)			
Whole	1 lb. (weighed with caps & seeds)	170	43.2
Flesh only	4 oz.	64	16.1
ROSE WINE:			
(Antinori) 12% alcohol	3 fl. oz.	84	6.3
Chateau Ste. Roseline, 11-14% alcohol	3 fl. oz.	84	6.3
(Chanson) *Rose des Anges,* 12% alcohol	3 fl. oz.	84	6.3
(Cruse) 12% alcohol	3 fl. oz.	72	D.N.A.
(Gallo) 13% alcohol	3 fl. oz.	55	1.8
(Gallo) *Gypsy,* 20% alcohol	3 fl. oz.	112	12.0
(Great Western) 12% alcohol	3 fl. oz.	88	4.7
(Great Western) Isabella, 12% alcohol	3 fl. oz.	84	3.8
(Italian Swiss Colony-Gold Medal) Grenache, 12.4 % alcohol	3 fl. oz.	69	2.2
(Italian Swiss Colony-Private Stock) Grenache, 12% alcohol	3 fl. oz.	61	.5
(Italian Swiss Colony-Gold Medal) Napa-Sonoma-Mendocino, 12% alcohol	3 fl. oz.	67	2.2
(Louis M. Martini) Gamay, 12½% alcohol	3 fl. oz.	90	.2
(Mogen David) 12% alcohol	3 fl. oz.	75	8.9
Nectarosé, vin rosé d'Anjou, 12% alcohol	3 fl. oz.	70	2.6
(Taylor) 12.5% alcohol	3 fl. oz.	69	Tr.
ROSE WINE, SPARKLING			
(Chanson)	3 fl. oz.	72	3.6
RUDESHEIMER SCHLOSSBERG, German Rhine wine (Deinhard) 11% alcohol	3 fl. oz.	72	4.5
RUM (See **DISTILLED LIQUOR**)			
RUSK:			
(USDA)	.5 oz.	59	10.1
Dutch (Hekman's)	1 piece	55	D.N.A.
Dutch (Sunshine)	1 piece (.5 oz.)	61	10.5
Holland (Nabisco)	1 piece (8 grams)	38	6.3

(USDA): United States Department of Agriculture
DNA: Data Not Available
*Prepared as Package Directs

Food and Description	Measure or Quantity	Calories	Carbo-hydrates (grams)
RUTABAGA:			
Raw, without tops (USDA)	1 lb. (weighed with skin)	177	42.4
Raw, diced (USDA)	½ cup (2.4 oz.)	32	7.7
Boiled, drained, diced (USDA)	½ cup (3 oz.)	30	7.1
Boiled, drained, mashed (USDA)	½ cup (4.3 oz.)	43	10.0
Canned (King Pharr)	½ cup	52	D.N.A.
RYE, whole grain (USDA)	1 oz.	95	20.8
RYE FLOUR (See **FLOUR**)			
RYE WAFER, Whole-grain:			
(USDA)	1 oz.	98	21.6
(USDA)	2 wafers (1⅞″ x 3½″)	44	9.9
RYE WHISKEY (See **DISTILLED LIQUOR**)			
RYE WHISKEY EXTRACT			
(Ehlers)	1 tsp.	14	D.N.A.
RYE-KRISP:			
Pizza	1 small cracker	8	D.N.A.
Seasoned	1 cracker (1⅞″ x 3½″)	25	4.5
Traditional	1 cracker (1⅞″ x 3½″)	21	4.8
RY-KING (Wasa):			
Brown rye	1 slice (12 grams)	43	8.4
Golden rye	1 slice (10 grams)	33	6.8
Lite rye	1 slice (8 grams)	30	6.2
Seasoned rye	1 slice (9 grams)	39	6.8

S

SABLEFISH, raw (USDA):			
Whole	1 lb.(weighed whole)	362	0.
Meat only	4 oz.	215	0.

(USDA): United States Department of Agriculture
DNA: Data Not Available
*Prepared as Package Directs

Food and Description	Measure or Quantity	Calories	Carbo-hydrates (grams)
SABRA, Israeli liqueur (Leroux)			
60 proof	1 fl. oz.	91	10.4
SACCHARIN (Dia-Mel)	1 tablet	0	0.
SAFFLOWER SEED KERNELS			
(USDA)	1 oz.	174	3.5
SAINT-EMILION WINE, French			
Bordeaux:			
(Barton & Guestier) 12% alcohol	3 fl. oz.	63	.7
(Cruse) 11.5% alcohol	3 fl. oz.	69	D.N.A.
SAINT JOHN'S-BREAD FLOUR			
(See **FLOUR,** Carob)			
SAINT-JULIEN WINE (Cruse)			
11.5% alcohol	3 fl. oz.	69	D.N.A.
SALAD DRESSING (See also **SALAD DRESSING, LOW CALORIE**):			
All purpose (Lawry's)	1 T.	59	1.5
Bleu or blue cheese:			
(USDA)	1 oz.	143	2.1
(USDA)	1 T.	81	1.2
(Kraft)	1 oz.	147	1.6
(Lawry's)	1 T.	57	.8
Roka (Kraft)	1 oz.	110	1.6
Caesar (Lawry's)	1 T.	70	.5
Caesar (Wish-Bone)	1 T.	62	.6
Canadian (Lawry's)	1 T.	72	.6
Cheese (Wish-Bone)	1 T.	67	1.2
Chef style, *Salad Bowl* (Kraft)	1 oz.	102	5.3
Coleslaw (Kraft)	1 oz.	124	6.7
Cuisine (Kraft)	1 oz.	98	4.7
French:			
Home recipe (USDA)	1 oz.	179	1.0
Commercial (USDA)	1 oz.	116	5.0
Commercial (USDA)	1 T.	66	2.8
(Best Foods) Family	1 T.	65	2.9
(Hellmann's) Family	1 T.	65	2.9
(Heinz)	1 T.	78	2.0
(Kraft)	1 oz.	129	3.7

(USDA): United States Department of Agriculture
DNA: Data Not Available
*Prepared as Package Directs

Food and Description	Measure or Quantity	Calories	Carbohydrates (grams)
(Kraft) Casino	1 oz.	119	6.0
(Kraft) Catalina	1 oz.	118	7.0
(Kraft) *Miracle*	1 oz.	123	5.1
(Lawry's) California	1 T.	60	1.5
(Marzetti's)	1 T.	74	D.N.A.
(Nalley's)	1 oz.	104	3.7
(Wish-Bone) Classic	1 T.	64	2.7
(Wish-Bone) Deluxe	1 T.	60	2.4
Garlic:			
(Best Foods) *Old Homestead*	1 T.	70	3.0
(Hellmann's) *Old Homestead*	1 T.	70	3.0
(Kraft) Salad Bowl	1 oz.	105	3.9
(Lawry's) San Francisco	1 T.	53	.8
(Wish-Bone)	1 T.	68	3.6
(Wish-Bone) Monaco	1 T.	84	3.6
Green Goddess:			
(Kraft)	1 oz.	149	1.5
(Lawry's)	1 T.	59	.7
(Wish-Bone)	1 T.	58	1.2
Hawaiian (Lawry's)	1 T.	77	5.8
Heinz Salad Dressing	1 T.	63	2.0
Herb & garlic (Kraft)	1 oz.	176	.9
Hickory Bits (Wish-Bone)	1 T.	78	.6
Italian:			
(USDA)	1 T.	83	1.0
(Hellmann's) True	1 T.	85	.8
(Kraft)	1 oz.	176	1.4
(Kraft) *Salad Bowl*	1 oz.	155	1.4
(Lawry's) with cheese	1 T.	60	4.7
(Marzetti's)	1 T.	74	D.N.A.
(Wish-Bone) Golden	1 T.	45	.9
(Wish-Bone) low oil	1 T.	80	.9
(Wish-Bone) Rosé	1 T.	64	.6
Mayonnaise (See **MAYONNAISE**)			
Mayonnaise-type salad dressing			
(USDA)	1 T.	65	2.2
Miracle Whip (Kraft)	1 oz.	138	3.6
Oil & vinegar (Kraft)	1 oz.	132	1.2
Onion, creamy (Wish-Bone)	1 T.	72	.9
Orleans (Wish-Bone)	1 T.	63	1.5
Roquefort (USDA)	1 oz.	143	2.1
Roquefort (Kraft) refrigerated	1 oz.	115	1.9

(USDA): United States Department of Agriculture
DNA: Data Not Available
*Prepared as Package Directs

Food and Description	Measure or Quantity	Calories	Carbo-hydrates (grams)
Russian:			
(USDA)	1 T.	74	1.6
(Kraft) pourable	1 oz.	109	8.6
(Wish-Bone)	1 T.	56	7.2
Salad Bowl (Kraft)	1 oz.	108	4.5
Salad Secret (Kraft)	1 oz.	112	3.7
Sherry (Lawry's)	1 T.	55	1.6
Slaw (Marzetti's)	1 T.	74	D.N.A.
Spin Blend (Hellmann's)	1 T.	55	2.6
Sweet & Sour (Kraft)	1 oz.	52	13.0
Tahitian Isle (Wish-Bone)	1 T.	56	7.2
Tang (Nalley's)	1 oz.	102	4.8
Thousand Island:			
(USDA)	1 T.	80	2.5
(Best Foods) pourable	1 T.	60	2.9
(Hellmann's) pourable	1 T.	60	2.9
(Kraft)	1 oz.	145	3.9
(Kraft) pourable	1 oz.	112	4.7
(Kraft) refrigerated	1 oz.	147	3.9
(Kraft) *Salad Bowl*	1 oz.	128	2.4
(Wish-Bone)	1 T.	72	2.7
Wine vinegar & oil (James H. Black)	1 T.	19	1.9

SALAD DRESSING, DIETETIC or LOW CALORIE:

Food and Description	Measure or Quantity	Calories	Carbo-hydrates (grams)
Bleu or blue:			
Low fat, 6% fat (USDA)	1 T.	11	.6
Low fat, 1% fat (USDA)	1 T.	3	.2
(Dia-Mel)	1 T.	12	.4
(Frenchette)	1 T.	6	D.N.A.
(Kraft)	1 T.	15	.3
(Tillie Lewis)	1 T.	12	.2
Caesar (Tillie Lewis)	1 T.	12	.2
Chef style (Kraft)	1 T.	16	2.6
Chefs (Tillie Lewis)	1 T.	1	.4
Cole slaw (Kraft)	1 oz.	42	6.0
Diet Whip (Dia-Mel)	1 T.	10	Tr.
Diet-Aise (Slim-ette)	1 T.	15	D.N.A.
French:			
Low fat (USDA)	1 T.	15	2.5
Low fat, with artificial sweetener (USDA)	1 T.	2	.3

(USDA): United States Department of Agriculture
DNA: Data Not Available
*Prepared as Package Directs

Food and Description	Measure or Quantity	Calories	Carbo-hydrates (grams)
Medium fat, with artificial			
sweetener (USDA)	1 T.	23	.2
(Dia-Mel)	1 T.	15	.2
(Dia-Mel) Green Garlic	1 T.	9	Tr.
(Frenchette)	1 T.	9	2.1
(Kraft)	1 T.	22	2.1
(Kraft) Fruit 'n Slaw	1 T.	22	3.1
(Marzetti's)	1 T.	24	3.6
(Tillie Lewis)	1 T.	4	1.0
(Wish-Bone)	1 T.	23	3.3
(Wish-Bone) Garlic	1 T.	16	2.7
Italian:			
(USDA)	1 T.	8	.4
(Dia-Mel)	1 T.	9	.4
Italianette (Frenchette)	1 T.	6	.6
(Kraft)	1 T.	10	.3
(Marzetti's)	1 T.	6	1.1
(Tillie Lewis)	1 T.	1	.3
(Wish-Bone)	1 T.	8	1.2
May-Lo-Naise (Tillie Lewis)	1 T.	9	.1
Mayonnaise, imitation (USDA)	1 T.	22	.8
Russian (Dia-Mel)	1 T.	24	1.4
Russian (Wish-Bone)	1 T.	27	5.4
Slaw (Marzetti's)	1 T.	30	3.0
Supreme (McCormick)	1 oz.	80	2.0
Thousand Island:			
(USDA)	1 T.	27	2.3
(Kraft)	1 oz.	28	1.0
(Marzetti's)	1 T.	24	3.3
(Tillie Lewis)	1 T.	10	.4
Whipped (Tillie Lewis)	1 T.	10	.2
SALAD DRESSING MIX, regular			
& low calorie:			
Bacon (Lawry's)	1 pkg. (.8 oz.)	69	11.9
Bleu or blue cheese:			
*(Good Seasons)	1 T.	85	.7
*(Good Seasons) thick, creamy	1 T.	89	.3
(Lawry's)	1 pkg. (.7 oz.)	79	4.5
Caesar garlic cheese (Lawry's)	1 pkg. (.8 oz.)	71	8.7
*Cheese garlic (Good Seasons)	1 T.	85	.7
*Coleslaw (Good Seasons) thick,			
creamy	1 T.	91	1.9

(USDA): United States Department of Agriculture
DNA: Data Not Available
*Prepared as Package Directs

Food and Description	Measure or Quantity	Calories	Carbo- hydrates (grams)
*French, old fashioned (Good Seasons)	1 T.	84	.7
French, old fashioned (Lawry's)	1 pkg. (.8 oz.)	72	16.8
*Garlic (Good Seasons)	1 T.	84	.7
*Green Goddess (Good Seasons) thick, creamy	1 T.	87	.8
Green Goddess (Lawry's)	1 pkg. (.8 oz.)	69	12.7
Italian:			
*(Good Seasons)	1 T.	84	.7
(Lawry's)	1 pkg. (.6 oz.)	44	9.6
(Lawry's) with cheese	1 pkg. (.8 oz.)	69	9.4
*Onion (Good Seasons)	1 T.	84	.7
*Parmesan (Good Seasons)	1 T.	84	.7
*Thousand Island (Good Seasons) thick, creamy	1 T.	85	.6
SALAD FRUIT, unsweetened, unseasoned (S and W) *Nutradiet*	4 oz.	43	9.8
SALAD SEASONING:			
(Durkee)	1 tsp.	4	.7
With cheese (Durkee)	1 tsp.	10	.4
SALAMI:			
Dry (USDA)	1 oz.	128	.3
Cooked (USDA)	1 oz.	88	.4
Cooked (Eckrich)	1 oz.	58	D.N.A.
(Vienna)	1 oz.	74	.5
Beef (Sugardale)	1-oz. slice	76	Tr.
Cotto (Oscar Mayer)	1 slice	54	D.N.A.
Cotto (Wilson)	1 oz.	84	.4
Hard (Oscar Mayer)	1 slice	38	D.N.A.
SALISBURY STEAK:			
Canned, with mushrooms (Morton House)	12¾-oz. can	835	D.N.A.
Frozen:			
(Banquet) buffet	2-lb. pkg.	1524	46.5
(Banquet) cookin' bag	5 oz.	239	7.2
(Holloway House)	1 steak	298	50.0
(Swanson)	5⁷⁄₁₀-oz. pkg.	329	35.4
Dinner, frozen:			
(Banquet)	11-oz. dinner	335	21.5

(USDA): United States Department of Agriculture
DNA: Data Not Available
*Prepared as Package Directs

Food and Description	Measure or Quantity	Calories	Carbo-hydrates (grams)
(Morton)	11-oz. dinner	394	16.4
(Swanson) 3-course	17-oz. dinner	520	50.2

SALMON:
  Atlantic (USDA):

Raw, whole	1 lb. (weighed whole)	640	0.
Raw, meat only	4 oz.	246	0.
Canned, solids & liq., including bones (USDA)	4 oz.	230	0.

  Chinook or King:

Raw, meat with bones (USDA)	1 lb. (weighed with bones)	640	0.
Raw, meat only (USDA)	4 oz.	252	0.
Canned, solids & liq.:			
Including bones (USDA)	4 oz.	238	0.
(Icy Point)	7¾-oz. can	460	0.
(Pillar Rock)	7¾-oz. can	460	0.
Chum, canned, solids & liq., including bones (USDA)	4 oz.	158	0.
Coho, canned, solids & liq., including bones (USDA)	4 oz.	174	0.
Coho, canned, dietetic (Silver Beauty)	4 oz.	187	0.

  Pink or Humpback:

Raw, steak (USDA)	1 lb. (weighed with bones)	475	0.
Raw, meat only (USDA)	4 oz.	135	0.
Canned, solids & liq.:			
Including bones (USDA)	4 oz.	160	0.
(Icy Point)	7¾-oz. can	310	0.
(Del Monte)	7¾-oz. can	310	0.
(Pink Beauty)	7¾-oz. can	310	0.
Sockeye or Red or Blueback, canned, solid & liq.:			
Including bones (USDA)	4 oz.	194	0.
(Icy Point)	3¾-oz. can	182	0.
(Pillar Rock)	3¾-oz. can	182	0.
Unseasoned (S and W) *Nutradiet*	3¾-oz. can	190	1.6
Unspecified kind of salmon, baked or broiled (USDA)	4-oz. steak (approx. 4″ x 3″ x ½″)	206	0.

(USDA): United States Department of Agriculture
DNA: Data Not Available
*Prepared as Package Directs

Food and Description	Measure or Quantity	Calories	Carbohydrates (grams)
SALMON RICE LOAF, home recipe (USDA)	4 oz.	138	8.3
SALMON, SMOKED (USDA)	4 oz.	200	0.
SALSIFY (USDA):			
Raw, without tops, freshly harvested	1 lb. (weighed untrimmed)	51	38.4
Raw, without tops, after storage	1 lb. (weighed untrimmed)	324	71.0
Boiled, drained solids, freshly harvested	4 oz.	14	17.1
Boiled, drained solids, after storage	4 oz.	79	17.1
SALT:			
Table (USDA)	any quantity	0	0.
Garlic (Lawry's)	1 pkg. (2.9 oz.)	116	22.9
Garlic (Lawry's)	1 tsp.	5	1.0
Imitation, butter flavored (Durkee)	1 tsp.	5	.2
Seasoned (Lawry's)	1 pkg. (3 oz.)	22	2.3
Seasoned (Lawry's)	1 tsp.	1	.1
Substitute (Adolph's)	1 gram	<1	Tr.
Substitute, seasoned (Adolph's)	1 gram	<1	.1
SALT PORK, raw (USDA):			
With skin	1 lb. (weighed with skin)	3410	0.
Without skin	1 oz.	222	0.
SALT STICK (See **BREAD STICK**)			
SANCERRE WINE, French white, Loire Valley:			
(Barton & Guestier) 12% alcohol	3 fl. oz.	61	.3
(Chanson) 12½% alcohol	3 fl. oz.	87	6.3
SAND DAB, raw (USDA):			
Whole	1 lb. (weighed whole)	118	0.
Meat only	4 oz.	90	0.

(USDA): United States Department of Agriculture
DNA: Data Not Available
*Prepared as Package Directs

Food and Description	Measure or Quantity	Calories	Carbo-hydrates (grams)
SANDWICH SPREAD:			
(USDA)	1 cup (8.7 oz.)	932	39.1
(USDA)	1 T.	57	2.4
(USDA) low calorie	1 T.	16	1.2
(Best Foods)	1 T.	60	2.4
(Hellmann's)	1 T.	60	2.4
Miracle (Kraft)	1 oz.	104	5.7
(Nalley's)	1 oz.	100	7.0
(Tillie Lewis) dietetic	1 T.	9	.2
SAPODILLA, raw (USDA):			
Whole	1 lb. (weighed whole)	323	79.1
Flesh only	4 oz.	101	24.7
SAPOTES, raw (USDA):			
Whole	1 lb. (weighed whole)	431	108.9
Flesh only	4 oz.	142	35.8
SARDINE:			
Atlantic, canned in oil (USDA):			
Solids & liq.	4 oz.	353	.7
Drained solids	3 oz.	175	0.
Moroccan, skinless & boneless, canned (Cresca):			
In olive oil	3¾-oz. can	341	D.N.A.
In water	3½-oz. can	165	D.N.A.
Norwegian, canned (Underwood):			
In mustard sauce	3 oz. sardines & 1 oz. sauce	134	1.6
In oil, drained solids	3 oz.	167	.7
In tomato sauce	3 oz. sardines & 1 oz. sauce	124	1.7
Pacific (USDA):			
Raw, meat only	4 oz.	181	0.
Canned in brine or mustard, solids & liq.	4 oz.	222	1.9
Canned in tomato sauce, solids & liq.	4 oz.	224	1.9
SARSAPARILLA SOFT DRINK:			
(Hoffman)	6 fl. oz.	84	21.0
(Yukon Club)	6 fl. oz.	90	22.5

(USDA): United States Department of Agriculture
DNA: Data Not Available
*Prepared as Package Directs

Food and Description	Measure or Quantity	Calories	Carbo-hydrates (grams)
SAUCE, regular and dietetic:			
Barbecue:			
(USDA)	1 oz.	26	2.3
(Good Seasons) *Open Pit*	1 T.	26	6.2
(Heinz) with onion	1 T.	20	4.7
(Kraft)	1 oz.	34	7.9
(Kraft) garlic	1 oz.	32	7.6
(Kraft) hot	1 oz.	31	7.0
(Kraft) smoked	1 oz.	34	7.9
Bolognaise (Crosse & Blackwell)	1 T.	24	1.4
Bordelaise (Crosse & Blackwell)	1 T.	18	1.4
Champignon (Crosse & Blackwell)	1 T.	12	1.4
Cheese (Kraft) *Deluxe Dinner*	1 oz.	77	2.0
Chili (See **CHILI SAUCE**)			
Cocktail, refrigerated (Kraft)	1 oz.	31	7.5
Enchilada (Rosarita)	1 oz.	8	1.2
Famous (Durkee)	1 T.	53	1.7
57 (Heinz)	1 T.	18	3.5
H.P. (Lea & Perrins)	1 T.	18	Tr.
Hard (Crosse & Blackwell)	1 T.	64	8.3
Hollandaise (Cresca)	1 oz.	39	D.N.A.
Horseradish (Kraft)	1 oz.	100	3.3
Hot tomato (Rosarita)	1 oz.	7	1.2
Marinara (Buitoni)	½ cup	84	11.4
Marinara (Chef Boy-Ar-Dee)	3¾ oz. (¼ of 15-oz. can)	62	10.9
Mint (Crosse & Blackwell)	1 T.	16	4.0
Mushroom steak (Green Giant)	1 oz.	9	D.N.A.
Newburg (Crosse & Blackwell)	1 T.	22	1.3
Polynesian (Crosse & Blackwell)	1 T.	16	3.6
Remoulade, dietetic (Tillie Lewis)	1 T.	11	.6
Savory (Heinz)	1 T.	74	1.5
Seafood cocktail (Crosse & Blackwell)	1 T.	22	4.9
Shrimp cocktail (Crosse & Blackwell)	1 T.	22	5.1
Soy (USDA)	1 oz.	19	2.7
Spaghetti (See **SPAGHETTI SAUCE**)			
Steak (Crosse & Blackwell)	1 T.	21	4.8
Sweet & sour (Kraft)	1 oz.	103	3.7
Tabasco (See individual listing)			
Tartar:			
(USDA)	1 oz.	151	1.2

Food and Description	Measure or Quantity	Calories	Carbo- hydrates (grams)
(USDA)	1 T.	74	.6
(Best Foods)	1 T.	75	.3
(Kraft)	1 oz.	145	1.4
(Kraft) spice blend	1 oz.	151	.9
White:			
Home recipe:			
Thin (USDA)	1 cup (8.8 oz.)	302	18.0
Medium (USDA)	1 cup (8.8 oz.)	413	22.4
Thick (USDA)	1 cup (8.7 oz.)	489	27.2
Canned, mushroom (Green Giant)	8 oz. (by wt.)	152	D.N.A.
Worcestershire:			
(Crosse & Blackwell)	1 T.	15	3.6
(Heinz)	1 T.	4	1.0
(Lea & Perrins)	1 T.	12	Tr.

SAUCE MIX:

Food and Description	Measure or Quantity	Calories	Carbo- hydrates (grams)
*a la King, without chicken (Durkee)	1⅛ cups (2-oz. dry pkg.)	306	18.9
*Barbecue (Kraft)	1 oz.	35	6.0
Cheese:			
*(Durkee)	1 cup (1½-oz. dry pkg.)	280	14.4
(French's)	1⅜-oz. pkg.	182	6.8
*(Kraft)	1 oz.	52	1.9
(McCormick)	1¼-oz. pkg.	170	4.8
*(McCormick)	1 oz.	40	2.0
*Chicken (Kraft)	1 oz.	15	2.3
*Cream (Kraft)	1 oz.	44	2.5
Enchilada (Lawry's)	1.6-oz. pkg.	144	27.3
Hollandaise:			
*(Durkee)	⅔ cup (1.7-oz. dry pkg.)	78	7.2
(French's)	1⅛-oz. pkg.	178	6.6
*(Kraft)	1 oz.	54	2.0
*(McCormick)	1 oz.	36	2.0
Newburg (French's)	1½-oz. pkg.	200	11.8
Seafood cocktail (Lawry's)	.6-oz. pkg.	43	9.7
Sloppy Joe (See **SLOPPY JOE MIX**)			
Sour cream:			
(French's)	1⅜-oz. pkg.	186	5.3
*(Kraft)	1 oz.	61	4.1

(USDA): United States Department of Agriculture
DNA: Data Not Available
*Prepared as Package Directs

Food and Description	Measure or Quantity	Calories	Carbo-hydrates (grams)
*(McCormick)	1 oz.	20	1.2
*With skim milk (Durkee)	⅔ cup (1½-oz. dry pkg.)	186	12.0
*With whole milk (Durkee)	⅔ cup (1½-oz. dry pkg.)	216	11.4
Stroganoff (French's)	1⅞-oz. pkg.	245	24.7
Tartar (Lawry's)	.6-oz. pkg.	64	9.8
*White sauce supreme (McCormick)	1 oz.	11	2.0
SAUERKRAUT, canned:			
Solids & liq. (USDA)	4 oz.	21	4.5
Solids & liq. (USDA)	1 cup (8.3 oz.)	42	9.4
Drained solids (USDA)	1 cup (5.2 oz.)	32	6.6
Drained solids (Steinfield's)	1 cup	33	6.6
SAUERKRAUT JUICE, canned (USDA)	½ cup (4.4 oz.)	12	2.8
SAUGER, raw (USDA):			
Whole	1 lb. (weighed whole)	133	0.
Flesh only	4 oz.	95	0.
SAUSAGE (See also individual kinds):			
Breakfast (Hormel)	8-oz. can	836	.7
Brown & serve, before browning (USDA)	1 oz.	112	.8
Brown & serve, after browning (USDA)	1 oz.	120	.8
Brown & serve, canned (Hormel)	8 oz.	925	2.3
Cocktail (Cresca)	1 oz.	71	D.N.A.
New England Brand (Wilson)	2 oz.	105	.5
In sauce (Prince)	4 oz.	214	4.5
SAUTERNES:			
(Barton & Guestier) French white Bordeaux, 13% alcohol	3 fl. oz.	95	7.6
(Barton & Guestier) haut, French white Bordeaux, 13% alcohol	3 fl. oz.	99	8.7
(Gallo) 12% alcohol	3 fl. oz.	50	.9
(Gallo) haut, 12% alcohol	3 fl. oz.	67	2.1
(Gold Seal) dry, 12% alcohol	3 fl. oz.	82	.4

(USDA): United States Department of Agriculture
DNA: Data Not Available
*Prepared as Package Directs

Food and Description	Measure or Quantity	Calories	Carbohydrates (grams)
(Gold Seal) semi-soft, 12% alcohol	3 fl. oz.	87	2.6
(Great Western) Aurora, 12% alcohol	3 fl. oz.	88	4.7
(Italian Swiss Colony-Gold Medal) 11.6% alcohol	3 fl. oz.	59	.6
(Louis M. Martini) dry, 12.5% alcohol	3 fl. oz.	90	.2
(Mogen David) cream, 12% alcohol	3 fl. oz.	35	6.2
(Mogen David) dry, American, 12% alcohol	3 fl. oz.	30	1.8
(Taylor) 12.5% alcohol	3 fl. oz.	81	2.9

SCALLION (See **ONION, GREEN**)

SCALLOP:

Raw, muscle only (USDA)	4 oz.	92	3.8
Cooked, steamed (USDA)	4 oz.	127	0.
Frozen:			
Breaded, fried, reheated (USDA)	4 oz.	220	11.9
Breaded, fried, reheated (Booth)	4 oz.	220	11.9
Breaded, fried (Mrs. Paul's)	4 oz.	222	12.0

SCHAV SOUP (Manischewitz) 8 oz. (by wt.)   11   2.1

SCHNAPPS, PEPPERMINT:

(Garnier) 60 proof	1 fl. oz.	83	8.4
(Hiram Walker) 60 proof	1 fl. oz.	78	7.2
(Leroux) 60 proof	1 fl. oz.	87	9.2
(Old Mr. Boston) 42 proof	1 fl. oz.	60	4.5
(Old Mr. Boston) 60 proof	1 fl. oz.	78	4.2

SCONE (Hostess)   1 pkg.   180   33.9

SCOTCH BROTH, condensed (Campbell)   8 oz. (by wt.)   168   19.5

SCOTCH WHISKEY (See **DISTILLED LIQUOR**)

SCRAPPLE (USDA)   4 oz.   244   16.6

SCREWDRIVER MIX (Bar-Tender's)   1 serving (⅝ oz.)   70   17.4

Food and Description	Measure or Quantity	Calories	Carbo-hydrates (grams)
SCREWDRIVER MIXER, soft drink (Canada Dry)	6 fl. oz.	75	19.3
SCUP (See **PORGY**)			
SEABASS, WHITE, raw, meat only (USDA)	4 oz.	109	0.
SEGO, diet food:			
*Instant mix with whole milk	1 cup	224	17.6
Liquid diet	1 cup	176	28.0
SEKT SPARKLING WINE (Deinhard)	3 fl. oz.	72	3.6
SENEGALESE SOUP (Crosse & Blackwell)	6½ oz. (½ can)	61	6.8
SESAME SEEDS, dry (USDA):			
Whole	1 oz.	160	6.1
Hulled	1 oz.	165	5.0
SESAME TAHINI (A. Sahadi)	1 T.	57	.8
SEVEN-UP, soft drink	6 fl. oz.	73	18.0
SHAD (USDA):			
Raw, whole	1 lb. (weighed whole)	370	0.
Raw, meat only	4 oz.	193	0.
Cooked, home recipe:			
Baked with butter & bacon slices	4 oz.	228	0.
Creole	4 oz.	172	1.8
Canned, solids & liq.	4 oz.	172	0.
SHAD, GIZZARD, raw (USDA):			
Whole	1 lb. (weighed whole)	299	0.
Meat only	4 oz.	227	0.
SHAKE 'N BAKE (Good Seasons):			
Chicken-coating mix, seasoned	2⅜-oz. pkg.	305	30.1
Fish-coating mix, seasoned	2-oz. pkg.	260	25.0
Pork-coating mix, seasoned	2⅜-oz. pkg.	234	45.1

(USDA): United States Department of Agriculture
DNA: Data Not Available
*Prepared as Package Directs

Food and Description	Measure or Quantity	Calories	Carbo-hydrates (grams)
SHALLOT, raw (USDA):			
With skin	1 oz.	18	4.2
With skin removed	1 oz.	20	4.8
SHAPE (Drackett):			
Liquid, any flavor	1 can (8 fl. oz.)	225	33.2
Powder:			
Chocolate	2 scoops (1 oz.)	109	19.3
Strawberry or vanilla	2 scoops (1 oz.)	109	20.0
SHEEFISH (See **INCONNU**)			
SHEEPSHEAD, Atlantic, raw (USDA):			
Whole	1 lb. (weighed whole)	159	0.
Meat only	4 oz.	128	0.
SHERBET & FRUIT ICE MIX, ORANGE (Junket)	6 serving pkg. (4 oz.)	388	108.8
SHERBET, ORANGE (See also individual brands):			
(USDA)	1 cup (6.8 oz.)	260	59.4
(USDA)	⅓ pint	174	39.8
(Carnation)	⅓ pint	158	D.N.A.
(Sealtest)	⅓ pint	152	35.6
SHERRY:			
(Gallo) 20% alcohol	3 fl. oz.	88	2.7
(Gallo) 16% alcohol	3 fl. oz.	76	3.3
(Gold Seal) 19% alcohol	3 fl. oz.	139	4.6
(Great Western) Solera, 19% alcohol	3 fl. oz.	143	8.5
(Taylor) 19.5% alcohol	3 fl. oz.	132	7.1
Cocktail (Gold Seal) 19% alcohol	3 fl. oz.	122	1.6
Cocktail (Petri)	3 fl. oz.	102	D.N.A.
Cream:			
(Gallo) 20% alcohol	3 fl. oz.	111	8.4
(Gallo) Old Decanter, Livingston, 20% alcohol	3 fl. oz.	117	12.8
(Gold Seal) 19% alcohol	3 fl. oz.	158	9.4
(Great Western) Solera, 19% alcohol	3 fl. oz.	154	11.6

(USDA): United States Department of Agriculture
DNA: Data Not Available
*Prepared as Package Directs

Food and Description	Measure or Quantity	Calories	Carbo-hydrates (grams)
(Italian Swiss Colony-Private Stock) 19.7% alcohol	3 fl. oz.	129	8.5
(Louis M. Martini) 19.5% alcohol	3 fl. oz.	138	1.2
(Taylor) 19.5% alcohol	3 fl. oz.	150	11.3
(Williams & Humbert) Canasta, 20½% alcohol	3 fl. oz.	150	5.4
Dry:			
(Gallo) 20% alcohol	3 fl. oz.	84	1.8
(Gallo) Old Decanter, very dry, 20% alcohol	3 fl. oz.	87	2.1
(Great Western) Solera, 19% alcohol	3 fl. oz.	128	4.2
(Italian Swiss Colony-Gold Medal) 19.7% alcohol	3 fl. oz.	104	1.7
(Italian Swiss Colony-Private Stock) 19.8% alcohol	3 fl. oz.	104	1.7
(Louis M. Martini) 19.5% alcohol	3 fl. oz.	138	1.2
(Williams & Humbert) Carlito Amontillado, 20½% alcohol	3 fl. oz.	120	4.5
(Williams & Humbert) Cedro, 20½% alcohol	3 fl. oz.	120	4.5
(Williams & Humbert) Dos Cortados, 20½% alcohol	3 fl. oz.	120	4.5
(Williams & Humbert) Pando, 17% alcohol	3 fl. oz.	120	4.5
Dry Sack (Williams & Humbert) 20½% alcohol	3 fl. oz.	120	4.5
Hartley (Italian Swiss Colony-Private Blend) 19.8% alcohol	3 fl. oz.	105	1.9
Medium:			
(Great Western) cooking, 19% alcohol	3 fl. oz.	135	7.5
(Italian Swiss Colony-Gold Medal) 19.7% alcohol	3 fl. oz.	106	2.6
(Italian Swiss Colony-Private Stock) 19.8% alcohol	3 fl. oz.	108	2.8

SHORTENING (See **FATS**)

SHREDDED OATS, cereal
(USDA)	1 oz.	107	20.4

(USDA): United States Department of Agriculture
DNA: Data Not Available
*Prepared as Package Directs

Food and Description	Measure or Quantity	Calories	Carbohydrates (grams)
SHREDDED WHEAT, cereal:			
(USDA) plain	1 cup (1.2 oz.)	124	28.0
(Kellogg's)	2 biscuits (1.3 oz.)	139	30.4
(Nabisco)	1 biscuit (.9 oz.)	92	18.8
(Nabisco) *Spoon Size*	1 biscuit (1 gram)	3	.8
(Quaker)	2 biscuits (1.3 oz.)	132	30.0
(Sunshine)	1 biscuit (1 oz.)	104	22.3
SHRIMP:			
Raw:			
Whole (USDA)	1 lb. (weighed in shell)	285	4.7
Meat only (USDA)	4 oz.	103	1.7
Peeled, deveined (Booth)	4 oz.	103	1.7
Canned:			
Solids & liq. (USDA)	4 oz.	91	.9
Drained solids (USDA)	4 oz.	132	.8
North Pacific, tiny, drained (Icy Point)	½ of 4½-oz. can	102	1.0
North Pacific, tiny, drained (Pink Beauty)	½ of 4½-oz. can	102	1.0
Cooked, fried (USDA)	4 oz.	255	11.3
Frozen:			
Raw:			
Breaded, not more than 50% breading (USDA)	4 oz.	158	22.6
Breaded (Booth)	4 oz.	158	22.6
Breaded (Chicken of the Sea)	4 oz.	158	22.6
Unbreaded (Chicken of the Sea)	4 oz.	103	D.N.A.
Fried (Chicken of the Sea)	4 oz.	255	D.N.A.
Fried, breaded (Mrs. Paul's)	4 oz.	158	22.8
SHRIMP COCKTAIL:			
(Sau-Sea)	4 oz.	80	18.0
(Sea Snack)	4 oz.	110	14.8
SHRIMP DINNER, frozen:			
(Morton)	7¾-oz. dinner	367	33.3
Fried (Swanson)	7½-oz. dinner	358	41.5
SHRIMP PASTE, canned (USDA)	1 oz.	51	.4
SHRIMP PUFF, hors d'oeuvres, frozen (Durkee)	1 piece	59	3.0

(USDA): United States Department of Agriculture
DNA: Data Not Available
*Prepared as Package Directs

Food and Description	Measure or Quantity	Calories	Carbo-hydrates (grams)
SHRIMP ROLL, frozen (Temple)	2½-oz. roll	117	20.7
SHRIMP SOUP, Cream of:			
Canned (Crosse & Blackwell)	8 oz. (by wt.)	113	8.0
Frozen:			
Condensed (USDA)	8 oz. (by wt.)	302	16.3
*Prepared with equal volume water (USDA)	8 oz. (by wt.)	150	7.9
*Prepared with equal volume milk (USDA)	8 oz. (by wt.)	225	14.1
Condensed (Campbell)	8 oz. (by wt.)	299	15.6
SILVER SATIN WINE (Italian Swiss Colony-Gold Medal):			
19.7% alcohol	3 fl. oz.	130	8.9
With bitter lemon, 19.7% alcohol	3 fl. oz.	130	8.9
SIMBA, soft drink	6 fl. oz.	78	21.0
SKATE, raw, flesh only (USDA)	4 oz.	111	0.
SLENDER (Carnation)	1 envelope	63	6.8
SLOE GIN (See **GIN, SLOE**)			
SLOPPY JOE:			
Canned, with beef (Morton House)	15-oz. can	860	D.N.A.
Frozen (Banquet) cookin' bag	5 oz.	251	11.0
SLOPPY JOE MIX:			
Sauce (French's)	1½-oz. pkg.	116	25.8
*With meat & tomato paste (Durkee)	3 cups (½-oz. dry pkg.)	1639	100.4
Seasoning (Lawry's)	1½-oz. pkg.	138	27.7
Seasoning (McCormick)	1⁵⁄₁₆-oz. pkg.	112	D.N.A.
Seasoning (Wyler's)	1¼-oz. pkg.	D.N.A.	20.0
SMELT, Atlantic, jack & bay (USDA):			
Raw, whole	1 lb. (weighed whole)	244	0.
Raw, meat only	4 oz.	111	0.
Canned, solids & liq.	4 oz.	227	0.

(USDA): United States Department of Agriculture
DNA: Data Not Available
*Prepared as Package Directs

[275]

Food and Description	Measure or Quantity	Calories	Carbohydrates (grams)
SMOKIE SAUSAGE:			
(Eckrich):			
Smoked, not bulk	4-oz. piece	344	D.N.A.
Smokee, from 12-oz. pkg.	1 link	115	D.N.A.
Smokee, from 1-lb. pkg.	1 link	150	D.N.A.
Smokette	1 piece	75	D.N.A.
Smok-Y-Links	1 piece	75	D.N.A.
(Oscar Mayer)	1 link	137	D.N.A.
Little sausage (Oscar Mayer)	1 link	30	D.N.A.
(Wilson)	3 oz.	242	1.5
SNACK (See **CRACKER, POP-CORN, POTATO CHIPS,** etc.)			
SNAIL, raw:			
(USDA)	4 oz.	102	2.3
Giant African (USDA)	4 oz.	83	5.0
SNAPPER (See **RED SNAPPER**)			
SNO BALL (Hostess)	1 cake	200	28.0
SOAVE WINE, Italian white (Antinori) 12% alcohol	3 fl. oz.	84	6.3
SODA or SOFT DRINK (See individual kinds listed by flavor or brand name)			
SOLE, raw (USDA):			
Whole	1 lb. (weighed whole)	118	0.
Meat only	4 oz.	90	0.
SORGHUM (USDA):			
Grain	1 oz.	94	20.7
Syrup	1 T.	51	13.6
SORREL (See **DOCK**)			
SOUP (See individual listing by kind)			
SOUR MIXER, soft drink (Canada Dry)	6 fl. oz.	71	18.4

(USDA): United States Department of Agriculture
DNA: Data Not Available
*Prepared as Package Directs

Food and Description	Measure or Quantity	Calories	Carbohydrates (grams)
SOURSOP, raw (USDA):			
Whole	1 lb. (weighed with skin & seeds)	200	50.3
Flesh only	4 oz.	74	18.5
SOUSE (USDA)	1 oz.	51	.3
SOUTHERN COMFORT, 100 proof	1 oz.	120	3.5
SOYBEAN (USDA):			
Young seeds:			
Raw	1 lb. (weighed in pods)	322	31.7
Boiled, drained solids	4 oz.	134	11.5
Canned, seeds & liq.	4 oz.	85	7.1
Canned, drained solids	4 oz.	117	8.4
Mature seeds, dry:			
Raw	1 lb.	1828	152.0
Raw	1 cup (7.4 oz.)	846	70.4
Cooked	4 oz.	147	12.2
SOYBEAN CURD:			
(USDA)	4 oz.	82	2.7
(USDA)	4.2-oz. cake (2¾″ x 2½″ x 1″)	86	2.8
SOYBEAN FLOUR (See **FLOUR**)			
SOYBEAN GRITS (USDA)	1 cup (4.8 oz.)	365	51.3
SOYBEAN MILK (USDA):			
Fluid	4 oz.	37	2.4
Powder	1 oz.	121	7.9
SOYBEAN PROTEIN (USDA)	1 oz.	91	4.2
SOYBEAN PROTEINATE (USDA)	1 oz.	88	2.2
SOYBEAN SPROUT (See **BEAN SPROUT**)			
SOY SAUCE (See **SAUCE**)			

(USDA): United States Department of Agriculture
DNA: Data Not Available
*Prepared as Package Directs

Food and Description	Measure or Quantity	Calories	Carbohydrates (grams)
SPACE FOOD:			
*Applesauce mix (Epicure)	1.5 oz.	191	40.5
*Banana pudding powder (Epicure)	2.5 oz.	299	49.7
*Beef bites (Epicure)	.6 oz.	73	.1
*Beef pot roast bars (Epicure)	1 oz.	121	0.
*Beef sandwich bites (Epicure)	.8 oz.	95	7.8
*Beef & vegetable bar (Epicure)	.9 oz.	170	5.8
*Brownie bites (Epicure)	1.1 oz.	184	23.6
*Butterscotch pudding powder (Epicure)	2.5 oz.	299	49.7
Caramel stick (Pillsbury)	1 oz.	118	19.8
*Caramel stick (Pillsbury)	1 piece	41	6.7
*Cheese sandwich bites (Epicure)	.8 oz.	168	3.0
*Chicken bites (Epicure)	.8 oz.	103	0.
*Chicken sandwich bites (Epicure)	.8 oz.	101	7.5
*Chicken & vegetable bar (Epicure)	.8 oz.	60	6.8
Chocolate malt stick (Epicure)	1 oz.	118	19.8
*Chocolate pudding powder (Epicure)	2.5 oz.	299	49.4
Chocolate stick (Pillsbury)	1 oz.	118	19.8
*Chocolate stick (Pillsbury)	1 piece	41	6.7
*Cinnamon toast bites (Epicure)	.8 oz.	117	14.9
*Cocoa beverage powder (Epicure)	1.5 oz.	180	27.4
*Corn bar (Epicure)	1 oz.	107	22.8
*Corn flake mix (Epicure)	1.3 oz.	143	31.0
*Fruit cocktail bar (Epicure)	.8 oz.	88	21.3
*Mushroom soup powder (Epicure)	1.1 oz.	184	12.2
*Orange beverage powder (Epicure)	.6 oz.	65	15.2
*Pea bar (Epicure)	.7 oz.	73	13.6
*Peach bar (Epicure)	.8 oz.	75	17.4
*Peanut butter sandwich bite (Epicure)	1.1 oz.	153	12.7
Peanut butter stick (Pillsbury)	1 oz.	118	19.8
Peanut butter stick (Pillsbury)	1 piece	41	6.7
*Pea soup powder (Epicure)	1.7 oz.	186	30.8
*Pineapple beverage powder (Epicure)	.6 oz.	60	15.0
*Potato salad bar (Epicure)	.9 oz.	113	10.0
*Shrimp cocktail bar (Epicure)	1.1 oz.	140	13.9

(USDA): United States Department of Agriculture
DNA: Data Not Available
*Prepared as Package Directs

Food and Description	Measure or Quantity	Calories	Carbohydrates (grams)
*Spaghetti & sauce (Epicure)	.7 oz.	96	7.3
*Tea (Epicure)	.4 oz.	37	9.2
*Toast bites (Epicure)	.6 oz.	76	8.2
SPAGHETTI. Plain spaghetti products are essentially the same in caloric value and carbohydrate content on the same weight basis. The longer the cooking, the more water is absorbed and this affects the nutritive value (USDA):			
Dry	1 oz.	105	21.3
Dry, broken	1 cup (2.5 oz.)	262	53.4
Cooked:			
8-10 minutes, "al dente"	1 cup (5.1 oz.)	216	43.9
8-10 minutes, "al dente"	4 oz.	168	34.1
14-20 minutes, tender	1 cup (4.9 oz.)	155	32.2
14-20 minutes, tender	4 oz.	126	26.1
SPAGHETTI DINNER:			
With meat balls:			
*(Chef Boy-Ar-Dee)	8¾-oz. pkg.	343	62.0
Frozen:			
(Banquet)	11½-oz. dinner	423	57.2
(Morton)	11-oz. dinner	530	85.8
(Swanson)	11½-oz. dinner	323	44.4
*With meat sauce (Chef Boy-Ar-Dee)	7-oz. pkg.	251	50.3
*With meat sauce (Kraft) *Deluxe Dinner*	4 oz.	151	23.1
*With mushroom sauce (Chef Boy-Ar-Dee)	7-oz. pkg.	229	51.5
SPAGHETTI & FRANKFURTERS in TOMATO SAUCE, canned:			
SpaghettiO's (Franco-American)	8 oz.	252	25.6
(Heinz)	8-oz. can	236	25.0
SPAGHETTI & GROUND BEEF in TOMATO SAUCE, canned:			
(Chef Boy-Ar-Dee)	7½ oz. (½ of 15-oz. can)	196	26.4
(Franco-American)	8 oz.	270	25.4
(Nalley's)	8 oz.	204	28.6

(USDA): United States Department of Agriculture
DNA: Data Not Available
*Prepared as Package Directs

SPAGHETTI & MEATBALLS IN TOMATO SAUCE

Food and Description	Measure or Quantity	Calories	Carbohydrates (grams)
SPAGHETTI & MEATBALLS in TOMATO SAUCE:			
Home recipe (USDA)	1 cup (8.8 oz.)	335	39.0
Canned:			
(USDA)	4 oz.	117	12.9
(Austex)	15½-oz. can	437	48.5
(Buitoni)	½ cup	130	12.1
(Chef Boy-Ar-Dee)	8 oz. (⅕ of 40-oz. can)	211	27.2
(Franco-American)	4 oz.	132	12.1
SpaghettiO's (Franco-American)	4 oz.	107	11.5
(Hormel)	15-oz. can	347	20.0
(Morton House)	4 oz.	288	D.N.A.
Frozen, (Banquet) buffet	2 lb.	1324	104.0
SPAGHETTI with MEAT SAUCE:			
Canned (Heinz)	8-oz. can	174	20.6
Frozen:			
(Banquet) cookin' bag	8 oz.	323	33.8
(Kraft)	8 oz.	202	30.2
(Morton)	1 pkg.	298	D.N.A.
(Swanson)	8-oz. pkg.	233	28.5
SPAGHETTI MIX:			
*American style (Kraft)	4 oz.	121	22.2
*Italiano (Golden Grain)	½ cup (3.5 oz.)	150	23.7
*Italian style (Kraft)	4 oz.	119	20.1
SPAGHETTI SAUCE:			
Clam, red (Buitoni)	½ cup	102	10.5
Clam, white (Buitoni)	½ cup	114	10.3
Marinara (See **SAUCE, Marinara**)			
Meat:			
(Buitoni)	½ cup	138	10.6
(Chef Boy-Ar-Dee)	3¾ oz. (¼ of 15-oz. can)	91	10.1
With ground meat (Chef Boy-Ar-Dee)	4⅐ oz. (⅐ of 29-oz. jar)	135	9.8
(Franco-American)	4 oz.	109	9.0
(Prince)	½ cup	135	10.4

(USDA): United States Department of Agriculture
DNA: Data Not Available
*Prepared as Package Directs

Food and Description	Measure or Quantity	Calories	Carbo-hydrates (grams)
Meatball (Chef Boy-Ar-Dee)	5 oz. (⅓ of 15-oz. can)	170	21.2
Meatless or plain:			
(Buitoni)	½ cup	88	11.1
(Chef Boy-Ar-Dee)	4 oz. (¼ of 16-oz. jar)	69	12.3
(Prince)	½ cup	88	13.0
(Ronzoni)	4 oz.	110	D.N.A.
Mushroom:			
(Buitoni)	½ cup	94	11.9
(Chef Boy-Ar-Dee)	3¾ oz. (¼ of 15-oz. can)	62	11.4
(Franco-American)	4 oz.	87	12.4
Arturo (Naas)	8-oz. can	132	D.N.A.
SPAGHETTI SAUCE MIX:			
*(Kraft)	1 oz.	15	2.2
(McCormick)	1½-oz. pkg.	147	D.N.A.
*(McCormick)	4-oz. serving	80	13.0
(Wyler's)	1½-oz. pkg.	D.N.A.	25.0
Italian (French's)	1½-oz. pkg.	105	23.3
*Prepared without oil (Spatini)	½ cup (4 oz.)	28	6.3
*Prepared with oil (Spatini)	½ cup (4 oz.)	51	6.0
With mushrooms (French's)	1½-oz. pkg.	118	12.3
With mushrooms (Lawry's)	1½-oz. pkg.	146	22.6
*With mushrooms, tomato paste (Durkee)	3 cups (1.2-oz. pkg.)	397	84.0
*Without meat (Durkee)	1½ cups (2¼-oz. pkg.)	148	31.9
SPAGHETTI with TOMATO SAUCE:			
Twists (Buitoni)	½ cup	99	16.2
(Franco-American)	4 oz.	92	17.7
SpaghettiO's (Franco-American)	4 oz.	92	17.2
SPAGHETTI in TOMATO SAUCE with CHEESE:			
Home recipe (USDA)	½ cup (4.4 oz.)	130	18.5
Canned:			
(USDA)	4 oz.	86	17.5
(Chef Boy-Ar-Dee)	8 oz. (⅕ of 40-oz. can)	158	31.8

(USDA): United States Department of Agriculture
DNA: Data Not Available
*Prepared as Package Directs

Food and Description	Measure or Quantity	Calories	Carbohydrates (grams)
Italian style (Franco-American)	4 oz.	87	15.4
(Heinz)	8-oz. can	204	35.2
SPAM (Hormel), canned:			
Regular	12-oz. can	1176	4.8
Spread	3-oz. can	216	2.8
SPANISH MACKEREL, raw (USDA):			
Whole	1 lb. (weighed whole)	490	0.
Meat only	4 oz.	201	0.
SPANISH-STYLE VEGE-TABLES, frozen (Birds Eye)	⅓ pkg. (3⅓ oz.)	86	6.6
SPEARMINT EXTRACT (Ehlers)	1 tsp.	12	D.N.A.
SPECIAL K, cereal (Kellogg's)	1 cup (⅔ oz.)	73	13.9
SPICE CAKE MIX:			
& apple (Betty Crocker)	1-lb. 3.5-oz. pkg.	2242	440.7
Chocolate flavor, New Orleans style (Betty Crocker)	1-lb. 2.5-oz. pkg.	2164	416.2
Honey:			
(USDA)	1 oz.	126	21.6
*Prepared with caramel icing (USDA)	2 oz.	200	34.5
(Betty Crocker)	1-lb. 2.5-oz. pkg.	2202	420.0
*(Duncan Hines)	1 cake	2317	384.0

SPICES. Most spices, such as cinnamon, saffron and allspice, are used in such small quantities that the contribution of calories and carbohydrates can be disregarded in diet planning.

SPINACH:			
Raw (USDA):			
Untrimmed	1 lb. (weighed with large stems & roots)	85	14.0
Trimmed	1 lb.	118	19.5

(USDA): United States Department of Agriculture
DNA: Data Not Available
*Prepared as Package Directs

Food and Description	Measure or Quantity	Calories	Carbohydrates (grams)
Trimmed, whole leaves	1 cup (1.2 oz.)	9	1.4
Trimmed, chopped	1 cup (1.8 oz.)	14	2.2
Boiled, drained whole leaves			
(USDA)	1 cup (5.5 oz.)	36	5.6
Canned, regular pack:			
Solids & liq. (USDA)	4 oz.	22	3.4
Solids & liq. (USDA)	½ cup (4.1 oz.)	22	3.5
Drained solids (USDA)	½ cup (3.4 oz.)	27	4.0
Drained liq. (USDA)	4 oz.	7	1.5
Drained solids (Stokely-Van			
Camp)	½ cup	27	4.0
(Hunt's)	4 oz.	22	3.4
Canned, dietetic pack:			
Solids & liq. (USDA)	4 oz.	24	3.7
Drained solids (USDA)	4 oz.	29	4.5
Drained liq. (USDA)	4 oz.	9	2.3
Solids & liq. (Blue Boy)	4 oz.	19	2.0
Frozen:			
Chopped:			
(USDA)	4 oz.	28	4.5
Boiled, drained solids			
(USDA)	4 oz.	26	4.2
(Birds Eye)	⅓ pkg. (3.3 oz.)	23	2.8
(Stokely-Van Camp)	4 oz.	28	4.5
Leaf:			
(USDA)	4 oz.	28	4.8
Boiled, drained solids			
(USDA)	4 oz.	27	4.4
(Birds Eye)	⅓ pkg. (3.3 oz.)	23	3.2
(Stokely-Van Camp)	4 oz.	28	4.8
In butter sauce (Birds Eye)	½ cup (3.3 oz.)	55	3.0
In butter sauce (Green Giant)	4 oz.	75	2.5
In cream sauce (Green Giant)	4 oz.	73	7.6

SPINACH, NEW ZEALAND (See
NEW ZEALAND SPINACH)

SPINACH SOUFFLE, frozen:
(Stouffer's)	12-oz. pkg.	484	29.0
(Swanson)	7½-oz. pkg.	260	15.9

SPINY LOBSTER (See
CRAYFISH)

(USDA): United States Department of Agriculture
DNA: Data Not Available
*Prepared as Package Directs

Food and Description	Measure or Quantity	Calories	Carbo-hydrates (grams)
SPLEEN, raw (USDA):			
Beef & calf	4 oz.	118	0.
Hog	4 oz.	121	0.
Lamb	4 oz.	130	0.
SPONGE CAKE, home recipe (USDA)	⅟₁₂ of 8″ cake (1.4 oz.)	119	21.6
SPORT COLA, soft drink (Canada Dry)	6 fl. oz.	77	20.0
SPOT, fillets (USDA):			
Raw	1 lb.	993	0.
Baked	4 oz.	335	0.
SPRITE, soft drink	6 fl. oz.	72	18.0
SQUAB, pigeon, raw (USDA):			
Dressed	1 lb. (weighed with feet, inedible viscera & bones)	569	0.
Meat & skin	4 oz.	333	0.
Meat only	4 oz.	161	0.
Giblets	1 oz.	44	.3
SQUASH SEEDS, dry (USDA):			
In hull	4 oz.	464	12.6
Hulled	4 oz.	627	17.0
SQUASH, SUMMER:			
Fresh (USDA):			
Crookneck & Straightneck, yellow:			
Whole	1 lb. (weighed untrimmed)	89	19.1
Boiled, drained solids, diced	½ cup (3.6 oz.)	14	3.2
Boiled, drained solids, slices	½ cup (3.1 oz.)	12	2.7
Scallop, white & pale green:			
Whole	1 lb. (weighed untrimmed)	93	22.7
Boiled, drained solids, mashed	½ cup (4.2 oz.)	19	4.5
Zucchini & Cocozelle, green:			
Whole	1 lb. (weighed untrimmed)	73	15.5

(USDA): United States Department of Agriculture
DNA: Data Not Available
*Prepared as Package Directs

Food and Description	Measure or Quantity	Calories	Carbohydrates (grams)
Boiled, drained solids, slices	½ cup (2.7 oz.)	9	1.9
Frozen:			
Not thawed (USDA)	4 oz.	24	5.3
Boiled, drained solids (USDA)	4 oz.	24	5.3
Slices (Birds Eye)	½ cup (3.3 oz.)	20	3.8
SQUASH, WINTER:			
Fresh (USDA):			
Acorn:			
Whole	1 lb. (weighed with skin & seeds)	152	38.6
Baked, flesh only, mashed	½ cup	64	16.2
Boiled, flesh only, mashed	½ cup (4 oz.)	39	9.7
Butternut:			
Whole	1 lb. (weighed with skin & seeds)	171	44.4
Baked, flesh only	4 oz.	77	19.8
Boiled, flesh only	4 oz.	46	11.8
Hubbard:			
Whole	1 lb. (weighed with skin & seeds)	117	28.1
Baked, flesh only	4 oz.	57	13.3
Baked, flesh only, mashed	½ cup (4.3 oz.)	77	18.8
Boiled, flesh only, diced	½ cup (4.2 oz.)	35	8.1
Frozen:			
(USDA)	4 oz.	43	10.4
Heated (USDA)	½ cup (4.2 oz.)	46	11.0
Cooked (Birds Eye)	½ cup (4 oz.)	43	9.0
SQUID, raw, meat only (USDA)	4 oz.	95	1.7
STARCH (See **CORNSTARCH**)			
***STARS,** cereal (Kellogg's)	1 cup (1 oz.)	110	25.0
***START,** instant breakfast drink	½ cup (4.7 oz.)	60	14.9
STAX, cereal (General Mills)	1 cup (1 oz.)	109	21.9
STEINWEIN REBENGOLD, Franconia wine (Deinhard) 11% alcohol	3 fl. oz.	60	1.0
STOMACH, PORK, scalded (USDA)	4 oz.	172	0.

(USDA): United States Department of Agriculture
DNA: Data Not Available
*Prepared as Package Directs

Food and Description	Measure or Quantity	Calories	Carbo-hydrates (grams)
STRAINED FOOD (See **BABY FOOD**)			
STRAWBERRY:			
Fresh, whole (USDA)	1 lb. (weighed with caps & stems)	161	36.6
Fresh, capped (USDA)	1 cup (5.1 oz.)	53	12.1
Canned, unsweetened or low calorie:			
Water pack, solids & liq. (USDA)	4 oz.	25	6.4
Solids & liq. (Blue Boy)	4 oz.	29	7.8
(White Rose)	4 oz.	26	5.8
Frozen:			
(USDA)	10-oz. pkg.	310	79.0
(USDA)	16-oz. can	495	126.0
Whole (Birds Eye)	¼ pkg. (4 oz.)	104	26.6
Halves (Birds Eye)	½ cup (5 oz.)	230	59.8
Quick thaw (Birds Eye)	½ cup (5 oz.)	179	45.7
STRAWBERRY CRISPS, dehydrated snack (Epicure)	1 oz.	85	19.2
***STRAWBERRY DANISH DESSERT** (Junket)	½ cup	138	33.8
***STRAWBERRY DRINK MIX:**			
Quik	2 heaping tsp.	62	15.9
*(Wyler's)	6 fl. oz.	63	15.8
STRAWBERRY FLAVORING, imitation:			
(Ehlers)	1 tsp.	12	D.N.A.
(No-Cal)	1 tsp.	<1	Tr.
STRAWBERRY ICE CREAM (Sealtest)	⅙ qt.	174	25.0
STRAWBERRY ICE CREAM MIX (Junket)	6 serving pkg. (4 oz.)	388	110.0
STRAWBERRY JAM, dietetic:			
(Diet Delight)	1 T.	3	.9
(Slenderella)	1 T.	21	5.4

(USDA): United States Department of Agriculture
DNA: Data Not Available
*Prepared as Package Directs

Food and Description	Measure or Quantity	Calories	Carbo-hydrates (grams)
STRAWBERRY LIQUEUR			
(Leroux) 50 proof	1 fl. oz.	110	8.3
STRAWBERRY PIE:			
(USDA)	⅙ of 9″ pie (5.6 oz.)	313	48.8
Creme (Tastykake)	4-oz. pie	356	50.7
Frozen:			
(Mrs. Smith's)	⅙ of 8″ pie	317	46.3
Cream (Banquet)	2½ oz.	187	27.5
Cream (Morton)	¼ of 14.5-oz. pie	235	30.9
Cream (Mrs. Smith's)	⅙ of 8″ pie	197	23.6
STRAWBERRY PIE FILLING,			
(Lucky Leaf)	8 oz.	248	60.0
STRAWBERRY PRESERVE,			
dietetic or low calorie:			
(Dia-Mel)	1 T.	22	5.4
Wild (Louis Sherry)	1 T.	24	6.0
(Tillie Lewis)	1 T.	9	2.1
*STRAWBERRY PUDDING MIX			
(Royal) *Shake-A-Pudd'n*	½ cup (5.8 oz.)	160	32.6
STRAWBERRY RENNET CUSTARD MIX:			
Powder:			
(Junket)	1 oz.	115	27.8
*Prepared with whole milk	4 oz.	108	14.6
Tablet:			
(Junket)	1 tablet	1	.2
*Prepared with whole milk & sugar	4 oz.	101	13.4
STRAWBERRY-RHUBARB PIE:			
(Tastykake)	4-oz. pie	399	63.5
Frozen (Mrs. Smith's)	⅙ of 8″ pie	312	45.8
STRAWBERRY-RHUBARB PIE FILLING (Lucky Leaf)	8 oz.	258	62.8
STRAWBERRY SOFT DRINK:			
Sweetened:			
(Canada Dry)	6 fl. oz.	85	22.2

(USDA): United States Department of Agriculture
DNA: Data Not Available
*Prepared as Package Directs

Food and Description	Measure or Quantity	Calories	Carbo-hydrates (grams)
Fanta	6 fl. oz.	90	24.0
(Shasta)	6 fl. oz.	80	20.3
(Yoo-Hoo)	6 fl. oz.	90	18.0
High-protein (Yoo-Hoo)	6 fl. oz.	114	24.6
Low calorie (Shasta)	6 fl. oz.	<1	<.1
STRAWBERRY SYRUP, dietetic:			
(Dia-Mel)	1 T.	22	5.5
(No-Cal)	1 tsp.	<1	Tr.
STRAWBERRY TURNOVER, frozen (Pepperidge Farm)	1 turnover	285	D.N.A.
STROGANOFF, BEEF:			
Canned (Hormel)	1-lb. can	643	9.5
Frozen (Swanson)	6.5-oz. pkg.	213	5.8
Dinner (Chef Boy-Ar-Dee)	6⅔-oz. pkg.	278	30.6
Mix (Lipton)	6¼-oz. pkg.	756	97.1
Noodle-Roni	½ cup	111	16.4
Sauce casserole base (Pennsylvania Dutch)	6¾-oz. pkg. (3 cups cooked)	860	126.0
Seasoning mix (Lawry's)	1½-oz. pkg.	118	23.4
STRUDEL, frozen (Pepperidge Farm):			
Apple	2″ x 3″ piece	299	D.N.A.
Blueberry	2″ x 3″ piece	311	D.N.A.
Cherry	2″ x 3″ piece	305	D.N.A.
Peach	2″ x 3″ piece	314	D.N.A.
Pineapple cheese	2″ x 3″ piece	305	D.N.A.
STURGEON (USDA):			
Raw, section	1 lb. (weighed with bones & skin)	362	0.
Raw, meat only	4 oz.	107	0.
Smoked	4 oz.	169	0.
Steamed	4 oz.	181	0.
SUCCOTASH, frozen:			
Not thawed (USDA)	4 oz.	110	24.4
Boiled, drained solids (USDA)	½ cup (3.4 oz.)	89	19.6
(Birds Eye)	½ cup (3.3 oz.)	82	18.5

(USDA): United States Department of Agriculture
DNA: Data Not Available
*Prepared as Package Directs

Food and Description	Measure or Quantity	Calories	Carbo-hydrates (grams)
SUCKER, CARP, raw (USDA):			
Whole	1 lb. (weighed whole)	196	0.
Meat only	4 oz.	126	0.
SUCKER, including **WHITE and MULLET,** raw:			
Whole (USDA)	1 lb. (weighed whole)	203	0.
Meat only (USDA)	4 oz.	118	0.
SUET (USDA)	1 oz.	242	0.
SUGAR, beet or cane (There is no difference in calories and carbohydrates among brands):			
Brown:			
(USDA)	1 lb.	1692	437.3
Firm-packed (USDA)	1 cup (7.5 oz.)	791	204.4
Firm-packed (USDA)	1 T.	49	12.8
Granulated:			
(USDA)	1 lb.	1746	451.3
(USDA)	1 cup (6.9 oz.)	751	194.0
(USDA)	1 T.	47	12.1
Lump (USDA)	1⅛" x ¾" x ⅜" piece (6 grams)	23	6.0
Confectioners':			
(USDA)	1 lb.	1746	451.3
Sifted (USDA)	1 cup	366	94.5
Sifted (USDA)	1 T.	23	5.9
Maple (USDA)	4 oz.	395	102.0
Maple (USDA)	1¾" x 1¼" x ½" piece	104	27.0
SUGAR APPLE, raw (USDA):			
Whole	1 lb. (weighed with skin & seeds)	192	48.4
Flesh only	4 oz.	107	26.9
SUGAR CRISP, puffed wheat cereal	1 cup (1⅓ oz.)	147	33.3
SUGAR FROSTED FLAKES, cereal	1 cup (1⅛ oz.)	143	33.9

(USDA): United States Department of Agriculture
DNA: Data Not Available
*Prepared as Package Directs

Food and Description	Measure or Quantity	Calories	Carbohydrates (grams)
SUGAR JETS, cereal	1 cup (1⅕ oz.)	128	28.9
SUGAR POPS, cereal	1 cup (1 oz.)	110	25.4
SUGAR RICE KRINKLES, cereal	1 cup (1½ oz.)	165	39.0
SUGAR SMACKS, cereal	1 cup (1 oz.)	110	25.0
SUGAR SUBSTITUTE:			
(Adolph's)	1 tsp.	0	0.
Sweetness & Light	1 tsp.	4	.9
Sweetnin (Tillie Lewis)	1 tsp.	0	0.
Sweet'n It, liquid (Dia-Mel)	1 tsp.	0	0.
Sweet'n It, powdered (Dia-Mel)	1 packet (1 gram)	3	.8
SUNFLOWER SEED (USDA):			
Hulls on	1 oz. (weighed in hull)	86	4.0
Hulled	1 oz.	159	5.6
SUNFLOWER SEED FLOUR (See **FLOUR**)			
SURINAM CHERRY (See **PITANAGA**)			
SUZY Q (Hostess)	1 cake	260	39.1
SWAMP CABBAGE (USDA):			
Raw, whole	1 lb. (weighed untrimmed)	107	19.8
Boiled, trimmed, drained solids	4 oz.	24	4.4
SWEETBREADS (USDA):			
Beef, raw	1 lb.	939	0.
Beef, braised	4 oz.	363	0.
Calf, raw	1 lb.	426	0.
Calf, braised	4 oz.	191	0.
Lamb, raw	1 lb.	426	0.
Lamb, braised	4 oz.	198	0.
SWEET POTATO:			
Raw (USDA):			
All kinds, unpared	1 lb. (weighed whole)	419	96.6

(USDA): United States Department of Agriculture
DNA: Data Not Available
*Prepared as Package Directs

Food and Description	Measure or Quantity	Calories	Carbohydrates (grams)
Jersey types, pared	4 oz.	116	25.5
Puerto Rico variety, pared	4 oz.	133	31.0
Baked, peeled after baking (USDA)	1 med. (5″ x 2″)	155	35.8
Boiled, peeled after boiling (USDA)	1 med. (5″ x 2″)	168	38.6
Candied, home recipe (USDA)	1 sweet potato (3½″ x 2¼″)	294	59.8
Canned, regular pack:			
In syrup, solids & liq. (USDA)	4 oz.	129	31.2
Vacuum or solid pack (USDA)	½ cup (3.8 oz.)	118	27.1
(King Pharr)	½ cup	118	22.5
Yam (King Pharr)	½ cup	114	27.0
Vacuum pack (Taylor's)	½ cup	135	32.0
Canned, dietetic pack, without added sugar & salt (USDA)	4 oz.	52	12.2
Dehydrated flakes, dry (USDA)	½ cup (2 oz.)	220	52.2
*Dehydrated flakes, prepared with water (USDA)	½ cup (4.4 oz.)	120	28.6
Frozen, candied (Mrs. Paul's)	4 oz.	196	39.2
Frozen, candied, yams (Birds Eye)	½ cup (4 oz.)	215	53.1
SWEET POTATO PIE:			
(USDA)	⅙ of 9″ pie (5.4 oz.)	324	36.0
(Tastykake)	4-oz. pie	359	50.0
SWEETSOP (See **SUGAR APPLE**)			
SWING (Shasta):			
Sweetened	6 fl. oz.	80	20.3
Low calorie	6 fl. oz.	<1	<.1
SWISS STEAK, frozen:			
(Stouffer's)	10-oz. pkg.	569	14.0
Dinner (Swanson)	10-oz. dinner	361	35.0
With gravy (Holloway House)	1 steak	291	32.0
SWISS UP WINE (Italian Swiss Colony-Gold Medal) 19.7% alcohol	3 fl. oz.	132	9.3
SWORDFISH (USDA):			
Raw, meat only	1 lb.	535	0.
Broiled with butter or margarine	4 oz.	197	0.

(USDA): United States Department of Agriculture
DNA: Data Not Available
*Prepared as Package Directs

Food and Description	Measure or Quantity	Calories	Carbohydrates (grams)
Broiled with butter or margarine	3″ x 3″ x ½″ steak (4.4 oz.)	218	0.
Canned, solids & liq.	4 oz.	116	0.
SYLVANER WINE (Louis M. Martini) 12.5% alcohol	3 fl. oz.	90	.2
SYRUP. (See also individual listings by kind, such as **PANCAKE & WAFFLE SYRUP** or by brand name, such as *LOG CABIN*):			
Cane and maple blend (USDA)	1 T.	50	13.0
All fruit flavors (Smucker's)	1 T.	44	D.N.A.

T

TABASCO (McIlhenny)	¼ tsp.	<1	0.
TACO, beef, frozen:			
Regular size:			
(Banquet)	1 taco	101	14.0
(Patio)	1 taco	190	D.N.A.
(Rosarita)	2-oz. taco	136	D.N.A.
Cocktail (Patio)	1 taco	38	D.N.A.
Cocktail (Rosarita)	½-oz. taco	30	D.N.A.
TACO FILLING, beef, canned (Rosarita)	1 oz.	61	D.N.A.
TACO SEASONING MIX (Lawry's)	1¼-oz. pkg.	117	22.3
TAHITIAN TREAT, soft drink (Canada Dry)	6 fl. oz.	100	26.2
TAMALE:			
Canned:			
(Hormel)	15-oz. can	583	41.2
(Rutherford)	4 oz.	161	D.N.A.
(Wilson)	4 oz.	155	16.4

(USDA): United States Department of Agriculture
DNA: Data Not Available
*Prepared as Package Directs

Food and Description	Measure or Quantity	Calories	Carbo-hydrates (grams)
Frozen:			
(Banquet) cookin' bag	2 tamales (3 oz. each)	219	17.5
(Rosarita)	3⅓-oz. tamale	256	D.N.A.
Hot, with gravy (Patio)	1 pkg.	1011	D.N.A.
With chili gravy (Patio)	1 pkg. (8 tacos)	1130	D.N.A.
TAMARIND, fresh (USDA):			
Whole	1 lb. (weighed with pods & seeds)	520	136.1
Flesh only	4 oz.	271	70.9
TANDY TAKE (Tastykake):			
Chocolate	1 cake (⅔ oz.)	147	21.0
Choc-o-mint	1 cake (.6 oz.)	102	13.0
Dandy Kake	1 cake (.6 oz.)	102	13.0
Karamel	1 cake (⅔ oz.)	100	12.2
Orange	1 cake (.6 oz.)	103	13.6
Peanut butter	1 cake (⅔ oz.)	194	32.1
***TANG,** instant breakfast drink	½ cup (4.7 oz.)	59	15.2
TANGELO, fresh (USDA):			
Fruit, whole	1 lb. (weighed with peel, membrane & seeds)	104	24.6
Juice	½ cup (4.4 oz.)	50	12.0
TANGERINE, fresh:			
Whole (USDA)	1 lb. (weighed with skin & seeds)	154	38.9
Whole (USDA)	4-oz. tangerine (2½″ dia.)	40	10.0
Sections, without membranes (USDA)	1 cup (6.8 oz.)	89	22.4
(Sunkist)	1 large tangerine	39	10.0
TANGERINE JUICE:			
Fresh (USDA)	½ cup (4.4 oz.)	53	12.4
Canned, unsweetened (USDA)	½ cup (4.4 oz.)	53	12.6
Canned, sweetened (USDA)	4 oz. (by wt.)	57	13.6
Frozen, concentrate, sweetened:			
Undiluted (USDA)	6-oz. can	340	80.0
*Diluted with 3 parts water by volume (USDA)	½ cup (4.4 oz.)	58	13.5

(USDA): United States Department of Agriculture
DNA: Data Not Available
*Prepared as Package Directs

Food and Description	Measure or Quantity	Calories	Carbohydrates (grams)
*(Minute Maid)	½ cup	58	13.5
*(Snow Crop)	½ cup	58	13.5
TAPIOCA, dry, quick cooking granulated:			
(USDA)	1 cup (5.4 oz.)	535	131.3
(USDA)	1 T.	35	8.6
(Minute)	1 T.	38	2.3
TAPIOCA PUDDING:			
Apple, home recipe (USDA)	4 oz.	133	33.3
Cream, home recipe (USDA)	4 oz.	152	19.4
Mix:			
*All flavors (Jell-O)	½ cup (5.1 oz.)	167	27.7
*(Minute Tapioca)	½ cup (5.8 oz.)	182	25.6
*Chocolate (Royal)	½ cup (5.1 oz.)	184	29.2
Vanilla (My-T-Fine)	1 oz.	84	19.5
*Vanilla (Royal)	½ cup (4.9 oz.)	170	28.1
TARO, raw:			
Tubers, whole (USDA)	1 lb. (weighed with skin)	373	90.3
Tubers, skin removed (USDA)	4 oz.	111	26.9
Leaves & stems (USDA)	1 lb.	181	33.6
TAUTOG or BLACKFISH, raw:			
Whole (USDA)	1 lb. (weighed whole)	149	0.
Meat only (USDA)	4 oz.	101	0.
TEA:			
Bag (Tender Leaf)	1 bag	1	Tr.
Instant:			
(USDA)	1 tsp.	1	.4
*(Lipton)	8 fl. oz.	3	Tr.
(Tender Leaf)	1 rounded tsp.	1	Tr.
TEAM FLAKES, cereal (Nabisco)	1 cup (¾ oz.)	83	18.6
TEA MIX, iced:			
All flavors, *Nestea*	3 tsp. (1 serving)	58	15.1
*All flavors (Salada)	1 cup	70	13.4
*(Tender Leaf)	1 cup	60	2.8
*(Wyler's)	1 cup	63	14.0

(USDA): United States Department of Agriculture
DNA: Data Not Available
*Prepared as Package Directs

Food and Description	Measure or Quantity	Calories	Carbo-hydrates (grams)
Lemon flavored:			
(Lipton)	3 tsp.	63	.6
Low calorie (Lipton)	8 fl. oz.	4	.6
Nestea	1 tsp.	2	.4
Lime flavored (Lipton)	3 tsp.	64	D.N.A.
*Low calorie (Tender Leaf)	1 cup	10	.4
Mint flavored (Lipton)	3 tsp.	60	D.N.A.
Orange flavored (Lipton)	3 tsp.	58	D.N.A.
Tropical punch flavored (Lipton)	3 tsp.	63	D.N.A.
TEE UP, soft drink (Kirsch)	6 fl. oz.	64	16.1
TEMPTYS (Tastykake):			
Butter creme	1 cake (⅔ oz.)	94	12.9
Chocolate	1 cake (⅔ oz.)	95	17.1
Lemon	1 cake (⅔ oz.)	95	17.3
TENDERGREEN (See **MUSTARD SPINACH**)			
TENDER MADE MAIN MEAL MEAT, canned (Wilson):			
Beef roast	3 oz.	100	0.
Corned beef brisket	3 oz.	135	.8
Ham	3 oz.	129	.8
Picnic	3 oz.	137	.8
Pork roast	3 oz.	133	0.
Pork loin, smoked	3 oz.	114	.8
Turkey & dressing	3 oz.	159	8.5
Turkey roast	3 oz.	87	0.
TEQUILA (See **DISTILLED LIQUOR**)			
TEQUILA SOUR (Calvert) 55 proof	3 fl. oz.	185	11.4
TERRAPIN, DIAMOND BACK, raw (USDA):			
In shell	1 lb. (weighed in shell)	106	0.
Meat only	4 oz.	126	0.
THUNDERBIRD WINE (Gallo):			
14% alcohol	3 fl. oz.	86	8.1
20% alcohol	3 fl. oz.	106	7.5

(USDA): United States Department of Agriculture
DNA: Data Not Available
*Prepared as Package Directs

Food and Description	Measure or Quantity	Calories	Carbohydrates (grams)
THURINGER, sausage (USDA)	1 oz.	87	.4
TIA MARIA, liqueur (Hiram Walker) 63 proof	1 fl. oz.	92	10.0
TIKI, soft drink (Shasta):			
Regular	6 fl. oz.	84	21.3
Diet	6 fl. oz.	<1	<.1
TILEFISH (USDA):			
Raw, whole	1 lb. (weighed whole)	183	0.
Baked, meat only	4 oz.	156	0.
TOASTER CAKE:			
Toast 'Em (General Foods):			
Animal	1 piece	181	33.3
Frosted	1 piece	198	37.1
Fruit flavors	1 piece	175	32.2
Toastette (Nabisco):			
Apple	1 piece (1¾ oz.)	197	34.4
Blueberry	1 piece (1¾ oz.)	199	34.3
Brown sugar, cinnamon	1 piece (1¾ oz.)	193	34.5
Cherry	1 piece (1¾ oz.)	196	34.8
Strawberry	1 piece (1¾ oz.)	198	34.7
Toast-r-Cake, bran (Thomas')	1 piece	118	17.0
Toast-r-Cake, corn (Thomas')	1 piece	140	20.5
TODDLER FOOD (See **BABY FOOD**)			
TOKAY WINE:			
(Gallo)	3 fl. oz.	107	7.5
(Gallo) 14% alcohol	3 fl. oz.	86	8.1
(Italian Swiss Colony-Gold Medal) 19.7% alcohol	3 fl. oz.	128	8.1
(Taylor) white, 18.5% alcohol	3 fl. oz.	144	11.3
TOMATO:			
Fresh, green (USDA)	4 oz.	27	5.8
Fresh, ripe (USDA):			
Whole	1 lb.	100	21.3
Whole	1 small (1¾" x 2¼")	24	5.2

(USDA): United States Department of Agriculture
DNA: Data Not Available
*Prepared as Package Directs

Food and Description	Measure or Quantity	Calories	Carbo-hydrates (grams)
Whole	1 med. (2″ x 2½″)	33	7.0
Peeled	1 lb. (weighed with skin, stem ends & hard core)	88	18.8
Sliced	1 cup (6.4 oz.)	40	8.5
Boiled (USDA)	4 oz.	29	6.2
Canned, regular pack:			
Solids & liq. (USDA)	4 oz.	24	4.9
Whole, solids & liq. (USDA)	½ cup (4.2 oz.)	25	5.1
Baby, sliced (Contadina)	14.5-oz. can (1⅔ cups)	131	29.1
Diced, in puree (Contadina)	14.5-oz. can (1⅔ cups)	148	30.5
Italian style (Hunt's)	4 oz.	24	4.9
Pear-shaped (Contadina)	14.5-oz. can (1⅔ cups)	95	19.8
Round, peeled (Contadina)	14.5-oz. can (1⅔ cups)	95	19.8
Stewed (Contadina)	14.5-oz. can (1⅔ cups)	115	23.3
Whole, peeled (Hunt's)	4 oz.	24	4.9
Canned, dietetic pack:			
Solids & liq. (USDA)	4 oz.	23	4.8
Solids & liq. (Blue Boy)	4 oz.	24	4.5
Whole, peeled (Diet Delight)	½ cup (4.2 oz.)	25	4.8
Whole, unseasoned (S and W)			
Nutradiet	4 oz.	24	4.6
(Tillie Lewis)	½ cup (4.2 oz.)	24	4.6
TOMATO COCKTAIL:			
(USDA)	4 oz. (by wt.)	24	5.7
(College Inn)	4 oz.	29	6.3
TOMATO JUICE:			
Canned, regular pack:			
(USDA)	4 oz.	22	4.8
(USDA)	½ cup (4.2 oz.)	23	5.2
(Campbell)	4 oz.	23	4.5
(Green Giant)	½ cup	25	5.2
(Heinz)	5½-oz. can	36	7.8
(Hunt's)	4 oz.	22	4.9
(Musselman's)	½ cup	25	D.N.A.
Canned, dietetic pack:			
(USDA)	4 oz. (by wt.)	22	4.9

(USDA): United States Department of Agriculture
DNA: Data Not Available
*Prepared as Package Directs

Food and Description	Measure or Quantity	Calories	Carbohydrates (grams)
(Blue Boy)	4 oz. (by wt.)	24	4.5
(Diet Delight)	½ cup (4.2 oz.)	24	5.0
(Stokely-Van Camp)	4 oz. (by wt.)	22	4.9
Unseasoned (S and W) *Nutradiet*	4 oz. (by wt.)	24	4.8
Concentrate, canned (USDA)	4 oz. (by wt.)	86	19.4
*Concentrate, canned, diluted with 3 parts water by volume (USDA)	4 oz. (by wt.)	23	5.1
Dehydrated (USDA)	1 oz.	86	19.3
*Dehydrated (USDA)	½ cup	24	5.5
TOMATO PASTE, canned:			
(USDA)	6 oz.	138	31.8
(Contadina)	6-oz. can	143	30.1
(Hunt's)	6-oz. can	138	31.8
TOMATO PUREE:			
Canned, regular pack:			
(USDA)	1 cup (8.8 oz.)	98	22.2
(Contadina)	15-oz. can (1⅔ cups)	170	36.2
(Hunt's)	1 oz.	11	2.5
Canned, dietetic pack (USDA)	1 oz.	11	2.5
TOMATO SALAD, jellied			
(Contadina)	15-oz. can (1⅔ cups)	187	41.4
TOMATO SAUCE:			
(Contadina)	8-oz. can (1 cup)	82	16.8
(Hunt's) plain or with cheese, mushrooms, onions or tomato bits	8-oz. can	64	12.8
TOMATO SOUP:			
Canned, regular pack:			
Condensed (USDA)	8 oz. (by wt.)	163	28.8
*Prepared with equal volume water (USDA)	1 cup (8.6 oz.)	88	15.7
*Prepared with equal volume milk (USDA)	1 cup (8.6 oz.)	169	22.0
Condensed (Campbell)	8 oz. (by wt.)	156	27.9
*(Heinz)	1 cup	97	16.1
*(Manischewitz)	8 oz. (by wt.)	60	9.6
Beef (Campbell) *Noodle-O's*	8 oz. (by wt.)	218	30.9

(USDA): United States Department of Agriculture
DNA: Data Not Available
*Prepared as Package Directs

Food and Description	Measure or Quantity	Calories	Carbo-hydrates (grams)
Bisque (Campbell)	1 cup	115	20.9
Rice, old fashioned (Campbell)	1 cup	99	16.7
*Rice (Manischewitz)	8 oz. (by wt.)	78	12.8
With vegetable (Heinz) *Great American*	1 cup (8¾ oz.)	126	17.6
Canned, dietetic pack:			
Low sodium (Campbell)	7¼-oz. can	121	15.8
*With rice (Claybourne)	8 oz.	72	14.6
(Tillie Lewis)	1 cup	70	14.1

TOMATO VEGETABLE SOUP MIX:

With noodles (USDA)	1 oz.	98	17.8
*With noodles (USDA)	1 cup (8 oz.)	62	11.6
*(Golden Grain)	1 cup	80	13.3
(Lipton)	1 pkg. (2.5 oz.)	276	48.2

TOMCOD, ATLANTIC, raw (USDA):

Whole	1 lb. (weighed whole)	136	0.
Meat only	4 oz.	87	0.

TOM COLLINS or COLLINS MIXER SOFT DRINK:

(Dr. Brown's)	6 fl. oz.	66	16.5
(Hoffman)	6 fl. oz.	66	16.5
(Key Food)	6 fl. oz.	66	16.5
(Kirsch)	6 fl. oz.	60	15.1
(Waldbaum)	6 fl. oz.	66	16.5
(Yukon Club)	6 fl. oz.	60	15.0

TONGUE (USDA):

Beef, medium fat, raw, untrimmed	1 lb.	714	1.4
Beef, medium fat, braised	4 oz.	277	.5
Calf, raw, untrimmed	1 lb.	454	3.1
Calf, braised	4 oz.	181	1.1
Hog, raw, untrimmed	1 lb.	741	1.7
Hog, braised	4 oz.	287	.6
Lamb, raw, untrimmed	1 lb.	659	1.7
Lamb, braised	4 oz.	288	.6
Sheep, raw, untrimmed	1 lb.	877	7.9
Sheep, braised	4 oz.	366	2.7

(USDA): United States Department of Agriculture
DNA: Data Not Available
*Prepared as Package Directs

Food and Description	Measure or Quantity	Calories	Carbo-hydrates (grams)
TONGUE, CANNED:			
Pickled (USDA)	1 oz.	76	.1
Potted or deviled (USDA)	1 oz.	82	.2
(Hormel)	12-oz. can	804	.7
TONIC WATER (See **QUININE SOFT DRINK**)			
TOPPING (See also **CHOCOLATE SYRUP**)			
Sweetened:			
Butterscotch:			
(Hershey's)	1 oz.	82	14.0
(Kraft)	1 oz.	84	18.9
(Smucker's)	1 T.	63	15.3
Caramel:			
(Kraft)	1 oz.	84	19.2
(Smucker's)	1 T.	55	D.N.A.
Chocolate (Kraft)	1 oz.	83	18.7
Chocolate or chocolate flavored:			
(Kraft)	1 oz.	73	18.0
Fudge (Hershey's)	1 oz.	96	15.8
Fudge, regular (Smucker's)	1 T.	53	12.6
Mint (Hershey's)	1 oz.	79	19.0
Peanut butter (Hershey's)	1 oz.	90	14.1
Marshmallow creme (Kraft)	1 oz.	89	22.9
Pineapple (Kraft)	1 oz.	80	19.7
Strawberry (Kraft)	1 oz.	80	19.7
Walnut (Kraft)	1 oz.	113	14.3
Dietetic, chocolate (Diet Delight)	1 T.	6	1.2
Dietetic, chocolate (Tillie Lewis)	1 T.	7	1.7
TOPPING, WHIPPED:			
(Birds Eye) *Cool Whip*	1 T.	16	1.1
(Kraft)	1 oz.	80	4.3
(Lucky Whip)	1 T. (4 grams)	12	.5
(Snow-Kist)	1 T.	15	D.N.A.
TOPPING, WHIPPED, MIX:			
*(D-Zerta)	1 T.	7	.3
*(Dream Whip)	1 T.	14	1.2
*(Lucky Whip)	1 T. (4 grams)	10	1.0
***TOTAL,** cereal (General Mills)	1 cup (1 oz.)	101	23.1

(USDA): United States Department of Agriculture
DNA: Data Not Available
*Prepared as Package Directs

Food and Description	Measure or Quantity	Calories	Carbo-hydrates (grams)
TORTILLA:			
(USDA)	.7-oz. tortilla (5″)	50	9.7
Corn, frozen (Patio)	1 tortilla	64	D.N.A.
TOWEL GOURD, raw (USDA):			
Unpared	1 lb. (weighed with skin)	69	15.8
Pared	4 oz.	20	4.6
TREET (Armour)	12-oz. can	996	4.1
TRIPE, beef (USDA):			
Commercial	4 oz.	113	0.
Pickled	4 oz.	70	0.
TRIPLE JACK WINE (Gallo)			
20% alcohol	3 fl. oz.	102	6.6
TRIPLE SEC LIQUEUR:			
(Bols) 78 proof	1 fl. oz.	101	8.8
(Garnier) 60 proof	1 fl. oz.	83	8.5
(Hiram Walker) 80 proof	1 fl. oz.	105	9.8
(Leroux) 80 proof	1 fl. oz.	102	8.9
(Old Mr. Boston) 42 proof	1 fl. oz.	97	10.1
(Old Mr. Boston) 60 proof	1 fl. oz.	105	10.1
TRIX, cereal (General Mills)	1 cup (1 oz.)	110	25.0
TROPICAL PUNCH SOFT DRINK (Yukon Club)	6 fl. oz.	90	22.5
TROUT:			
Brook, fresh, whole (USDA)	1 lb. (weighed whole)	224	0.
Brook, fresh, meat only (USDA)	4 oz.	115	0.
Lake (See **LAKE TROUT**)			
Rainbow (USDA):			
Fresh, meat with skin	4 oz.	221	0.
Canned	4 oz.	237	0.
Frozen (1000 Springs):			
Dressed	4 oz.	106	0.
Boned	4 oz.	124	0.
Boned & breaded	4 oz.	185	D.N.A.

(USDA): United States Department of Agriculture
DNA: Data Not Available
*Prepared as Package Directs

Food and Description	Measure or Quantity	Calories	Carbo-hydrates (grams)
TUNA:			
Raw, bluefin, meat only (USDA)	4 oz.	165	0.
Raw, yellowfin, meat only (USDA)	4 oz.	151	0.
Canned in oil:			
Solids & liq.:			
(USDA)	4 oz.	327	0.
(Breast O'Chicken)	6½-oz. can	540	0.
(Star-Kist)	7-oz. can	577	0.
Chunk (Star-Kist)	6½-oz. can	535	0.
Chunk (Star-Kist)	3¼-oz. can	268	0.
Chunk, light (Chicken of the Sea)	6½-oz. can	405	0.
Chunk, light (Icy Point)	6½-oz. can	530	0.
Chunk, light (Pillar Rock)	6½-oz. can	530	0.
White (Icy Point)	6½-oz. can	570	0.
White (Pillar Rock)	6½-oz. can	570	0.
Drained solids:			
(USDA)	4 oz.	223	0.
(Del Monte)	7 oz.	340	0.
Chunk, light (Chicken of the Sea)	6½-oz. can	294	0.
Chunk, white (Bumble Bee)	3 oz.	210	0.
White (Icy Point)	7-oz. can	388	0.
White (Pillar Rock)	7-oz. can	388	0.
Canned in water:			
Solids & liq. (USDA)	4 oz.	144	0.
(Breast O'Chicken)	6½-oz. can	240	0.
(Deep Blue)	7-oz. can	215	0.
Solids & liq. (Star-Kist)	7-oz. can	210	0.
Canned, dietetic:			
Drained solids (Chicken of the Sea)	⅓ of 6½-oz. can	75	0.
Solids & liq. (Star-Kist)	6½-oz. can	207	0.
Solids & liq. (Star-Kist)	3¼-oz. can	112	0.
TUNA & NOODLE DINNER			
(Star-Kist)	15-oz. can	364	D.N.A.
TUNA PIE, frozen:			
(Banquet)	8-oz. pie	479	40.2
(Star-Kist)	8-oz. pie	450	D.N.A.
(Swanson)	8-oz. pie	453	38.1
TUNA SALAD, home recipe			
(USDA)	4 oz.	193	4.0

(USDA): United States Department of Agriculture
DNA: Data Not Available
*Prepared as Package Direct

Food and Description	Measure or Quantity	Calories	Carbo-hydrates (grams)
TUNA SOUP, Creole, canned (Crosse & Blackwell)	6½ oz. (½ can)	57	6.6
TURKEY:			
Raw, ready-to-cook (USDA)	1 lb. (weighed with bones)	722	0.
Roasted (USDA):			
Flesh & skin	4 oz.	253	0.
Meat only:			
Chopped	1 cup (5 oz.)	268	0.
Diced	1 cup (4.8 oz.)	257	0.
Light	4 oz.	200	0.
Dark	4 oz.	230	0.
Canned, meat only, boned (USDA)	4 oz.	229	0.
Canned, boned (Lynden)	5-oz. jar	317	0.
Frozen, with giblet gravy (Banquet) cookin' bag	5 oz.	129	5.8
Frozen (Swanson)	9½-oz. pkg.	314	33.7
TURKEY DINNER, frozen:			
Sliced turkey, mashed potato, peas (USDA)	12 oz.	381	43.2
(Banquet)	11-oz dinner	280	28.2
(Morton)	11-oz. dinner	334	25.7
(Swanson)	12¼-oz. dinner	401	43.7
(Swanson) 3-course	17½-oz. dinner	557	67.6
TURKEY GIZZARD (USDA):			
Raw	4 oz.	178	1.3
Simmered	4 oz.	222	1.2
TURKEY PIE:			
Home recipe, baked (USDA)	4 oz.	269	21.0
Frozen:			
Commercial, unheated (USDA)	8 oz.	448	45.6
(Banquet)	8-oz. pie	398	45.2
(Morton)	8¼-oz. pie	441	39.5
(Swanson)	8-oz. pie	442	40.1
(Swanson) deep dish	1-lb. pie	608	53.1
TURKEY PRIMAVERA, dinner (Lipton)	1 pkg.	781	86.5

(USDA): United States Department of Agriculture
DNA: Data Not Available
*Prepared as Package Directs

Food and Description	Measure or Quantity	Calories	Carbo-hydrates (grams)
TURKEY SOUP:			
Noodle:			
Condensed (USDA)	8 oz. (by wt.)	148	15.9
*Prepared with equal volume water (USDA)	1 cup (8.8 oz.)	82	8.8
Condensed (Campbell)	8 oz. (by wt.)	143	15.0
*(Heinz)	1 cup	88	8.6
(Heinz) *Great American*	1 cup	89	11.1
Low sodium (Campbell)	8¼-oz. can	82	9.0
Vegetable, condensed (Campbell)	8 oz. (by wt.)	145	15.9
TURKEY TETRAZZINI, frozen (Stouffer's)	12-oz. pkg.	694	68.7
TURNIP (USDA):			
Fresh, without tops	1 lb. (weighed with skins)	117	25.7
Boiled, drained solids, diced	½ cup (2.8 oz.)	18	3.8
Boiled, drained solids, mashed	½ cup (4 oz.)	27	5.8
TURNIP GREENS, leaves & stems:			
Fresh (USDA)	1 lb. (weighed untrimmed)	107	19.0
Boiled, in small amount water, short time, drained solids (USDA)	½ cup (2.6 oz.)	14	2.6
Boiled, in large amount water, long time, drained solids (USDA)	½ cup (2.6 oz.)	14	2.4
Canned, solids & liq. (USDA)	½ cup (4 oz.)	20	3.7
Frozen:			
Uncooked (USDA)	4 oz.	26	4.5
Boiled, drained solids (USDA)	4 oz.	26	4.4
Boiled, drained solids (USDA)	½ cup (2.8 oz.)	19	3.2
Chopped (Birds Eye)	½ cup (3.3 oz.)	22	2.7
TURNOVER (See individual kinds)			
TURTLE, GREEN (USDA):			
Raw, in shell	1 lb. (weighed in shell)	97	0.
Raw, meat only	4 oz.	101	0.
Canned	4 oz.	120	0.

(USDA): United States Department of Agriculture
DNA: Data Not Available
*Prepared as Package Directs

Food and Description	*Measure or Quantity*	*Calories*	*Carbo-hydrates (grams)*
TV DINNER (See individual listing such as: **BEEF DINNER, CHICKEN DINNER, CHINESE DINNER, ENCHILADA DINNER,** etc.)			
20-20 WINE (Mogen David) 20% alcohol	3 fl. oz.	105	9.8
TWINKIE (Hostess)	1 cake	187	26.3
TWINKLES, cereal (General Mills)	1 cup (1⅐ oz.)	126	27.2
TWISTER, wine (Gallo) 20% alcohol	3 fl. oz.	109	8.4

V

Food and Description	*Measure or Quantity*	*Calories*	*Carbo-hydrates (grams)*
VALPOLICELLA WINE, Italian red (Antinori)	3 fl. oz.	84	6.3
VANDERMINT, Dutch liqueur, (Leroux) 60 proof	1 fl. oz.	90	10.2
VANILLA CAKE, layer, frozen (Pepperidge Farm)	1″ x 3″ piece	179	D.N.A.
VANILLA CAKE MIX, French (Betty Crocker)	1-lb. 2.5-oz. pkg.	2202	423.6
VANILLA DRINK MIX, *Quik*	2 heaping tsp.	60	15.6
VANILLA EXTRACT (Ehlers)	1 tsp.	8	D.N.A.
VANILLA ICE CREAM (See also individual brand names):			
(Sealtest)	1 slice (⅛ qt.)	133	15.5
(Sealtest) 10.2% fat	⅙ qt.	176	20.5
(Sealtest) 12.1% fat	⅙ qt.	186	20.2
French (Prestige)	⅙ qt.	247	21.0
Fudge royale (Sealtest)	⅙ qt.	183	23.4
VANILLA ICE CREAM MIX (Junket)	6 serving pkg. (4 oz.)	388	110.0

(USDA): United States Department of Agriculture
DNA: Data Not Available
*Prepared as Package Directs

Food and Description	Measure or Quantity	Calories	Carbo-hydrates (grams)
VANILLA ICE MILK (Sealtest)	⅙ qt.	135	23.4
VANILLA PIE FILLING MIX:			
*(Jell-O)	½ cup (5.3 oz.)	179	31.0
(My-T-Fine)	1 oz.	123	27.0
*With whole milk (D-Zerta)	½ cup (4.5 oz.)	107	12.0
*With nonfat milk (D-Zerta)	½ cup (4.5 oz.)	71	12.0
VANILLA PUDDING:			
Blancmange, home recipe, with starch base (USDA)	4 oz.	126	18.0
Canned (Betty Crocker)	1-lb. 2-oz. can	666	117.0
Canned, French vanilla (Bounty)	4 oz.	127	21.3
VANILLA PUDDING MIX:			
Sweetened:			
*(Jell-O)	½ cup (5.3 oz.)	179	31.0
*Instant (Jell-O)	½ cup (5.3 oz.)	177	30.5
*French, instant (Jell-O)	½ cup (5.3 oz.)	177	30.5
(My-T-Fine)	1 oz.	123	27.0
Instant (My-T-Fine)	1 oz.	82	20.7
*(Royal)	½ cup (4.9 oz.)	165	26.6
*Instant (Royal)	½ cup (4.9 oz.)	185	30.3
*Shake-A-Pudd'n (Royal)	½ cup (5.6 oz.)	165	32.3
*(Thank You)	½ cup	169	29.2
Low calorie:			
*With whole milk (Dia-Mel)	4 oz.	90	8.1
*With nonfat milk (Dia-Mel)	4 oz.	53	8.2
*With whole milk (D-Zerta)	½ cup (4.5 oz.)	107	12.0
*With nonfat milk (D-Zerta)	½ cup (4.5 oz.)	71	12.0
VANILLA RENNET CUSTARD MIX:			
Powder:			
(Junket)	1 oz.	116	28.0
*Prepared with whole milk	4 oz.	108	14.7
Tablet:			
(Junket)	1 tablet	1	.2
*Prepared with whole milk & sugar	4 oz.	101	13.4
VANILLA SOFT DRINK:			
(Yoo-Hoo)	6 fl. oz.	90	18.0
High-protein (Yoo-Hoo)	6 fl. oz.	114	24.6

(USDA): United States Department of Agriculture
DNA: Data Not Available
*Prepared as Package Directs

Food and Description	Measure or Quantity	Calories	Carbo-hydrates (grams)
VEAL, medium fat (USDA):			
Chuck, raw	1 lb. (weighed with bone)	628	0.
Chuck, braised, lean & fat	4 oz.	266	0.
Flank, raw	1 lb. (weighed with bone)	1410	0.
Flank, stewed, lean & fat	4 oz.	442	0.
Foreshank, raw	1 lb. (weighed with bone)	368	0.
Foreshank, stewed, lean & fat	4 oz.	245	0.
Loin, raw	1 lb. (weighed with bone)	681	0.
Loin, broiled, chop, lean & fat	4 oz.	265	0.
Plate, raw	1 lb. (weighed with bone)	828	0.
Plate, stewed, lean & fat	4 oz.	344	0.
Rib, raw, lean & fat	1 lb. (weighed with bone)	723	0.
Rib, roasted, lean & fat	4 oz.	305	0.
Round & rump, raw	1 lb. (weighed with bone)	573	0.
Round & rump, broiled, steak or cutlet, lean & fat	4 oz.	245	0.
VEAL PARMIGIANA DINNER, frozen (Swanson)	12¼-oz. dinner	492	47.7
VEGETABLE BOUILLON CUBE:			
(Herb-Ox)	1 cube	6	.5
(Wyler's)	1 cube	8	.3
VEGETABLE FAT (See **FAT**)			
VEGETABLE JUICE COCKTAIL, canned:			
(USDA)	4 oz. (by wt.)	19	4.1
Unseasoned (S and W) *Nutradiet*	4 oz.	24	4.8
V-8 (Campbell)	4 oz.	22	4.1
Vegemato (College Inn)	4 oz.	22	4.7
VEGETABLE, MIXED:			
Canned (Veg-All)	4 oz.	39	7.8
Frozen:			
(USDA)	4 oz.	74	15.5

(USDA): United States Department of Agriculture
DNA: Data Not Available
*Prepared as Package Directs

VEGETABLE, MIXED (Continued)

Food and Description	Measure or Quantity	Calories	Carbo-hydrates (grams)
Boiled, drained solids (USDA)	½ cup (3.2 oz.)	58	12.2
(Birds Eye)	½ cup (3.3 oz.)	53	11.8
Jubilee (Birds Eye)	½ cup	138	18.7
(Blue Goose)	4 oz.	60	12.8
In butter sauce (Birds Eye)	½ cup (3.3 oz.)	83	11.3
With onion sauce (Birds Eye)	½ cup (2.7 oz.)	120	11.0

VEGETABLE OYSTER (See **SALSIFY**)

VEGETABLE SOUP:
Canned, regular pack:

Beef, condensed (USDA)	8 oz. (by wt.)	148	17.9
*Prepared with equal volume water (USDA)	1 cup (8.8 oz.)	80	9.8
With beef broth, condensed (USDA)	8 oz. (by wt.)	145	25.0
*With beef broth, prepared with equal volume water (USDA)	1 cup (8.8 oz.)	80	13.8
Condensed (Campbell)	8 oz. (by wt.)	154	25.2
Condensed (Campbell) old fashioned	8 oz. (by wt.)	120	16.3
Beef, condensed (Campbell)	8 oz. (by wt.)	150	14.5
& beef stockpot (Campbell)	8 oz. (by wt.)	179	17.0
& noodles (Campbell) Noodle-O's	8 oz. (by wt.)	141	19.3
*Beef (Heinz)	1 cup	82	11.1
Beef (Heinz) Great American	1 cup	116	11.2
With beef broth (Heinz) Great American	1 cup	132	16.9
*With beef stock (Heinz)	1 cup	78	12.9
With ground beef (Heinz) Great American	1 cup	127	11.0
Vegetarian:			
Condensed (USDA)	8 oz. (by wt.)	145	24.1
*Prepared with equal volume water (USDA)	1 cup	80	13.5
Condensed (Campbell)	8 oz. (by wt.)	141	23.6
*(Heinz)	1 cup	82	12.8
(Heinz) Great American	1 cup	119	17.1
*(Manischewitz)	8 oz. (by wt.)	63	10.1
Canned, dietetic pack:			
Low sodium (Campbell)	8¼-oz. can	72	11.0
Beef, low sodium (Campbell)	8¼-oz. can	77	7.5

(USDA): United States Department of Agriculture
DNA: Data Not Available
*Prepared as Package Directs

[308]

Food and Description	Measure or Quantity	Calories	Carbo-hydrates (grams)
*Condensed (Claybourne)	1 cup	105	21.0
(Tillie Lewis)	1 cup	68	13.2
Frozen:			
With beef, condensed (USDA)	8 oz. (by wt.)	159	15.9
*With beef, prepared with equal volume water (USDA)	8 oz. (by wt.)	79	7.7
With beef, condensed, old fashioned (Campbell)	8 oz. (by wt.)	154	15.0
VEGETABLE SOUP MIX:			
(Croyden House)	1 tsp.	12	2.3
*(Wyler's)	6 fl. oz.	42	7.0
Beef (Lipton)	1 pkg.	159	22.0
VENISON, raw, lean meat only (USDA)	4 oz.	143	0.
VERMOUTH:			
Dry & extra dry:			
(C & P) 19% alcohol	3 fl. oz.	90	3.0
(Gallo) 18% alcohol	3 fl. oz.	75	1.8
(Gancia) 21% alcohol	3 fl. oz.	126	D.N.A.
(Lejon) 18.5% alcohol	3 fl. oz.	99	2.2
(Noilly Pratt) 19% alcohol	3 fl. oz.	101	1.6
(Taylor) 17% alcohol	3 fl. oz.	102	.9
Rosso, (Gancia) 21% alcohol	3 fl. oz.	153	6.9
Sweet:			
(C & P) 16% alcohol	3 fl. oz.	120	14.4
(Gallo) 18% alcohol	3 fl. oz.	118	2.3
(Lejon) 18.5% alcohol	3 fl. oz.	134	11.4
(Noilly Pratt) 16% alcohol	3 fl. oz.	128	12.1
(Taylor) 17% alcohol	3 fl. oz.	132	10.4
White (Gancia) 16.8% alcohol	3 fl. oz.	132	7.8
White (Lejon) 18.5% alcohol	3 fl. oz.	101	2.6
VICHYSSOISE SOUP (Crosse & Blackwell)	6½ oz. (½ can)	94	9.4
VIENNA SAUSAGE, canned:			
(USDA)	1 oz.	68	Tr.
(Armour Star)	5-oz. can	390	0.
(Armour Star)	1 sausage (.6 oz.)	29	0.
(Hormel)	4-oz. can	324	.6
(Wilson)	1 oz.	86	.1

(USDA): United States Department of Agriculture
DNA: Data Not Available
*Prepared as Package Directs

VILLA ANTINORI

Food and Description	Measure or Quantity	Calories	Carbo-hydrates (grams)
VILLA ANTINORI, Italian white wine, 12½% alcohol	3 fl. oz.	87	6.3
VINEGAR:			
Cider:			
(USDA)	1 T.	2	.8
(USDA)	½ cup (4 oz.)	16	7.0
(Hunt's)	1 oz.	4	1.7
Distilled:			
(USDA)	1 T.	2	.8
(USDA)	½ cup (4 oz.)	14	6.0
(Hunt's)	1 oz.	3	1.4
VINESPINACH or BASELLA, raw (USDA)	4 oz.	22	3.9
VINO PRIMO WINE (Italian Swiss Colony-Gold Medal) 12% alcohol	3 fl. oz.	66	1.6
VIN ROSE (See **ROSE WINE**)			
VODKA, unflavored (See **DISTILLED LIQUOR**)			
VODKA COCKTAIL:			
Martini (Calvert) 75 proof	3 fl. oz.	188	Tr.
Screwdriver (Old Mr. Boston) 25 proof	3 fl. oz.	117	10.5
VODKA, FLAVORED (Old Mr. Boston):			
Wild cherry, grape, lemon, lime or orange, 70 proof	1 fl. oz.	100	8.0
Peppermint, 70 proof	1 fl. oz.	90	5.0
VOIGNY WINE (Chanson) 13% alcohol	3 fl. oz.	96	7.5

W

WACKIES, cereal (General Mills)	1 oz.	110	23.2
WAFER (See **COOKIE or CRACKER**)			

(USDA): United States Department of Agriculture
DNA: Data Not Available
*Prepared as Package Directs

[310]

Food and Description	Measure or Quantity	Calories	Carbo-hydrates (grams)
WAFFLE:			
Home recipe (USDA)	2.6-oz. waffle (½" x 4½" x 5½")	209	28.1
Frozen:			
(USDA)	1 waffle (8 in 13-oz. pkg.)	116	19.3
(USDA)	1 waffle (6 in 5-oz. pkg.)	61	10.1
Country (Aunt Jemima)	2 sections (1.5 oz.)	116	16.0
WAFFLE MIX (USDA) (See also **PANCAKE & WAFFLE MIX**):			
Dry	1 oz.	130	18.5
*Prepared with water	1 waffle (½" x 4½" x 5½")	229	30.2
WAFFLE SYRUP (See **SYRUP**)			
WALNUT:			
Black:			
In shell, whole (USDA)	1 lb. (weighed in shell)	627	14.8
Shelled, whole (USDA)	4 oz.	712	16.8
Chopped (USDA)	½ cup (2.1 oz.)	374	8.8
Kernel (Hammons)	1 lb.	2985	46.3
English or Persian:			
In shell, whole (USDA)	1 lb. (weighed in shell)	1329	32.2
Shelled, whole (USDA)	4 oz.	738	17.9
Chopped (USDA)	½ cup (2.1 oz.)	391	9.5
Chopped (USDA)	1 T.	49	1.2
Chopped (Diamond)	1 T.	49	1.2
Halves (USDA)	½ cup (1.8 oz.)	326	7.9
Halves (Diamond)	½ cup	327	7.8
Halves (Diamond)	8-15 halves	98	2.3
WALNUT, BLACK, EXTRACT (Ehlers)	1 tsp.	4	D.N.A.
WALNUT CAKE MIX, BLACK (Betty Crocker)	1-lb. 2.5-oz. pkg.	2202	423.6
WATER CHESTNUT, CHINESE, raw (USDA):			
Whole	1 lb. (weighed unpeeled)	272	66.4
Peeled	4 oz.	90	21.5

(USDA): United States Department of Agriculture
DNA: Data Not Available
*Prepared as Package Directs

Food and Description	Measure or Quantity	Calories	Carbo-hydrates (grams)
WATERCRESS, raw (USDA):			
Whole	½ lb. (weighed untrimmed)	40	6.3
Trimmed	½ cup (.6 oz.)	3	.5
WATERMELON, fresh:			
(USDA)	1 lb. (weighed with rind)	54	13.4
(USDA)	1 piece (4″ x 8″ measured with rind)	115	27.0
Diced (USDA)	1 cup (5.6 oz.)	42	10.2
WATERMELON RIND (Crosse & Blackwell)	1 T.	38	9.3
WAX GOURD, raw (USDA):			
Whole	1 lb. (weighed with skin & cavity contents)	41	9.4
Flesh only	4 oz.	15	3.4
WEAKFISH (USDA):			
Raw, whole	1 lb. (weighed whole)	263	0.
Broiled, meat only	4 oz.	236	0.
WELSH RAREBIT, home recipe (USDA)	4 oz.	203	7.1
WEST INDIAN CHERRY (See **ACEROLA**)			
WHALE MEAT, raw (USDA)	4 oz.	177	0.
WHEAT CHEX, cereal (Ralston)	½ cup (1 oz.)	102	23.3
*WHEATENA, cereal	½ cup	88	18.1
WHEAT FLAKES, cereal:			
Crushed (USDA)	1 cup (2.4 oz.)	248	56.4
Dietetic (Van Brode)	1 oz.	109	23.0
WHEAT GERM, crude, commercially milled (USDA)	1 oz.	103	13.2

(USDA): United States Department of Agriculture
DNA: Data Not Available
*Prepared as Package Directs

Food and Description	Measure or Quantity	Calories	Carbo-hydrates (grams)
WHEAT GERM, CEREAL:			
(USDA)	¼ cup (1 oz.)	110	14.0
(Kretschmer)	1 oz.	106	12.6
With sugar & honey (Kretschmer)	1 oz.	107	26.9
WHEAT HONEYS, cereal	1 cup (1⅓ oz.)	152	32.7
WHEATIES, cereal	1 cup (1 oz.)	101	23.1
WHEAT OATA, cereal, dry	¼ cup (1 oz.)	104	19.6
WHEAT, PUFFED, cereal:			
(USDA)	1 cup (.4 oz.)	44	9.4
Frosted (USDA)	.5 oz.	53	12.5
(Checker)	.5-oz. serving	51	11.0
(Kellogg's)	1 cup (.5 oz.)	56	.2
(Quaker)	1 cup (⅜ oz.)	38	8.3
WHEAT, SHREDDED, cereal (See **SHREDDED WHEAT**)			
***WHIP'N CHILL** (Jell-O):			
*With whole milk	½ cup (2 oz.)	138	19.3
*With skim milk	½ cup (2 oz.)	130	19.2
WHISKEY or WHISKY (See **DISTILLED LIQUOR**)			
WHISKEY SOUR:			
(Calvert) 60 proof	3 fl. oz.	190	9.5
(Hiram Walker) 52.5 proof	3 fl. oz.	177	12.0
WHISKEY SOUR MIX:			
(Bar-Tender's)	1 serving (⅝ oz.)	70	17.2
Low calorie, *Sip 'n Slim*	1 serving (¾ oz.)	2	.5
WHISKEY SOUR SOFT DRINK:			
(Canada Dry)	6 fl. oz.	71	18.4
(Shasta)	6 fl. oz.	65	16.5
WHITEFISH, LAKE (USDA):			
Raw, whole	1 lb. (weighed whole)	330	0.
Raw, meat only	4 oz.	176	0.
Baked, stuffed, home recipe	4 oz.	244	6.6
Smoked	4 oz.	176	0.

(USDA): United States Department of Agriculture
DNA: Data Not Available
*Prepared as Package Directs

Food and Description	Measure or Quantity	Calories	Carbo-hydrates (grams)
WHOOPEE PIE (Berwick)	1 pie	300	45.0
WIENER (Oscar Mayer):			
Regular	1 link	161	D.N.A.
Little	1 link	30	D.N.A.
WILD BERRY, fruit drink (Hi-C)	6 fl. oz.	92	22.7
WILD RICE, raw:			
(USDA)	4 oz.	400	85.4
(USDA)	½ cup (2.8 oz.)	288	61.4
WINE (Most wines are listed by kind, brand, vineyard, region or grape name):			
Dessert (USDA) 18.8% alcohol	3 fl. oz.	120	6.9
Dessert (Petri)	3 fl. oz.	124	D.N.A.
Flavored (Petri)	3 fl. oz.	124	D.N.A.
Red (Great Western) *Pleasant Valley*, 12% alcohol	3 fl. oz.	88	4.7
Table:			
(USDA) 12.2% alcohol	3 fl. oz.	75	3.6
(Petri)	3 fl. oz.	59	D.N.A.
White (Great Western) *Pleasant Valley*, 12% alcohol	3 fl. oz.	88	4.7
WINK, soft drink (Canada Dry)	6 fl. oz.	89	23.2
WINTERGREEN EXTRACT (Ehlers)	1 tsp.	11	D.N.A.
WONTON SOUP, frozen (Temple)	8-oz. serving (with 2 wontons)	76	D.N.A.
WORCESTERSHIRE SAUCE (See **SAUCE,** Worcestershire)			
WRECKFISH, raw, meat only (USDA)	4 oz.	129	0.

(USDA): United States Department of Agriculture
DNA: Data Not Available
*Prepared as Package Directs

Food and Description	Measure or Quantity	Calories	Carbo-hydrates (grams)

Y

YAM (USDA):
Raw, whole	1 lb. (weighed with skin)	394	90.5
Raw, flesh only	4 oz.	115	26.3
Canned and frozen (See **SWEET POTATO**)			

YAM BEAN, raw (USDA):
Unpared	1 lb. (weighed unpared)	225	52.2
Pared	4 oz.	62	14.5

YANKEE DOODLES (Drake's)	1 cake	125	18.0

YEAST:
Baker's:			
Compressed (USDA)	1 oz.	25	3.0
Compressed (Fleischmann's)	⅗-oz. cake	18	1.9
Dry (USDA)	1 oz.	80	11.0
Dry (USDA)	1 T.	25	3.5
Dry (Fleischmann's)	¼-oz. (pkg. or jar)	24	2.9
Brewer's dry, debittered (USDA)	1 oz.	80	10.9
Brewer's dry, debittered (USDA)	1 T.	25	3.0

YELLOWTAIL, raw, meat only (USDA)	4 oz.	157	0.

YOGURT:
Made from whole milk (USDA)	½ cup (4.3 oz.)	76	6.0
Made from partially skimmed milk (USDA)	½ cup (4.3 oz.)	61	6.3
Plain:			
Swiss style (Borden)	5-oz. container	81	9.9
Swiss style (Borden)	8-oz. container	129	15.9
(Breakstone)	8-oz. container	141	12.7
(Breakstone)	1 T. (.5 oz.)	10	.8
(Dannon)	8 oz. container	136	14.1
Apple, Dutch (Dannon)	8-oz. container	258	51.1
Apricot (Breakstone)	8-oz. container	220	37.4
Apricot (Breakstone) _Swiss Parfait_	8-oz. container	249	42.9

(USDA): United States Department of Agriculture
DNA: Data Not Available
*Prepared as Package Directs

[315]

YOGURT (Continued)

Food and Description	Measure or Quantity	Calories	Carbo-hydrates (grams)
Apricot (Dannon)	8-oz. container	258	51.1
Black cherry (Breakstone) *Swiss Parfait*	8-oz. container	256	44.9
Blueberry (Breakstone)	8-oz. container	252	46.3
Blueberry (Breakstone) *Swiss Parfait*	8-oz. container	286	53.1
Blueberry (Dannon)	8-oz. container	258	51.1
Blueberry (Sealtest) *Light n' Lively*	8-oz. container	257	50.6
Boysenberry (Dannon)	8-oz. container	258	51.1
Cherry (Dannon)	8-oz. container	258	51.1
Cinnamon apple (Breakstone)	8-oz. container	229	39.9
Coffee (Dannon)	8-oz. container	198	33.3
Danny (Dannon):			
Cuplet:			
Blueberry	4-oz. container	129	25.5
Red raspberry	4-oz. container	129	25.5
Strawberry	4-oz. container	129	25.5
Frozen pops	2½-oz. pop	127	18.0
Honey (Breakstone) *Swiss Parfait*	8-oz. container	277	51.5
Lemon (Breakstone) *Swiss Parfait*	8-oz. container	254	44.9
Lemon (Sealtest) *Light n' Lively*	8-oz. container	229	43.4
Lime (Breakstone) *Swiss Parfait*	8-oz. container	243	40.1
Mandarin orange:			
(Borden)	5-oz. container	142	28.7
(Borden)	8-oz. container	227	45.9
(Breakstone) *Swiss Parfait*	8-oz. container	263	48.3
Peach:			
(Borden)	5-oz. container	138	27.8
(Borden)	8-oz. container	221	44.5
(Breakstone) *Swiss Parfait*	8-oz. container	254	47.4
(Sealtest) *Light n' Lively*	8-oz. container	252	49.3
Peach Melba (Breakstone) *Swiss Parfait*	8-oz. container	268	49.4
Pineapple (Breakstone)	8-oz. container	220	37.9
Pineapple (Sealtest) *Light n' Lively*	8-oz. container	241	47.2
Pineapple-orange (Dannon)	8-oz. container	258	51.1
Prune Whip (Breakstone)	8-oz. container	231	41.1
Prune Whip (Dannon)	8-oz. container	258	51.1

(USDA): United States Department of Agriculture
DNA: Data Not Available
*Prepared as Package Directs

Food and Description	Measure or Quantity	Calories	Carbo-hydrates (grams)
Raspberry:			
(Borden)	5-oz. container	147	29.5
(Borden)	8-oz. container	236	47.2
(Breakstone)	8-oz. container	249	45.8
(Sealtest) *Light n' Lively*	8-oz. container	225	41.8
Red (Breakstone) *Swiss Parfait*	8-oz. container	263	46.5
Red (Dannon)	8-oz. container	258	51.1
Strawberry:			
(Borden)	5-oz. container	142	27.8
(Borden)	8-oz. container	227	44.5
(Breakstone)	8-oz. container	225	43.5
(Breakstone) *Swiss Parfait*	8-oz. container	259	50.6
(Dannon)	8-oz. container	258	51.1
(Sealtest) *Light n' Lively*	8-oz. container	234	44.3
Vanilla:			
(Borden)	5-oz. container	148	28.4
(Borden)	8-oz. container	235	45.4
(Breakstone)	8-oz. container	195	29.5
(Dannon)	8-oz. container	198	33.3

YOUNGBERRY, fresh (See
BLACKBERRY, fresh)

Z

ZELTINGER ANGLERWEIN,
German Moselle wine (Deinhard)
11% alcohol · 3 fl. oz. · 60 · 1.0

ZINFANDEL WINE:
(Italian Swiss Colony-Gold
Medal) 12.3% alcohol · 3 fl. oz. · 63 · .7
(Louis M. Martini) 12.5%
alcohol · 3 fl. oz. · 90 · .2

ZUCCHINI (See **SQUASH,
SUMMER**)

ZWIEBACK:
(USDA)	1 oz.	120	21.1
(Nabisco)	1 piece (7 grams)	31	5.4
(Sunshine)	1 piece (7 grams)	30	5.3

(USDA): United States Department of Agriculture
DNA: Data Not Available
*Prepared as Package Directs

BIBLIOGRAPHY

Dawson, Elsie H., Gilpin, Gladys L., and Fulton, Lois H., *Average weight of a measured cup of various foods.* U.S.D.A. ARS 61–6, February 1969. 19 pp.

Merrill, A. L. and Watt, B. K., *Energy value of foods — basis and derivation.* U.S.D.A. Handb. 74, 105 pp. 1955.

Pecot, Rebecca K., Jaeger, Carol M., and Watt, Bernice K., *Proximate composition of beef from carcass to cooked meat: Method of derivation and tables of values.* U.S.D.A. Home Economics Research Report 31, 32 pp. 1965.

Pecot, Rebecca K. and Watt, Bernice K., *Food yields: Summarized by different stages of preparation.* U.S.D.A. Handb. 102, 93 pp. 1956.

U.S.D.A. Nutritive value of foods. Home and Garden Bul. 72, 36 pp. 1964 and revised edition, 1970. 41 pp.

U.S.D.A. Unpubl. Data 1969.

Watt, Bernice K., Merrill, Annabel L., et. al., *Composition of foods: Raw, processed, prepared.* U.S.D.A. Agriculture Handb. 8, 190 pp. 1963.

Visual Meat Portions and Their
Calories and Carbohydrates
(Source: USDA)

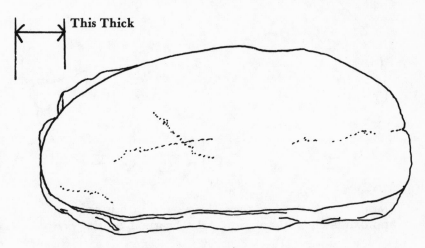

One piece of *round steak* (lean only) of this size is approximately 160 calories and 0. carbohydrates (See also p. 35).

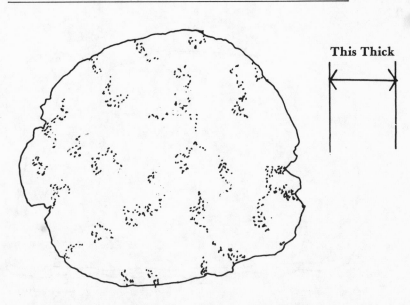

One *hamburger* (lean only) of this size is approximately 185 calories and 0. carbohydrates (See also p. 33).

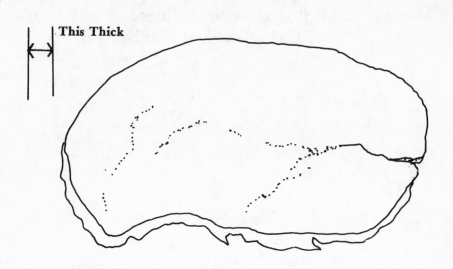

This Thick

Two slices of *roast beef round* (lean only) of this size are approximately 140 calories and 0. carbohydrates (See also p. 34)

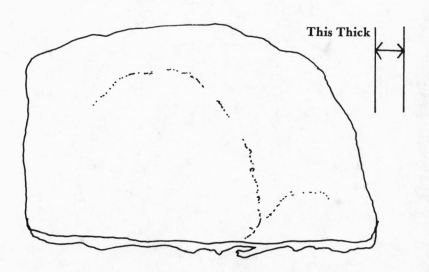

This Thick

Two slices of *cured ham* (lean only) of this size are approximately 160 calories and 0. carbohydrates (See also p. 237).

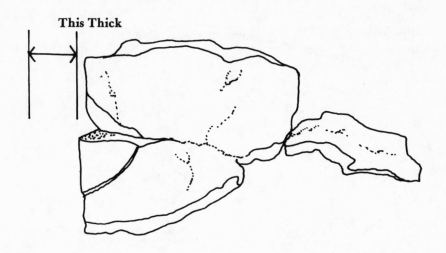

This Thick

Two *lamb chops* (lean only) of this size are approximately 160 calories and 0. carbohydrates (See also p. 175).

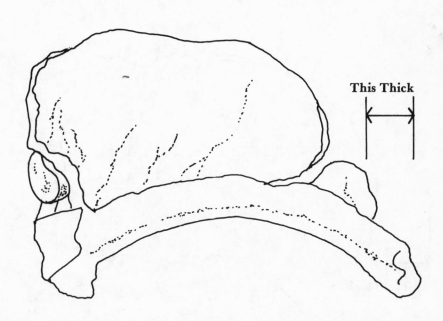

This Thick

Two *pork chops* (lean only) of this size are approximately 230 calories and 0. carbohydrates (See also p. 236).

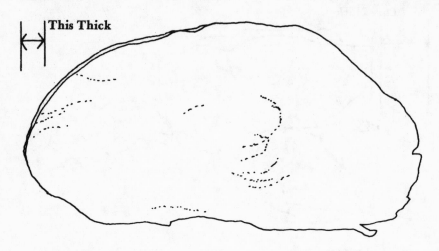

This Thick

Two slices of this size of the light meat of a *roast turkey* are approximately 150 calories and 0. carbohydrates. Two slices of this size of the dark meat of a *roast turkey* are approximately 175 calories and 0. carbohydrates (See also p. 303).

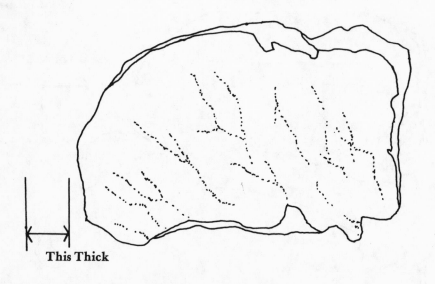

This Thick

One *veal cutlet* (trimmed) of this size is approximately 185 calories and 0. carbohydrates (See also p. 307).